SPORTS MEDICINE

Prevention of Athletic Injuries

Alfred F. Morris

*University of Illinois
at Urbana-Champaign*

SPORTS MEDICINE

Prevention of Athletic Injuries

wcb
Wm. C. Brown Publishers
Dubuque, Iowa

Book Team
Edward G. Jaffe *Senior Editor*
Lynne M. Meyers *Associate Developmental Editor*
Kevin J. Pruessner *Designer*
Colleen A. Yonda *Production Editor*
Faye M. Schilling *Visual Research Editor*
Mavis M. Oeth *Permissions Editor*

wcb group

Wm. C. Brown *Chairman of the Board*
Mark C. Falb *President and Chief Executive Officer*

wcb

Wm. C. Brown Publishers, College Division
Lawrence E. Cremer *President*
James L. Romig *Vice-President, Product Development*
David Wm. Smith *Vice-President, Marketing*
David A. Corona *Vice-President, Production and Design*
E. F. Jogerst *Vice-President, Cost Analyst*
Marcia H. Stout *Marketing Manager*
Linda M. Galarowicz *Director of Marketing Research*
Marilyn A. Phelps *Manager of Design*
William A. Moss *Production Editorial Manager*
Mary M. Heller *Visual Research Manager*

Consulting Editor: Aileene Lockhart (Texas Woman's University)

Interior photos by Anna Moore Butzner: 103; David A. Corona: 52, 193, 194, 196, 201; Cybex Division of Lumex: 68; Allen Ruid: 24, 110, 270, 273; U Conn Photo: 6, 77

Library of Congress Catalog Card Number: 83-071289

ISBN 0-697-00087-7

2-00087-01

Printed in the United States of America

Dedicated to Ann and V. D. B.

Contents

Part Two Basic Concepts of Human Skeletal Muscle 31

Part **T**hree **Athletic Training and Conditioning for Sports 49**

Contents

Contents

Preface

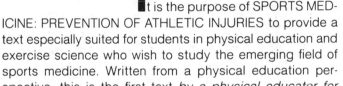

It is the purpose of SPORTS MEDICINE: PREVENTION OF ATHLETIC INJURIES to provide a text especially suited for students in physical education and exercise science who wish to study the emerging field of sports medicine. Written from a physical education perspective, this is the first text *by a physical educator for physical education and other allied health profession students.*

As the only sports medicine book of its kind written by a single author, this text is an integration between the two main areas of sports medicine: the *training and preparation for sport,* and the *injury aspects of sports competition.* Other texts available in the sports medicine area either concern themselves exclusively with the physical fitness and training aspect of sport, or are written by orthopedic physicians, or other clinical people, who stress the injury or clinical aspect of sport.

This book is intended for students who are interested in learning about the new field of sports medicine. Undergraduate students who are thinking of majoring in physical education, exercise science, athletic training, physical therapy, or one of the other allied health or fitness areas, should be interested in this text. It is ideally suited for the beginning student in that it defines the area of sports medicine, covers the field accurately, and also includes a discussion of the types of personnel currently working within the field. Its treatment of training and conditioning for sport is unique. Pertinent questions and comments from over one thousand students, who have taken an introductory sports medicine course from the author over a period of several years, are included to make the book particularly appropriate to the beginning student.

The book is organized into five main areas. The first part is an introduction to sports medicine, including definitions of the field, the concept of wellness, and what types of individuals currently comprise the field. Part Two concerns basic concepts of human skeletal muscle. These concepts enable the student to better understand Part Three, which is training and conditioning for sports. This is the major area that the beginning student in physical education or athletics is concerned with. Specific content areas within this part include strength, endurance, and flexibility training for sports competition. Part Four deals with the injury aspect of sports, listing definitions, degrees of severity, and immediate first aid and rehabilitation for many common athletic injuries. Part Five covers other topics intimately related to sports medicine, such as nutrition, drugs, and environmental concerns—each of which is integrated into the concept of total preparation for the sport activity. The remaining chapters deal with individuals relatively new to the sporting experience. These include female athletes, children, and older individuals involved in sport, and the topic of psychological preparation for sport activity.

The author wishes to acknowledge the reviewers whose comments have helped in the preparation of this manuscript. They include Charles J. Redmond (Springfield College), Earlene Durrant (Brigham Young University), Michael D. Aitken (SUNY Cortland), Thomas G. Manfredi (University of Rhode Island), and Michael J. Welch (United States Military Academy).

The author also wishes to acknowledge the assistance of Peggy Swanson, who has helped during all phases of the preparation of the manuscript, and the illustrator, Bret Dye. ■

SPORTS MEDICINE

Prevention of Athletic Injuries

Sports, the Athlete, And Total Health

Part 1

Introduction to Sports Medicine

1

Outline

Introduction

This first chapter presents a general overview of the entire field of sports medicine, which has shown tremendous growth during the past few years. It explains the increase in popularity of sports and exercise in the 1970s and 1980s, defines the terms used in the area of sports medicine, and presents a brief history of sports medicine in this country and in Europe. A major portion of this introductory chapter covers personnel active in the field—allied health professionals, athletic trainers, therapists, and physicians—and the specialized areas in which they work. Finally, it presents the concept of health and total wellness as it relates to fitness and sports medicine.

The tremendous growth of sports medicine within the last decade has been largely due to the increase in the numbers of women, older adults, and youth involved in athletic activities. This increased participation in organized and nonorganized sports activities is especially evident in North America, Western Europe, and Scandinavia. Participation figures in running, swimming, cycling, skiing, and other athletic events, show a two- to tenfold increase over recent years. Major running, cycling, swimming, and skiing events in several countries routinely attract several thousand entrants of all ages. Some of the reasons for this increase in sports activity will be explored in this chapter.

Along with the increase in the number of athletic participants, a concomitant increase in sports medicine professionals has occurred. A variety of athletic trainers, exercise physiologists, allied health professionals, and physicians have become involved—contributing to this rapid growth in the sports medicine field.

The objectives of this chapter are to examine developments that have caused the sports medicine field to grow, to define and describe the content area of sports medicine, to present a brief history of sports medicine, and to list some of the professionals working in the sports medicine area. This chapter is a brief state-of-the-art examination of the emerging sports medicine discipline.

Developments That Have Promoted an Increase in Sports Participation

Women Sports

A major impetus for increasing the involvement of women in sports in the United States was the passage of federal legislation (Title IX) during the 1970s. This federal law opened the doors for many female athletes to compete in sports which were previously restricted to males. The number of athletic teams which represent the various secondary schools, colleges, and universities in the United States has doubled since women have started competing.

On the international scene, the number of events for female athletes added to Olympic and world-class competition has increased. One example of expanded athletic opportunity for women is the ruling to permit female long distance runners to compete in the Olympic marathon. All these developments lead to more sports opportunities for female athletes.

Youth Sports

Parallel to the increasing involvement by women in sports has been the growth of youth athletics. Age-group baseball, football, and swimming have been popular activities for some time in the United States. Additional opportunities in other sports, such as track and field

5

Federal legislation (Title IX) has enabled many women to experience the benefits of sport training and competition.

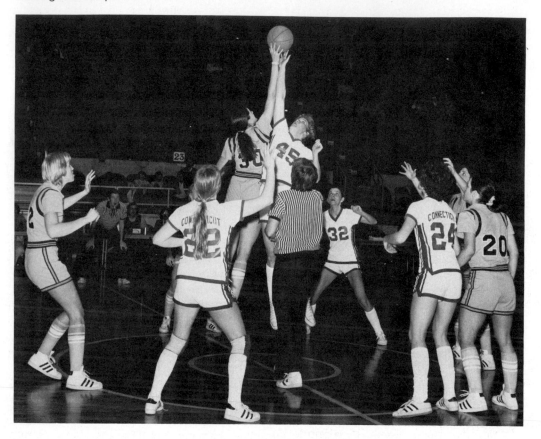

athletics, gymnastics, wrestling, and soccer (world football) are now becoming available for both girls and boys. Youth age-group competition—properly organized and conducted—provides youngsters with a wholesome outlet for their youthful energies. If fun and skill development are properly stressed, and winning is intelligently viewed by adults and youngsters alike, youth sports activity can be a very positive experience for any child.

Masters Sports

A third impetus for the increase in the number of people involved in sports is the implementation of "masters" or "veteran" divisions of competition. Older athletes may now participate in various organized sports on a regional, national, and world level. Swimming was one of the first sports to hold national and international meets in the masters division and now other sports are offering senior age-group activities. Typically, athletes over age forty are grouped into five- or ten-year age brackets and compete against age-matched

Figure 1.1 A Health/Fitness Continuum. As one's health habits (diet, rest, etc.) and physical activity improve, one can move to a higher level of wellness. With detraining, one moves to the left on the continuum and further inactivity can lead to sickness. An injury may temporarily move a person to the left on the scale. Note that aging tends to move *all* people to the left. Movement along the scale continues throughout life, ending with death at the extreme left.

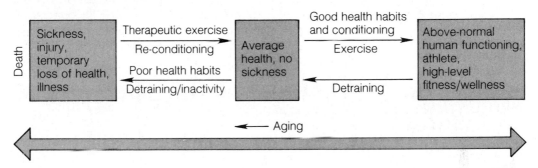

colleagues. In some sports, such as swimming, a master athlete may be a competitor who is twenty-five years young! The camaraderie and achievement of these gifted athletes are outstanding.

All three of the above listed developments—women, youth, and masters sports—have greatly increased the number of athletes participating worldwide in many sporting activities. Along with this increased participation comes the necessity for physicians to conduct pretraining physicals, to work as team physicians, and to aid in the treatment and rehabilitation of sports injuries. In addition, various team and individual trainers and coaches are necessary to conduct conditioning programs for these new athletes.

Preventive Medicine and Total Fitness

Another recent development leading to increased recreational sports participation is new emphasis in medical writings on the point that individuals must take increasing responsibility for their own health (Pelletier, 1977; Surgeon General, 1979). This has lead people to select better diets and be aware of the role of physical activity in preventing degenerative diseases that may accompany aging. In fact, some authors think that the decline in the rate of coronary heart disease (CHD) in the late 1970s is a reflection of the fact that people have become more aware of better patterns of eating and physical activity (Pollock, Wilmore & Fox, 1978).

For a better portrayal of this total health/fitness concept and the role physical activity plays in it, refer to figure 1.1. In this illustration the average individual is located at about the center of the health/fitness continuum. As this individual's diet, rest, and physical activity patterns improve, they may move to the right on the continuum to more positive health and a higher fitness level. The extremely fit athlete might be placed to the extreme right point, indicating supranormal human functioning.

The average person, who has a poor diet, receives much negative stress, and gets little or no physical activity, may move to the left to the unfit/unhealthy category on the continuum. Obviously, other poor health habits, like smoking, also tend to move a person to the left on this scale. A factor which tends to move *all individuals* to the left on this continuum is *aging.* An accident, illness, or athletic injury would also take the person to the left on this health/fitness scale. Finally, death could be represented at the extreme left point on this life scale. Everyone can be represented at some point on this fitness continuum, regardless of age.

An important final consideration of figure 1.1 is that therapeutic exercise (Morris, 1977, 1978) can lead a person from subaverage health to normal functioning, or certainly to better health. Proper, intelligent training or conditioning exercises can lead most persons to higher levels of fitness than they may possess at the outset. Van Aaken (1972), a leading German physician, has also noted that therapeutic exercise is similar to training exercises, except that the dosages (intensity and duration) differ (Morris, 1977, 1978). Of necessity, all of the above factors indicating increased sports participation involve sports medicine. The next section will examine the definitions used by the leading sports medicine individuals in this emerging discipline.

Expert Definitions of the Field

Sports medicine can mean many things to many people. However, to get a better grasp on this new medical discipline, it is important to look at how the leaders in the field define sports medicine.

Dr. David R. Lamb, Past President of The American College of Sports Medicine

Dr. David R. Lamb, a past president of the ten thousand member organization dealing with the area of sports medicine in North America, defines sports medicine as

> . . . the scientific and medical aspects of exercise and athletics. More specifically, sports medicine is the study of the physiological, biomechanical, psychosocial and pathological phenomena associated with exercise and athletics and the clinical application of the knowledge gained from the study to the improvement and maintenance of functional capacities or physical labor, exercise and athletics, and to the prevention and treatment of disease and injuries related to exercise and athletics (Lamb, 1981).

Although Lamb's second definition is much more involved, the first is very sufficient. It adequately covers sports medicine in that *sports medicine is essentially the scientific and medical aspects of sports.*

Dr. Vojin N. Smodlaka, Physiatrist

A practicing physiatrist (specialist in physical medicine), Dr. Vojin N. Smodlaka is a clinical professor of rehabilitation medicine at the State University of New York at Brooklyn, and one of the original members of The American College of Sports Medicine. Dr. Smodlaka was originally trained in Europe, where sports medicine is recognized as a specialty. He has given a somewhat different definition of sports medicine. Smodlaka's definition of sports medicine is

> . . . the investigation of the positive and negative influences of physical exercise, training and competition on the body. Further, the practical obligations of the sports physician include prevention, treatment and rehabilitation of traumatized and diseased athletes and the supervision of training (Smodlaka, 1980).

This second definition differs from Dr. Lamb's view in that it is a somewhat more clinical definition from a trained sports medicine physician.

Dr. Allan J. Ryan, Editor

Dr. Allan J. Ryan, M.D., is the editor-in-chief of the journal, *The Physician and Sportsmedicine.* Dr. Ryan, in an article entitled "Sports Medicine Today" (Ryan, 1978), which appeared in *Science* magazine, detailed what he thought were the major categories of sports medicine. Dr. Ryan has had extensive experience as a team physician for the University of Wisconsin, and is the editor of one of the most prominent sports medicine journals in the world. In a 1978 article describing sports medicine, Dr. Ryan gave the following description of the field of sports medicine.

> Sports medicine is generally conceived to include not only the medical and paramedical supervision of the training and competition of the individual or team athlete, or participant in recreational sports, but also the identification and the provision of sports for those who are physically or mentally disadvantaged, the prescription and supervision of exercise programs to achieve and maintain physical fitness in the apparently unhealthy, and the use of exercise as a means of therapy for those who are not well.

Dr. Ryan's description of the field of sports medicine is limited to four major areas; (1) conditioning for sports participation which involves the effective development of strength, speed, endurance, flexibility, coordination, and power for the athlete, (2) prevention of illness and injury, which begins with a discussion and the preseason examination, and goes on to cover the day-to-day maintenance and evaluation of the health of the athlete, (3) discussion of the treatment of injuries, in which the physician is involved in the diagnosis and immediate treatment of athletic trauma, and (4) rehabilitation after sports injuries, in which the physician, athletic trainer, physical therapist, coach, and athlete might all be members of the team involved in the process of seeing that the athlete is returned to athletic competition safely and efficiently.

Dr. Ernest Jokl, Physician, Researcher, Writer

Dr. Ernest Jokl, M.D., wrote a text entitled *What is Sports Medicine* nearly twenty years ago (Jokl, 1964). This world-renowned researcher, teacher, writer, and lecturer divided sports medicine into three areas: (1) clinical medicine, (2) applied physiology, and (3) sports surgery. Dr. Jokl also noted that sports medicine was a major discipline of medicine which could be justified conceptually because of its integrative influence and empirically because of its diagnostic and therapeutic importance in clinical practice (Jokl, 1964).

Somewhat later, Jokl (1974) included *four* major areas in his definition of sports medicine. Those areas were: (1) applied physiology, (2) clinical medicine, (3) traumatology, and (4) rehabilitation. Rehabilitation was added to his initial three areas. It is interesting to observe that (1) and (4) apply to training and/or reconditioning for sports.

There appears to be a common thread in these definitions. Regardless of whether an exercise physiologist (Lamb, 1981) or a physician (Ryan, Jokl, Smodlaka) is defining the area of sports medicine, most of these prominent individuals have noted the twin areas of training and conditioning for the sport experience. Secondly, they have mentioned the clinical aspects of sports—the proper prevention, diagnosis, treatment, and rehabilitation of the injured athlete. The definitions offered by the physician emphasize the clinical or medical aspects of sports medicine, whereas the athletic trainer, the coach, the athlete, or most especially, the exercise physiologist, emphasizes the area of training and conditioning for athletic participation. Both of these areas of training and injuries are crucial in sports medicine. It is important that the many individuals working in the sports medicine field realize that proper conditioning of the athlete for sports competition may reduce the number of particular athletic injuries or render them less severe (O'Donoghue, 1976; Williams & Sperryn, 1976; Strauss, 1979), demonstrating the interrelationship of these twin areas of concentration within the sports medicine field. These areas of *training and preparation for sports* and *injury prevention, recognition, and rehabilitation* are the two main areas within the overall field of sports medicine (fig. 1.2).

We have looked at the two major areas of sports medicine—training and injury aspects. Turning our attention to other related content areas in the field, we will next examine the writings of prominent individuals in the sports medicine field, looking in detail at how these experts have subdivided the areas of study.

Content Areas

Dr. Lamb (1981) noted that sports medicine encompasses the following fields: exercise physiology, motor control, sports psychology and sociology, biomechanics of exercise and athletics, athletic training, athletic medicine, adult fitness, cardiac rehabilitation, and some aspects of athletic coaching. This is an all-encompassing list and certainly would cover the practices of many sports medicine professionals.

Dr. Allan Ryan noted that there are four major areas in the sports medicine field: conditioning and preparation for sports competition, prevention of illness and injury to the athlete, diagnosis and treatment of illness and injury, and rehabilitation and return of the athlete to sports activity. The training and conditioning aspect is emphasized together with the injury recognition and treatment phase.

Smodlaka (1980) noted that there are several areas of study which could contribute to the sports medicine field: biology, anatomy, anthropology, biomechanics, kinesiology, physiology, hygiene, medical control, traumatology, rehabilitation, first aid, massage, and psychology. All these areas relate to physical education, games, sports training, and competition for everyone. This description of the subareas in the field emphasizes that sports medicine draws upon many subdisciplines.

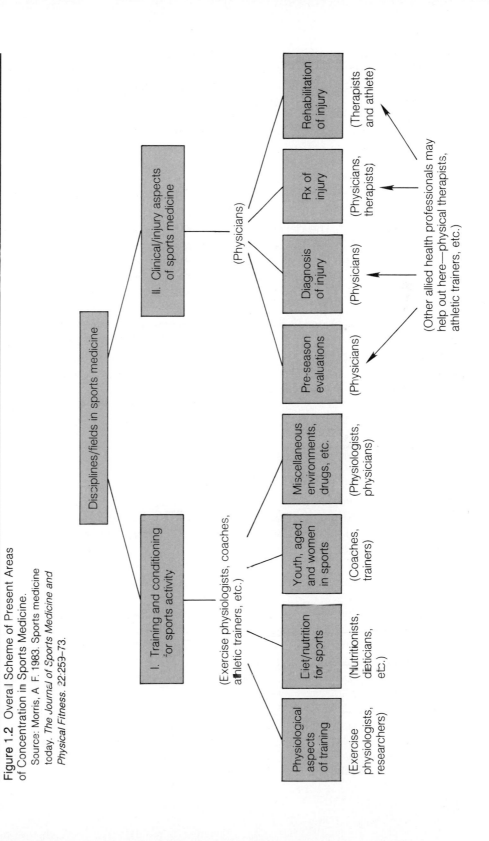

Figure 1.2 Overall Scheme of Present Areas of Concentration in Sports Medicine.

Source: Morris, A. F. 1983. Sports medicine today. *The Journal of Sports Medicine and Physical Fitness.* 22:259–73.

Table 1.1 Major Areas of Study Within the Field of Sports Medicine

Area of study	Title	Description
1. Physiology	Exercise Physiology	Function of the human body during brief exercise or accumulated effects of long-term exercise.
2. Anatomy	Applied Anatomy Kinesiology	Kinesiological aspects of sports; study of the body in motion.
3. Anthropology	Physical Anthropology	Classification of various body types as applied to sports competition.
4. Hygiene	Personal Health	Work and recreation schedules as related to health; effects of diet, alcohol, and tobacco on human performance.
5. Pathology	Sports Pathology	Relation of structural pathology (disfigurement or disability) to participation in various sports; pathology of trauma.
6. Clinical	Clinical Sports Medicine	Methodology of the health examination, diagnosis, and suggested treatments for rehabilitation.
7. Rehabilitation	Physical Rehabilitation	Exercise therapy for rehabilitation of the injured athlete; also includes therapeutic exercise.
8. Surgery	Orthopedic and Corrective Surgery	Use of surgical correction for athletic trauma.
9. Exercise	Therapeutic Exercise	Application of exercise to improve strength, flexibility, or endurance after an athletic injury.
10. Psychology	Sport Psychology	Principles of motor skill learning; effects of personality on sports selection and participation.

Source: McCloy, C. H. 1958. What is sports medicine? *Journal of Health, Physical Education and Recreation*. 29:45–48.

LaCava (1977) defined sports medicine as medical knowledge applied to sport with the aim of preserving the health of the athlete while improving the athlete's performance. Dr. LaCava noted that sports medicine is an applied science concerned with six major areas. These subdisciplines are:

1. *Sports biotypology*—establishing the athlete's biotype or somatotype by each sport discipline.
2. *Sports physiopathology*—studying human adaption to physical effort.
3. *Medical evaluation of sport*—relating the athlete's conditioning to the effort required.
4. *Sports traumatology*—evaluating and preventing typical sport injuries.
5. *Hygiene of sports*—fixing the hygienic behavior of the athlete and the sport environment.
6. *Sport therapeutics*—using sport for the prevention and treatment of diseases.

One of the earlier articles describing the field (McCloy, 1958) shows several important areas of study within sports medicine. McCloy noted seventeen such important areas which are listed in table 1.1.

Area of Study	Title	Description
11. Individual Sports	Women and Youth in Sports	Effect of sex in certain athletic activities; special considerations of athletic competition for women and youth.
12. Training	Conditioning for Sports	General and specific principles regarding athletic training and conditioning.
13. Pedagogy	Motor Learning and Teaching	Methods of teaching or instructing; best practice procedures for skill development.
14. Trainer	Athletic Trainer	Responsibilities of the certified athletic trainer; relationship of the trainer to the coach and athlete.
15. Measurement	Tests and Measurement in Sports	Measurement of physiological capacities, achievement, performance; application of measurements to training and conditioning.
16. Research	Clinical and Physiological Research	Research investigations in training and conditioning; research into the numbers, types, and severity of various athletic injuries.
17. Miscellaneous	General and Miscellaneous Topics	References to sports medicine found in the medical literature; publication of textbooks and journals specifically related to the sports medicine field; publication of year-to-year bulletins and other avenues of information available to the sports medicine professionals.

The importance of table 1.1 is in showing the extreme variety of the topic areas that an early pioneer in the area of sports medicine listed as vital in the field. The table indicates that the areas of training and preparation for sports are equally balanced with those areas representing the clinical and medical aspects of sports. This emphasizes the two major subdivisions in this important area of sports medicine as noted in the previous section. To further understand this emerging field of sports medicine, we will look at some of its early historical developments.

Early History of Sports Medicine

In the early history of sports medicine, the first references were made to this discipline in the early parts of the twentieth century. The first congress of sports medicine took place during the World Hygienic Exposition in Dresdin in 1911. There was a special program during that exhibition entitled "The Hygiene of Physical Exercise." This is probably the first official reference to a formal sports medicine meeting.

A second meeting was a gathering of French physicians which was held in Paris in 1913. The discussion centered on the physiology and kinesiology of physical exercise. In addition, particular sports medicine problems were discussed. This was probably the first formal world congress of sports medicine.

During the First World War, there was a standstill in many of these sports activities, as in many other things. However, in preparation for the winter Olympics in St. Moritz in 1928, physicians from Europe called a meeting of thirty-two Olympic team physicians. These physicians met prior to the winter Olympic Games in 1928, and as such, they formed another congress on sports medicine. That same year, at the summer Olympics in Amsterdam, another meeting and general assembly for an international sports congress was held. It was at this time that the Fédération Internationale of Médecine in Sport (FIMS) was developed. This federation still exists, and is recognized as the international governing body for sports medicine physicians. The FIMS attempts to meet prior to both the winter and summer Olympic Games. First published in 1961, the official journal of this organization is *The Journal of Sports Medicine and Physical Fitness.* Now published in Torino, Italy, Dr. Guiseppe LaCava, internationally known orthopedic surgeon, is its editor. In the mid-1950s, Dr. Joseph B. Wolfe, an American physician, came up with the idea of establishing an American counterpart to the FIMS, founding the American College of Sports Medicine (ACSM) in 1954. As its first president, Dr. Wolfe acted as a representative to the international body for the ACSM.•The official journal of the ACSM is *Medicine and Science in Sports and Exercise,* first published in 1969. The American College of Sports Medicine is probably the largest single sports medicine organization in the world and represents many physicians, exercise scientists, and other related sports medicine personnel from North America.

A final section of this chapter will take a look at some of the professionals who work in the sports medicine field. Since training for sports and the injury aspects of sports are the two main areas of sports medicine (fig. 1.2), it is likely that we would find sports medicine people involved in preparing athletes for sport competition and clinical professionals interested in preventing and treating sport injuries.

Personnel in the Sports Medicine Field

Sometimes students will ask how they can study the field of sports medicine. A typical response is that most of the professionals in this area are physicians, therapists, athletic trainers, and exercise physiologists. Therefore, if they wish to go the medical route, they must go to medical school, or if they are interested in exercise physiology, they should apply to graduate school in that area. The only critical concern is that they have an interest in the care and treatment of athletes (Morris, 1982).

Examining the roster of the American College of Sports Medicine gives an idea of the various groups and percentages of people represented in the general sports medicine field. In the early 1980s, there were approximately ten thousand members in the ACSM. Of this group, about 35–40% were physicians and another 35–40% were exercise physiologists; the remaining 20–30% were therapists, athletic trainers, nurses, and other allied health professionals.

Any person who is interested and works in the scientific and medical aspects of exercise and sports may be said to be sports medicine personnel. Including athletes and their coaches, this group involves many people.

Physicians in Sports Medicine

Before we look at the individual **medical doctor (MD)** involved in the field of sports medicine, let's examine the three primary medical specialists in the United States. The first general medical doctor is the **family practitioner,** or the general medicine specialist. The second category is the **internal medicine specialist.** The last, and final, primary care physician is the **pediatric physician,** who is involved with the care and diagnosis of the young child. In many geographic locations, these three primary care physicians may also function in a sports medicine capacity. One of these primary care medical doctors may be the first physician the athletes see to be cleared for school athletics. In addition to these three primary categories are roughly twenty-two to twenty-four recognized medical specialties in the United States.

It is important to point out that sports medicine, per se, is not an officially recognized medical specialty in North America. There is no board certification at this time in sports medicine. In Europe and other areas there may be some specialized sports medicine physicians. Although there are residency programs at some university and clinical centers, and other institutions in certain areas of the United States which may provide fellowships in the general field of sports medicine, at this time it is not recognized as one of the legitimate medical specialties. The next section will provide a list of certain medical specialties in which physicians function in the capacity of sports medicine physicians. A list of certain board-certified medical specialists who practice in the general area of sports medicine follows. This listing of physicians involved in sports medicine is in approximate order of the number of each of these types of doctors who are found in sports medicine centers.

Major Medical Specialties

Orthopedist

Since most athletic injuries involve the musculoskeletal system, the **orthopedist** is most often consulted. Many major college, university, club, and professional teams have an orthopedic specialist as the team physician. This medical doctor is often a surgeon and is qualified to make minor and major repairs to the musculoskeletal system. Several outstanding physicians, who are or have been university athletic surgeons, are Dr. Peter Jokl of Yale, Dr. Don O'Donoghue of Oklahoma, and Dr. Allan Ryan of Wisconsin. All have written excellent texts on sports medicine (Mangi, Jokl & Dayton, 1979; O'Donoghue, 1976; Ryan, 1962).

Cardiologist

A second category of medical specialist in sports medicine is the **cardiologist.** This medical doctor functions in the diagnosis, treatment, and rehabilitation of people who have cardiovascular problems. The young athlete who has a heart murmur or a congenitally weak heart may be examined and cleared for sports participation by a cardiologist. The physician who works in the area of exercise stress test evaluations for determining the factors of primary or secondary cardiac pathology is generally a cardiac specialist. The cardiac physician may be the screening physician for individuals who are coming out for athletic teams.

Physiatrist or the Physical Medicine Specialist

The third type of medical practitioner most often involved in seeing sports participants is the physical medicine specialist. Because these physicians are intimately involved in the rehabilitation and treatment of individuals who have suffered neuromuscular, musculoskeletal, or other medical problems, they are frequently involved in the treatment of injured athletes. Dr. Vojin Smodlaka, of New York, a European-trained sports medicine physiatrist, is one of the leading world experts in this medical specialty (Smodlaka, 1968).

Neurologist

The **neurologist** becomes involved in the practice of sports medicine when an athlete suffers severe trauma involving the nervous system. Many injuries to the athlete involve the musculoskeletal system, however, if the injury is severe enough, it may also damage soft nervous tissue. When nerve tissue is stretched, jarred, cut, or inflamed in some way, the neurologist becomes involved in sports injuries. Also, in many traumatic injuries, the athlete may suffer a head, back, neck, limb, or spinal cord injury due to a fall from a height, (pole vaulting, dancing, or gymnastics), resulting in neurological damage to the back and spinal cord. When this is the case, the neurologist is called in to help with the athlete's neurological diagnosis, treatment, and rehabilitation.

Obstetrician and Gynecologist

This medical specialist becomes involved in sports medicine cases in situations where young girls or women are participating in athletics. Very often these medical specialists are called in to perform the pre-season medical exams and/or to work with female athletes in their overall preparation for sports activities. Certain female athletic considerations, such as amenorrhea, dysmenorrhea, or pregnancy may suggest to female athletes that they should modify certain activities to some extent. Certain changes (primarily amenorrhea) that she should talk over with the **gynecologist** may occur in the female athlete as she engages in strenuous athletic competition. Additionally, the gynecologist can counsel these athletes on the various dietary and nutritional practices which may help them in their performance. More information concerning women and sports participation will be covered in chapter seventeen.

Ophthalmologist

Another physician who may be involved in the treatment of the athlete is the **ophthalmologist** or eye specialist. Any time the athlete suffers an eye injury or needs improved vision for sports, the ophthalmologist may become involved.

16

Physician Specialties

There are several other physician specialists who may be involved in the care and the treatment of the injured athlete. Very often, the athlete submits blood samples as part of a preseason examination and the **hematology** (the study of blood and blood diseases) **specialist** becomes involved. The **radiologist** or the **nuclear medicine specialist** may be called in as a consultant to the orthopedist to examine X rays, to read arthrograms (joint evaluations), or to examine the result of a bone scan to determine if a stress fracture is present.

Still other physician specialists may be involved in the treatment of athletes. One of these physicians may be the **psychiatrist,** who is a medical doctor trained in neurology, mental health, and proper mental functioning. It has been implicated that there is an indivisible nature involving mind and body when dealing with the athlete. Certain changes may occur in the athlete's psyche when forced into inactivity as a result of an injury or illness. Certain types of athletic activities, primarily endurance in nature, may actually seem to reduce anxiety and, to some degree, reduce depression. There are several prominent psychiatrists, at major universities in the West and Midwest, who have dealt with the problem of depression and anxiety in various groups of athletes and sedentary people. Some very interesting findings have come forth in this area which indicate that long-term endurance activities (running, cycling, walking, skiing, swimming, or other continuous, vigorous, physical activity) appear to be beneficial in reducing mild anxiety and depression in certain individuals. Very often, the psychiatrist is part of a total medical team, which is involved in this area of sports medicine.

Other Doctors in Sports Medicine

Some other categories of medical specialists who become involved in the total overall care and treatment of the athlete include the following.

Osteopath

Another particular type of physician is called the doctor of osteopathy (D.O.). In many cases these doctors study the same things that M.D.s do. The **osteopath** must be licensed in order to practice, just as a regular physician does. Osteopaths often perform surgery and may prescribe drugs (a unique function of the medical doctor). Most doctors of osteopathy can legally practice anywhere within the United States. The main difference between the doctor of osteopathy (D.O.) and the M.D. is that the D.O. places a great deal of emphasis on the neuromusculoskeletal system. In many instances the D.O. looks at the person as a holistic entity, and not really as a person with a particular disease or problem which happens to be affecting just one organ or tissue at any given time. Some individuals in the practice of osteopathic medicine contribute a great deal to the sports medicine field. The training that the D.O. receives is similar to that of the M.D. In addition, the D.O. uses manipulation of muscles and bones to treat special problems. Dr. Keith Peterson, at the University of Washington in Seattle, is a leading sports medicine osteopath who is also on the editorial board of *The Physician and Sportsmedicine.*

Podiatrist

There is another group of doctors who have greatly aided athletes, especially running athletes. This group of doctors is called **podiatrists.** The podiatrist, or foot doctor, is responsible for proper foot care and foot function. Since many sports, especially team sports, involve running, many professional athletic teams consult podiatrists. With the great boom in distance running, there are more and more podiatrists becoming interested in the field of sports medicine. As we learn more about this growing field of podiatry, we realize that, in many instances, an athlete's knee, hip, or even back problems may be related to improper foot care and improper foot placement. Therefore, the podiatrist is assuming a larger and larger role in the care of the athlete. Podiatrists may perform surgery; however, their practice of medicine is generally restricted to the foot.

It must be pointed out here that the orthopedic surgeon may also be involved in foot care for the athlete, since the orthopedist is involved in total musculoskeletal care of the athlete. Both podiatrists and orthopedists may prescribe orthotics or other assists for the athlete in an attempt to aid performance.

Chiropractor

Still another medical person involved in sports medicine is the **chiropractor,** who is skilled in body manipulation and massage. Many athletes today are putting their bodies in the care of certified chiropractors and letting these allied health professionals render them treatment. The person who is well-trained in massage techniques has always been an important medical member of European national sport teams. It is interesting to note that the last United States Olympic team included a chiropractic doctor as a member of the sports medicine team. This may indicate an increasing role for this type of allied health professional in the total scheme of athletic injury care.

Therapists

Athletic Trainer

Many types of therapists in the allied health profession are also involved in the area of sports medicine. Perhaps one of the larger groups of professionals involved in athletic injury care is the **athletic trainer.** The National Athletic Trainers Association (NATA) is the professional organization for all certified athletic trainers who work in the capacity of athletic trainer for a high school, college, or professional team. They work directly with the coach in establishing conditioning and training programs for the athletes, with the hope of preventing many athletic injuries. In addition, realizing that many athletes will be injured in athletic competition, these athletic trainers work closely with team physicians in the care and rehabilitation of these injured athletes. Athletic trainers generally work their way up through physical education curriculums which have been specifically modified to give them certain classroom and practicum experiences in athletic situations.

Physical Therapist

Another group of therapists who are involved in athletic care are registered **physical therapists,** who may work in sports medicine institutes or in medical schools which have sports medicine centers. Again, this is a licensed/certified professional person who has received specific baccalaureate training, and who, in many instances must go through an extensive practicum experience with an athletic team or in a hospital ward situation, treating and aiding in the rehabilitation of ill or injured athletes. These physical therapists must pass a rigorous written and practical exam, in addition to obtaining clinical experience, before being licensed or certified.

Occupational Therapist

Another type of individual involved in therapy is the **occupational therapist.** The occupational therapist is mostly involved with rehabilitation of the hand and development of other work skills in order to get the athlete or patient to function more independently after a major injury or illness. Since many team sports involve hand skills, the athlete may often need proper hand rehabilitation so as to return to participation in that sport. The occupational therapist may work closely in this aspect of injury rehabilitation.

Corrective Therapist

Another therapist who could be involved in the sports medicine field is the **corrective therapist.** These people often have an undergraduate degree in physical education or similar type background. They then do hospital (e.g. veterans) or other clinical affiliation, and practicum or experiential work. They generally seek basic employment in a hospital or a rehabilitation setting.

Nurse Practitioner and Physician's Assistant

There is a new group of **nurse practitioners** who work with primary care physicians. The nurse practitioner is a registered nurse (R.N.) and may aid the physician with the physical exam and/or be in charge of taking a patient's history. The **physician's assistant** often has a similar function to that of the nurse practitioner and helps the physician in more routine work.

Other Professionals

The last major group of professionals in the sports medicine field are the exercise physiologists who are often involved in the educational and research aspects of sports medicine. Exercise physiologists typically teach, do research, and may provide a service function at universities. They are most often involved in the training aspect of the sports medicine discipline. Kinesiologists and applied anatomists are intimately interested in basic human, anatomical, or structural function, and also in using and analyzing that structural basis for human performance.

There are many individuals involved in the study of biomechanics, which is the study of mechanical principles as they are applied to the human body. These individuals also make an important contribution to analyzing athletic movement and, in many cases, analyzing incorrect movement with the hope of detecting a potential problem area in terms of injury recognition or prevention.

Typically, exercise physiologists have at least one advanced graduate degree. Undergraduate degrees are in the biological sciences or physical education. Graduate degrees are in biomechanics or exercise physiology.

Other groups of scientists involved in the study of athletes are the behavioral scientists. Psychology plays an important part in the total preparation of the athlete for competition. Individuals who teach psychology of sport and psychology of coaching classes or who counsel athletes directly or indirectly may be considered sports medicine professionals. Also, there are sport sociologists who study the broad social strata as it affects athletes and their levels of participation in various sports.

Many coaches are involved in the improvement and evaluation of training and conditioning programs for their athletes. Any person who goes about the systematic and intelligent study of the athlete in training in order to determine optimal strategies of conditioning in preparing athletes for competition could be considered to be affiliated with the sports medicine field.

Finally, there are adaptive physical education specialists, who are in charge of designing courses and activities for individuals who may be physically or mentally disabled. Adaptive physical education specialists provide sports opportunities for these disabled individuals. These educators, and other similar professionals, would comprise still another category of allied health professionals involved in the sports medicine field.

There are many professionals in the sports medicine field. In fact, there are almost as many different categories of sports medicine professionals as content areas. Figure 1.2 gives a graphic representation of the sports medicine field and its two major categories: (1) *training and conditioning for sports activity,* and (2) *clinical/injury aspects of sports participation.* Beneath each of these major categories are listings of these important individual areas of study within the major groups, along with a partial listing of sports medicine personnel for each respective subject area. ■

Summary

This first chapter is an introduction to the general sports medicine area. A definition is used for sports medicine, which includes the scientific and medical aspects of exercise and sports. Several prominent sports medicine figures are listed with their definitions of the field. A brief early history of the field shows that the sports medicine movement began in the late 1920s. The international sports medicine society (FIMS) organized in 1928, exists today as the major international body, holding meetings prior to both the winter and summer Olympics.

The variety of personnel involved in sports medicine includes physicians, exercise physiologists, athletic trainers, therapists, and other people involved in preparing the athlete for sport.

The two major areas in sports medicine are: (1) the training and conditioning for sport activity, and (2) the clinical/injury aspect of sports participation. Table 1.1 lists the major subtopical areas within the two major categories of sports medicine.

References

Jokl, E. ed. 1964. *What is sportsmedicine?* Springfield, IL: Charles C. Thomas.

Jokl, E. 1974. Sports medicine. *American Corrective Therapy Journal.* 28:172–82.

LaCava, G. 1977. What is sports medicine: definition and tasks. *Journal of Sports Medicine and Physical Fitness.* 17:1–3.

Lamb, D. R. 1981. Sports medicine—what is it? *Sports Medicine Bulletin.* (ACSM) 16:2–3.

Mangi, R., E. Jokl, & O. W. Dayton. 1979. *The runner's medical guide.* New York: Summit Books.

McCloy, C. H. 1958. What is sports medicine? *Journal of Health, Physical Education and Recreation.* 29:45–48.

Morris, A. F. 1977. What is adapted physical education? *American Corrective Therapy Journal.* 31:75–79.

Morris, A. F. 1978. Comparing and contrasting two similar individual sports: swimming and track. *The Journal of Sports Medicine and Physical Fitness.* 18:409–15.

Morris, A. F. 1982. Sports medicine today. *The Journal of Sports Medicine and Physical Fitness.* 22:259–73.

O'Donoghue, D. H. 1976. *Treatment of injuries to athletes.* 3d ed. Philadelphia: Saunders.

Pelletier, K. R. 1977. *Mind as healer, mind as slayer.* New York: Dell.

Pollock, M. L., J. H. Wilmore, & S. M. Fox, III. 1978. *Health and fitness through physical activity.* New York: John Wiley & Sons.

Ryan, A. J. 1962. *Medical care of the athlete.* Hightstown, NJ: McGraw-Hill.

Ryan, A. J. 1978. Sports medicine today. *Science.* 200:919–24.

Smodlaka, V. N. 1968. Sports medicine in the world today. *Journal of the American Medical Association.* 205:762–63.

Smodlaka, V. N. 1980. Specializing in sportsmedicine. *The Physician and Sportsmedicine.* 8:29.

Smodlaka, V. N. 1980. History of sports medicine (FIMS). *Sports Medicine Bulletin. (ACSM).* 15:11–12.

Strauss, R. H. ed. 1979. *Sports medicine and physiology.* Philadelphia: Saunders.

Surgeon General's Report on Health. *Healthy People.* Washington, DC: U. S. Department of Health, Education and Welfare, Public Health Service, Pub. No. 79-55071, 1979.

Van Aaken, E. 1972. *The Van Aaken method.* Mountain View, CA: World Publications.

Williams, J. Q. P., & P. N. Sperryn, eds. 1976. *Sports medicine* 2d ed. Baltimore: Williams & Wilkins.

Contribution of Sport and Physical Activity to Total Health and Well-Being

Introduction

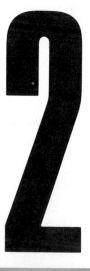

This brief chapter serves as an introduction to several terms and topics that run throughout this text. Initially, a brief discussion of the words *exercise, play,* and *sport* is given. Since many authors use these terms to denote different contexts, it is important to have an *operational definition* of these concepts before getting into the main chapters in the text.

A section follows on the contributions of physical activity and exercise to human health and well-being. In this section, some of the major physical, as well as psychological, benefits of physical activity are described. Later chapters on training and psychological well-being also cover some of these concepts.

The contributions of physical activity to life quality are also discussed. Morris and colleagues (1978, 1982) have done several studies regarding the relationship between life quality and physical activity and their results are briefly mentioned. The relationship of sports competition and the quality of lifestyle (Walker, 1980; Burt, 1976) is mentioned.

Finally, the concept of the unified athlete (deVries, 1980) is detailed. The importance of the integrated association of mental health with physical health is emphasized in this section. In fact, this text is based upon the premise that the human being has an indivisible mind/body nature.

Definitions of Exercise, Play, and Sport

Before starting this chapter on the contributions of physical activity to well-being, it might be well to pause and look at several possible definitions of the words **exercise, play,** and **sport.** These words will be used throughout the text and this is a good place to give them operational definitions.

Exercise

Dr. Robert N. Butler, a former director of the National Institute on Aging, and now the head of the only geriatric department in a medical school, has noted that the word exercise, derived from Latin, means "to drive on" or "to keep busy." It is Dr. Butler's contention that activity, especially physical activity, is a definition of life itself; that is, to be active, to be reconditioned, to be involved. Dr. Butler has written a Pulitzer Prize winning book on aging, and is considered an expert on the aging process. Of course, physical activity is one of the major factors in promoting healthful aging.

Another term for exercise that is used synonymously in many exercise physiology texts is "to work." In a recent article, Sheehan (1982) notes that exercise has become an exact science that can be measured very carefully in a laboratory with many sophisticated devices. Therefore, one working definition that we can use for exercise is *physical work which can be accurately measured* as in a human performance laboratory. The American College of Sports Medicine has also suggested that exercise can be measured in terms of intensity, duration, and frequency. These are noted in an appendix (ACSM Position Statement on Exercise).

Play

Play, at its simplest, is any self-rewarding activity that is not necessary to the daily function of life. It is, generally, self-initiated and participated in during leisure or nonworking circumstances. Most authors agree that play allows complete freedom. We will use play here to refer to *unstructured total-body activities engaged in during leisure time.* Sheehan (1982) notes that play liberates people from the necessity of everyday tasks and is completely *unserious* in its nature. Play seems to restore the individual for the next work cycle.

Sport

Sport is a highly complex term. Sport activity involves *organized, structured competition.* Sport activity takes place within definite boundaries within certain time periods. Within the structure of sports there are many rules which the competitors must abide by. There is, generally, something at risk in sports; that is, the competition or the winning and losing

Physically active play is a voluntary, self-rewarding activity, which enhances the human spirit and serves as a further preparation for life.

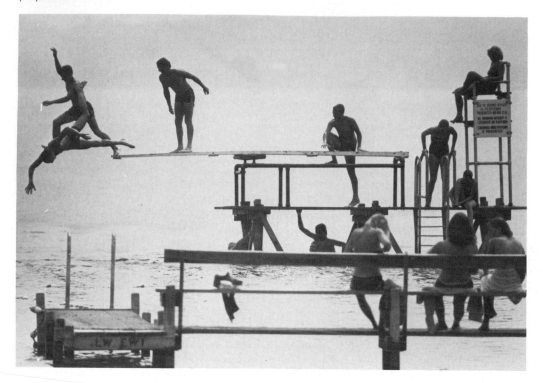

(Walker, 1980). In highly-organized, professional sports, the winning and losing aspect and the competition seem to be of paramount importance. As one descends from that pinnacle of professional sport participation to the collegiate, amateur, and scholastic ranks, the emphasis placed on the competitive and winning aspects of sports should diminish. But, always, there will be the aspect of competition in sports. The desire to exert oneself to the fullest in athletic competition or sports has been present from our earliest beginnings. It is good that sports serve as an outlet for this competitive striving (Walker, 1980; Sheehan, 1980; Stewart, 1979).

This book concerns itself with the large muscle sports activities. The team sports of football, basketball, baseball, and track have long been considered the big-three, team-participant American sports. Today, individual sports, such as running, cycling, swimming, and skiing are becoming increasingly popular. Sedentary activities, such as chess and card playing, *will not* be considered as sports for our purposes in this text.

The Contributions of Physical Activity to Health and Well-Being

In many of my presentations to both scientific and general audiences regarding the value of physical activity, exercise, or sports, I begin by emphasizing the *physical* aspects or benefits of physical activity. I then go on to list a series of changes which may occur within the individual as physical fitness increases. Even though this sounds like I have described a drug with magical qualities, documented pieces of evidence show the amazing contributions that exercise and physical activity can make to physical **well-being** (Stewart, 1979; Morris, 1983; Massie & Shephard, 1971; deVries, 1982).

Many physicians and exercise physiologists are convinced that proper physical activity and exercise not only can increase the length of life, but most certainly can improve the quality of life. There have been many epidemiologic studies (studies of the trends of disease within whole populations) that have shown the relationships between exercise and disease. These longitudinal and cross-sectional studies have indicated that individuals who are physically active in their jobs or in their leisure time generally have a lower risk of cardiac disease, as well as other diseases (Paffenbarger, Wing, & Hyde, 1978; Hartung, 1980). Following are some of the specific ways in which physical activity has a beneficial physiological effect.

Lower resting heart rate and more efficient heart and cardiovascular system.
Lower levels of both circulating cholesterol and triglycerides (fats in the blood) brought about by endurance-type training.
Reduced incidence of smoking.
Reduction in certain electrocardiographic abnormalities, both at rest and during maximal exercise tests.
Favorable changes in body weight and body composition (decrease in percent of fat and increase in lean body weight).
More energy and greater capacity for work.
Greater resistance to stress, anxiety, and fatigue, leading to a much better outlook on life.
Increased stamina in the individual who engages in an endurance exercise program.
Reduced risk of heart attack.
Better sleep habits with endurance exercise.

Some suggested references for these findings are McArdle, Katch & Katch, 1981; Wilmore, 1981; Morris, 1983; Cooper, 1983; Massie & Shepard, 1971.

The previous list of potential benefits that accrue to the individual undertaking an exercise program shows that there are many outstanding physiological benefits which the exercise adherent may derive. In addition to this list of physiological changes that occur to the human organism with exercise, there is a myriad of changes which have been suggested to occur to the *mental* health or mental functioning of the exercising individual.

A positive correlation has been shown between physical fitness and academic success.
Exercise has been shown to increase total circulation, as well as circulation to the brain and other vital organs.

Prolonged physical exercise has been shown to enhance the ability to do mental work during and after the physical exercise.

Exercise tends to increase resistance to both mental and physical fatigue.

Exercise tends to produce arousal, which in turn increases alertness and the speed and efficiency of certain perceptual and psychomotor processes.

Exercise appears to have a positive effect on creativity.

Exercise has been shown to aid in relieving many of the stresses of the twentieth century.

Exercise has been shown to reduce anxiety following certain bouts of physical activity.

A west coast physician has indicated that running may be used as a form of psychotherapy.

Exercise, in conjunction with certain relaxation techniques, has been shown to be effective in coping with acute emotional stress.

Exercise may provide the physiological basis for mystical awareness (deep inner feeling of self-knowledge through physical activity).

Many of these relationships between physical fitness and mental health were discussed during a conference held at the University of Nebraska in the late 1970s (Fuenning et al., 1981). An excellent publication, Proceedings of the Research Seminar on Physical Fitness and Mental Health, can be obtained from the University of Nebraska Press. Other references noting the relationships between physical fitness and mental functioning are found in Kostrubala, 1976; Glasser, 1976; deVries, 1980; Morris & Husman, 1978; Fuenning, et al, 1981.

The Contributions of Physical Activity to the Quality of Life

Several research investigators at Purdue University have found that highly fit individuals tend to be "intellectually inclined, emotionally stable, secure, unconventional, and adventurous." Their report indicates that the most outstanding differences between these fit individuals and their more sedentary contemporaries are factors such as emotional stability and security. Generally, as fitness increases, so does emotional stability and, according to Young and Ismael (1976), this was a fairly typical finding in their investigations. Many other studies have indicated that in extremely fit endurance athletes, self-confidence and self-esteem increase. Morris, Vaccaro, and Clarke (1979) have shown that this increase in self-confidence and self-esteem has manifested itself even in young children. Work with older runners, both male and female, has also found this increased self-confidence and self-esteem.

Other studies, using paper and pencil inventories, have also shown an improvement in **life quality** associated with endurance exercise programs. Morris and Husman (1978) reported that college adults who participated in an endurance conditioning program over the fifteen weeks of a semester significantly improved on measures of life quality. Harris and Morris (1983), in a study of adults in the Baltimore metropolitan area, also showed an

Table 2.1 Total Life Quality Changes During Twelve-Week Activity Programs

Subjects	Pre X	S.D.	Post X	S.D.	Change
Group 1 (Ballroom) dancing	150.53 +	13.90	153.53 +	11.35	3.0
Group 2 (Ballet) dancing	150.46 +	13.63	156.33 +	12.30	5.9
Group 3 (Slimnastics and aerobics)	151.26 +	12.96	158.80 +	10.13	7.5
Group 4 (Control)	153.00 +	15.46	153.33 +	14.62	0.3

Source: Harris, R., & A. F. Morris. 1983. Life quality changes of adult participants during a 12-week physical activity program. Paper submitted for publication.

increase in life quality among physical activity program participants. This latest study indicates that individuals who are involved in more vigorous exercise programs appear to increase more significantly in certain reported life quality outlooks as indicated in table 2.1. Many Americans today are concerned about a high-quality lifestyle.

The Relationship Between Sports Competition and Quality of Lifestyle

Dr. John Burt, Chairman of the Department of Health Education at the University of Maryland, addressed the American Academy of Physical Education at a recent annual meeting and spoke about the relationship between sports competition and life quality. He contended in this national address that people cannot participate in sports without learning something of value about their own personal limits and *their own* responsibility for success and failure within those limits. Sport is one of the few arenas in which humans can experience those conditions of success and failure. A point repeatedly emphasized by Dr. Burt in his presentation is that athletic experiences and competition have as much or more power than most other human experiences to promote self-realization; that is, within discovered limits, people are responsible for their own success or failure. Burt emphasizes that, having learned this, an individual may take a major step toward a quality lifestyle.

Sheehan (1978, 1980) also indicates that many people need a physical challenge in their lives. Sport, and in particular, running, seems to be a test for Sheehan. Here, people can learn whether they are better suited to an endurance event or a speed event. They can learn their amount of tolerance for pain. In sport, they can learn which work/rest cycles they are best suited for. They can attempt very rigorous tests of their athletic ability, or seek out minor confrontations with friends or relatives. They can learn about bodily function and get an idea of their own levels of fitness and performance. Athletes can seek excellence (Stewart, 1979).

Walker, in his excellent text, *Winning in Sports* (1980), notes that the contestant seeks out a sport or competition for the inherent risk involved. Walker tells of the delight the athlete takes in the uncertainty, the challenge, the surprise of the contest. Further, he notes that the athlete accepts the risk, even the possibility of failure, in order to attempt the improbability of a perfect performance. The athlete wishes to be distinguishable—to be able to risk being a winner or loser!

Sheehan, Walker, and Burt realize that competition at its best is the greatest of the performing arts. Winning is the object of the sport, game, or contest, but the *striving* to win is the ultimate experience in sport.

Both Sheehan and Burt emphasize that an absence of competition in the lives of individuals would be a very serious deficiency. They note that through pushing themselves to the limits in their sport or activity, people learn about their own growth and self-esteem. As Sheehan has stated (1980), "through doing what we do best, we attain maturity."

The Unified Athlete

Dr. Herbert A. deVries, of the University of California, has coined the concept of "the unified athlete" (1980). In his discussion of the unified athlete, deVries describes the training, conditioning, and other aspects of preparing the athlete for competition, and the athletic competition itself. DeVries talks about the pressures of training and practice and the stress that accompanies the effort that the athletes are making. He cautions the athletes to continue to monitor their training programs. There are many ways that they can do this. One of the ways is for the athletes to get in-tune with their bodies, as has been suggested above, by monitoring the daily resting pulse rate. When this is taken upon wakening in the morning, it gives the athlete a good physiological indicator of the amount and quality of rest that has been received during the preceeding night or since the last workout. If the true, resting pulse rate is six to eight to ten beats higher than usual, the athlete has not had sufficient rest or sleep and should curtail the training program.

DeVries also cautions the athlete to closely monitor and record daily body weight. Fluctuations in weight can indicate the severity of the training regime, as well as the adequacy of the rest and relaxation schedule. Finally, deVries makes the caution that the athlete should constantly evaluate performance data. This performance data may be obtained from a laboratory test on a bicycle ergometer, or it may be the feedback that the athlete can gather from performance on the daily workout. Other aspects of the unified athlete concept are also important, such as diet and nutrition. The athlete must make sure that adequate calories are being taken in and that the quality of those calories is extremely high. The athlete may be one of the few people in our society who is striving to get the maximum performance out of his or her body, since there are few arenas of human endeavor in which one can try to function at maximum or near-maximum levels of physical activity. Athletes have this opportunity on a regular (weekly, monthly, or, at least, yearly) basis. Athletes should attempt to know themselves thoroughly—to know their bodies and analyze the effects of the stress of training and competition. It is by seeking a balance between training/competition and rest/relaxation cycles that athletes can "get it all together" and perform up to their maximum physiological capacities (Appenzeller & Atkinson, 1981; White, 1982).

Summary

This chapter on the contributions of sport and physical activity to total health and well-being is a brief introduction to the relationship of sports and activity to healthful living. Definitions and descriptions of the terms *exercise, play,* and *sport* are noted.

Exercise is carefully measured human work or physical activity. Exercise can be very accurately measured and prescribed in a laboratory. Exercise is a very purposeful human activity, designed to improve certain aspects of fitness (strength, endurance, and flexibility).

Play, in its simplest form, is any self-rewarding activity that is not necessary to the daily function of life. Play is completely unstructured and free. It is unserious in its nature and seems to restore humans for their next work cycle.

Sport is a highly-complex, organized, structured physical activity. There are rigorous time and space constraints to the sporting activity. Finally, the characteristic of competition is always present in sport. Competition serves to promote excellence and a striving for a high level of human performance in total-body muscular activities.

Physical activity contributes to a high level of life quality. Several studies indicate that as people improve their cardiovascular endurance, positive changes occur to their life quality.

The concept of the unified athlete, as defined by deVries, refers to the individual who continually monitors all aspects of physical performance. Diet and nutrition, rest and relaxation, as well as the intricacies of the training regime, are all scheduled into appropriate segments of the daily, weekly, and yearly training cycles of the athlete.

References

Appenzeller, O., & R. Atkinson. 1981. *Sports medicine.* Baltimore, MD: Urban & Schwarzenberg.

Burt, J. J. 1976. The contributions of physical education to high quality lifestyle. Paper presented to the American Academy of Physical Education, 48th Annual Meeting, Milwaukee, WI, April.

Cooper, K. H. 1983. Aerobic update. *Runner's World.* 18:47.

deVries, H. A. 1980. *Physiology of exercise.* 3d ed. Dubuque IA: Wm. C. Brown.

deVries, H. A. 1982. On exercise for relieving anxiety and tension. *Executive Health.* 18:1–5.

Fuenning, S. I., et al. 1981. Physical fitness and mental health. Proceedings of the Research Seminar on Physical Fitness and Mental Health, University of Nebraska Foundation, Lincoln, Nebraska.

Glasser, W. 1976. *Positive addiction.* New York: Harper & Row

Harris, R., & A. F. Morris, 1983. Life quality changes of adult participants during a 12-week physical activity program. Paper submitted for publication.

Hartung, G. H. 1980. Jogging—the potential for prevention of heart disease. *Comprehensive Therapy.* 6, 28–32.

Kostrubala, T. 1976. *The joy of running.* Philadelphia: Lippincott.

Massie, J. F., & R. J. Shephard. 1971. Physiological and psychological effects of training. *Medicine and Science in Sports.* 3:100–17.

McArdle, W. D., V. Katch, & F. I. Katch. 1981. *Exercise physiology.* Philadelphia: Lea & Febiger.

Morris, A. F., & B. F. Husman. 1978. Life quality changes following an endurance conditioning program. *American Corrective Therapy Journal.* 32:3–6.

Morris. A. F., P. Vaccaro, & D. H. Clarke. 1979. Psychological characteristics in age group competitive swimmers. *Perceptual and Motor Skills.* 43:1265–66.

Morris, A. F. 1982. Sleep disturbances in athletes. *The Physician and Sportsmedicine.* 10:75–78, 83–85, 192.

Morris, A. F., et al. 1982. Life quality characteristics of national class women masters long distance runners. *Annals of Sports Medicine.* 1:23–26.

Morris, A. F. 1983. Training for the elite athlete. Invited address to the 1st International Symposium on Sports Medicine, San Sebastian, Spain, March.

Paffenbarger, R. S., A. L. Wing, & R. T. Hyde. 1978. Physical activity as an index of heart attack risk in college alumni. *American Journal of Epidemiology.* 108:161–75.

Sheehan, G. 1978. *Running and being: the total experience.* New York: Simon & Schuster.

Sheehan, G. 1980. *This running life.* New York: Simon & Schuster.

Sheehan, G. 1982. Exercise sport playfully. *The Physician and Sportsmedicine.* 10:33.

Stewart, M. J. 1979. Presidential address. *American Journal of Sports Medicine.* 7:1.

Walker, S. H. 1980. *Winning.* New York: W. W. Norton.

White, S. W. 1982. Sports: barriers to participation. *The National Forum.* 62:2.

Wilmore, J. 1981. *The Wilmore fitness program.* New York: Simon & Schuster.

Young, R. J., & A. H. Ismail. 1976. Personality differences of adult men before and after a physical fitness program. *Research Quarterly.* 47:513–19.

Basic Concepts of Human
Skeletal Muscle

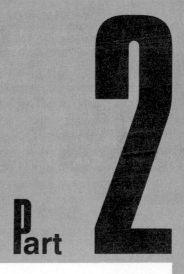

Part 2

Human Skeletal Muscle

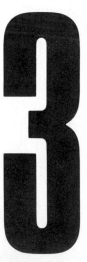

Outline

Introduction

The first two chapters present a brief introduction to the field of sports medicine. These next few chapters set the stage for study of a major area within sports medicine: proper training and preparation for sports competition. Before we approach this, we must examine skeletal muscle. Because movement is so vital to all human endeavors, we must obtain an understanding of how we move and the muscles responsible for this movement. Therefore, this chapter looks in some detail at the more than six hundred skeletal muscles that allow the athlete the range of movement necessary in today's sporting activity.

Muscle Types

Human beings were made for movement. An individual moves by contracting the skeletal muscles. When physical activity begins, other types of muscle tissue begin to speed up or slow down their activity. There are essentially three types of muscle tissue in the body: **smooth muscle, cardiac muscle,** and striated or **skeletal muscle.**

Smooth, Non-Striated Muscle

is found in the blood vessels and throughout the walls of the hollow visceral organs (stomach, intestines, etc.). Smooth muscle receives its innervation from the autonomic (automatic) nervous system. This is mostly an involuntary control system whereby nervous impulses reach smooth muscle via the autonomic nervous system, and contraction is of an involuntary nature. One does not have to think about this muscle contraction in order for it to occur. More will be presented about nervous system innervation later.

Cardiac Muscle

is a specialized type of muscle found in the heart. Cardiac muscle is found in all vertebrates and appears as a lattice-work of striated fibers. This network of fibers is the major difference between cardiac muscle and the other two types of muscle tissue. Cardiac muscle has another unique characteristic in that it contracts rhythmically and automatically, without outside or voluntary stimulation. This rhythmic contraction continues, generally uninterrupted, throughout an individual's lifetime.

Striated Skeletal Muscle

provides a force for movement of the skeletal system. This muscle gives form and shape to the body. In skeletal muscle, the innervation is through the voluntary motor system. The striations of skeletal muscle are due to their interlacing bands of actin and myosin filaments, which give it the dark and light appearance. Each fiber within the striated muscle system is composed of a large cell, which may have several hundred nuclei. Each cell is structurally independent of its neighboring cell or fiber. Therefore, in the skeletal muscle system, *each muscle fiber is equivalent to a single muscle cell.* A person is born with a certain number of muscle cells and these cells must last and function throughout life. Occasionally, it is said that top-class, gifted athletes picked their parents wisely—they started with good athletic genes and good muscle fibers!!

Gross Structure of Skeletal Muscle

In order to effectively study the area of exercise, which includes muscular contraction, we must become more familiar with the various components of skeletal muscle. It is important in our study of muscular contraction to understand the nature of the individual muscle cell, which is the basic functional unit in the skeletal muscle system. Skeletal muscle is essentially organized as shown in figure 3.1. In general, if the total muscle is taken from the limb and then dissected further, it can be seen how this muscle is broken into its parts. The first major subdivision of the entire skeletal muscle is called the muscle fasciculus. The fasciculus is a group of muscle cells surrounded by connective tissue. Skeletal muscles are composed of many fasciculi. A single fasciculus generally lies along the long axis of the muscle, and probably lies parallel to other fasciculi. When this fasciculus is broken down further, the individual muscle cells can be seen (fig. 3.1). The subunits of the muscle cell (fibers) reveal many myofibrils. The myofibril is the contractile component of the skeletal muscle cell. A further breakdown of the myofibril shows the individual actin and myosin protein filaments (myofilaments), which compose the different myofibrils. Generally, the actin filaments are thin and less highly-developed when viewed under a microscope. The myosin filaments are thicker and lie adjacent to the actin filaments. These alterations of thick and thin filaments in the muscle give the skeletal muscle its striations, or alternating light and dark bands. It is believed that when skeletal muscle increases in size as the result of strength training, the size and number of myofibrils increase. This increase in muscle fiber size is termed **hypertrophy.** However, recent animal work (Ho, et al., 1980) shows that rat muscle fibers may increase in number by fiber splitting with heavy strength training. This would also cause an increase in skeletal muscle girth.

Components of the Muscle Cell

In addition to these general considerations of the muscle, you should become familiar with other specific components of the muscle cell.

The Cell Membrane

The muscle cell is surrounded by a cellular membrane. This membrane consists of two parts: an inner membrane (the plasma membrane) and an outer membrane. The outer membrane plays a minor role and is less critical to the maintenance of cell life, when compared to the plasma membrane. Within this outer membrane is the cytoplasm. Strictly defined, the cytoplasm consists of all the constituents outside the nucleus of the cell, but bordered within the plasma membrane. One other major component of the muscle cell is the nucleus, which is the major control center of the cell. The genetic material is contained within the nucleus, which is surrounded by its own membrane.

Figure 3.1 A Skeletal Muscle *(a)* and Its Components—fasciculus *(b)*, muscle cell or fiber *(c)*, and myofibril *(d)*.

From Hole, John W., Jr., Human Anatomy and Physiology, 2d ed. © 1978, 1981 Wm. C. Brown Publishers, Dubuque, Iowa. All Rights Reserved. Reprinted by Permission.

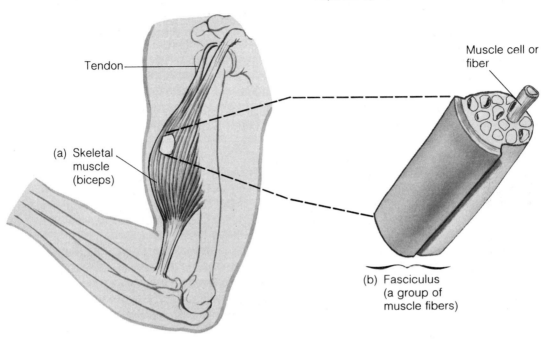

Tendon

(a) Skeletal muscle (biceps)

Muscle cell or fiber

(b) Fasciculus (a group of muscle fibers)

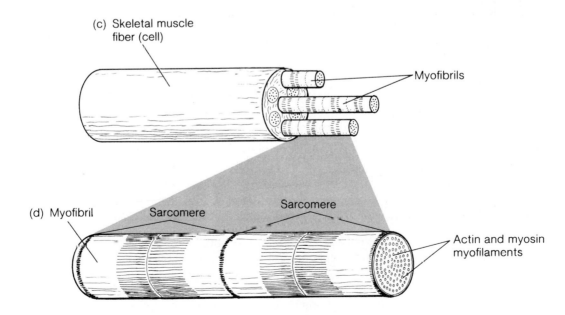

(c) Skeletal muscle fiber (cell)

Myofibrils

(d) Myofibril

Sarcomere

Sarcomere

Actin and myosin myofilaments

Mitochondria

Another major component of the muscle cell is the **mitochondria.** The mitochondria are small, specialized organelles that serve as the major site of energy production within the cell. These small "energy units" are sometimes referred to as the powerhouse of the cell. They are small in size, but large in quantity, within the cell. It is known that athletes undergoing endurance training can increase the size and number of mitochondria contained in their muscle cells (Edington & Edgerton, 1976; Strauss, 1979). These changes in size and/or number of mitochondria within the cell are some of the primary subcellular adaptations that the athlete undergoes in an endurance training program.

Among the other particular components of the muscle cell may be found glycogen particles, as well as lipid granules. These are small types of foodstuffs that are available as energy for the muscle cell.

Blood Supply to the Muscle

Skeletal muscle tissue is profusely supplied with blood and blood vessels. In the adult college male, approximately 40–45 percent of body weight is skeletal muscle tissue (Fox, 1979; deVries, 1980). In the average adult female athlete there is approximately 35–40 percent muscle tissue. (These are standard or average values.) In highly-conditioned athletes who have reduced their percentage of body fat, skeletal muscle tissue may involve a larger percentage of total tissue. In fact, in the well-trained male, 50 percent or more of body tissue may be composed of skeletal muscle tissue. In the highly-trained female athlete, muscle mass may be as much as 40 or 50 percent of the total body weight. A very profuse blood supply to the area is needed to support this muscular tissue, which is highly metabolically active. It has been estimated that in every excess pound of fat carried, there may be an extra two hundred miles of capillaries. If that is the case for fat tissue, which generally does not have many blood vessels within it, then you could expect more vascularization in muscle tissue. If you look at muscular tissue, you generally notice its pink or red color. This is due to the many blood vessels and blood that circulates through this type of tissue. In fact, some skeletal muscle tissue appears darker than others because of its increased blood supply. This type of tissue is generally called "red" muscle tissue, or slow muscle tissue. Other muscle tissue, somewhat more pink, is considered fast muscle tissue. These two particular muscle fibers, the fast type and the slow type, will be discussed later. It is important to remember that there is a heavy blood supply to the muscle tissues. This explains why the athletic trainer or coach first tries to retard the massive loss of blood that occurs in the muscle immediately after an injury.

Neuromuscular Considerations

With some understanding of the basic structure of skeletal muscle, we will now turn our attention to the neurological organization, as it relates to muscular tissue. The attempt here is not to make you a neuroanatomist or neurophysiologist. However, you must learn certain basic concepts involving neuromuscular considerations to more fully understand muscular contraction. We will discuss the motor unit and proprioception.

36

Figure 3.2 A Motor Unit. One motor neuron *(a)* is shown along with all of the muscle fibers *(b)* innervated by that single motor nerve cell.

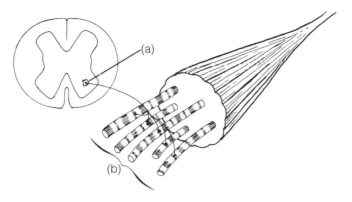

The Motor Unit

It was noted earlier that the basic functional unit in the skeletal muscle system is the muscle cell or fiber. In the nervous system, the basic functional unit is the **motor unit.** *A motor unit may be defined as a single nerve cell* (lower motor neuron) *and all of the terminal muscle fibers that are innervated by that single nerve cell.* Another name for the nerve cell is the neuron. Because these neurons are located in the spinal cord, below the level of the brain, they are often referred to as lower motor neurons. Another synonym for the lower motor neurons is alpha motor neurons, because they are often large nerve cells of motor origin. Therefore, the singular motor nerve cell, and all of the terminal muscle cells that are innervated by it, comprise the motor unit. This can be seen in figure 3.2.

Motor units may be large or small. In a large motor unit, one motor nerve cell could innervate as many as two thousand terminal muscle fibers, while in a small motor unit a single nerve cell might only innervate two to six muscle fibers. For example, in larger muscles of the lower limb, like the gastrocnemius (the large muscle of the calf), the innervation ratio may be one nerve cell to several thousand muscle cells or fibers. The reason for this extremely low ratio of motor nerve innervation to muscle cells is that, when the muscle cells of the gastrocnemius contract, large forces are required to make the gastrocnemius muscle function in getting the athlete moving or running. Typically, small motor units are found in smaller muscles which are used for example in small, precise eye, or hand and finger movements.

Proprioception

In addition to our consideration of motor units and the structure and function of the motor neuron in relation to the muscle cells, we must also be concerned with **proprioception** that occurs within the muscles. *Proprioception may be briefly defined as the individual's awareness of joint positions and the movement occurring at those joints.* Obviously, proprioception is an important mechanism in the physical performance of many motor skills.

The main organ of proprioception in the muscular system is the **muscle spindle.** *The muscle spindle is a highly developed sensory organ that is responsible for recording muscle stretch and contraction of the muscle.* Essentially, when a muscle stretches, due either to a voluntary contraction or an outside impulse, a signal is picked up by the muscle spindle. This signal is sent back into the nervous system, resulting in a reflex contraction of the muscle. An example of the workings of the muscle spindle and a basic proprioceptive reflex is the simple patella tendon tap, or the common knee jerk response elicited by a physician doing a basic neuromuscular test. This simple type of nervous system test informs the physician of the basic state of the involuntary nervous system. When an individual is being tested for the patella tendon jerk reflex, the person is asked to relax, perhaps with eyes closed, and the physician delivers a slight blow to the patella tendon (located immediately below the kneecap). This tendon tap stretches the quadriceps muscle. The muscle spindle, located within the quadriceps muscle, records this stretch and, in turn, sends an impulse back into the spinal cord. After a synapse (space between nerve cells) is passed, the same impulse returns via a motor neuron to the same quadriceps muscle,

Figure 3.3 Basic Stretch Reflex. The sensory neuron *(a)* receives input to the system. The motor neuron *(b)* then fires, resulting in a muscle contraction. This example illustrates a reflexive quadriceps contraction.

From Hole, John W., Jr., Human Anatomy and Physiology, 2d ed. © 1978, 1981 Wm. C. Brown Publishers, Dubuque, Iowa. All Rights Reserved. Reprinted by Permission.

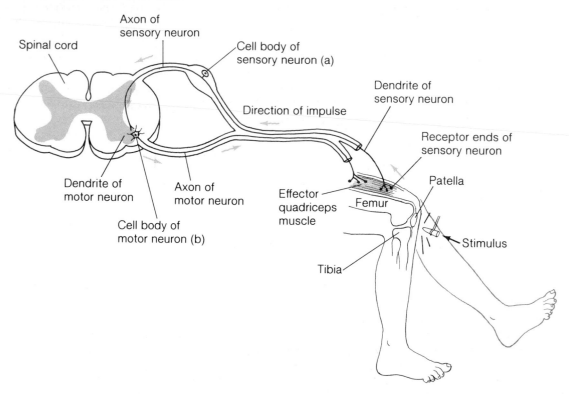

initiating a muscle contraction. This results in a reflex contraction of the quadriceps muscle, causing the foot to kick forward in the knee jerk movement. This is diagrammed simply in figure 3.3. The importance of this muscle spindle mechanism will become obvious when we discuss various methods of training, especially strength and flexibility training. Certain strength training programs capitalize on the mechanism of the stretch reflex with this type of muscle stretch training in an attempt to seek increases in strength. This simple reflex is also called **myotatic** reflex, *a simple stretch reflex of the muscle.* The tendon jerk is, therefore, an example of a myotatic reflex.

Fiber Types and Skeletal Muscle Function

It is important for several reasons that the exercise scientist understand skeletal muscle fiber types. First of all, there has been a myth present in athletics that anyone who works hard enough at a particular athletic event can become a champion. This is a half truth, in that we now know that an individual who does not have an appropriate genetic makeup, or possess certain types of muscle cells, may not be successful in some athletic events. Another reason for the importance of muscle fiber typing is in understanding the relationship between certain athletic events and the propensity of athletes with certain body types to go into those events. For example, if we look at the athletes entered in the 100-meter dash in the Olympics, we are likely to see very powerful, muscular individuals. On the other hand, if we examine the body types of the Olympic marathon runners we are likely to find smaller, leaner types of individuals. The different muscle fiber types are generally responsible for the different characteristics that are displayed by these superior athletes. Predicting which fiber types are predominant in an athlete or a particular athletic group is important in channeling young people into events in which their particular muscular fiber compositions may be best suited. For example, the high school coach who finds a rather small individual with mostly slow twitch leg muscle fibers coming out for an activity may encourage this individual to participate in a middle- or long-distance event, rather than a speed or power type event. Simple tests, such as vertical jumping or the standing long jump, may help the coach determine if an athlete is a mostly fast twitch or slow twitch athletic type.

Classification of Muscle Fiber Types

Fast/Slow Twitch Classification System

There are several different methods for classifying skeletal muscle fiber types. Perhaps the earliest classification system simply described the muscle as either dark red or mostly pink. Somewhat later, another classification system came into being, characterizing the muscle fiber in terms of twitch characteristics. This classification scheme is shown diagrammatically in figure 3.4. In this classification scheme, the force or tension characteristics of the muscle are examined with regard to the duration of contraction of that particular fiber. In a **fast twitch muscle fiber,** the muscle is capable of generating *more tension in a shorter period of time* than a slow twitch muscle fiber. In figure 3.4, this ratio of contraction and relaxation of the particular fast muscle fiber is displayed by the dotted line.

Figure 3.4 Contraction/Relaxation Curves For Fast Twitch (FT) and Slow Twitch (ST) Mammalian Skeletal Muscles. This classification scheme is based on individual muscle twitch contraction speeds.

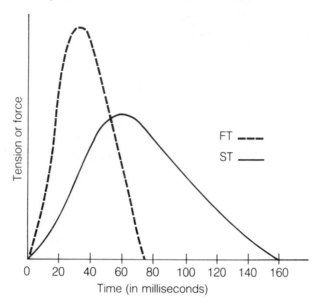

The **slow twitch muscle fiber,** on the other hand, develops tension very slowly over time, and it also develops a lesser amount of tension than the fast twitch muscle fiber. This ratio is represented in figure 3.4 by the solid line. Two other general distinctions between these particular fast twitch and slow twitch fibers are that the slow twitch fibers are (1) generally red and (2) less fatiguable than the fast twitch fibers. The fast twitch fibers tend to be pale or somewhat whiter than the red slow twitch muscle fibers. (Observe this for yourself at Thanksgiving time, when you see the leg musculature of the turkey at the dinner table. The legs, or drumsticks, appear more red than the white of the breast and wings because the turkey used its legs more than its other musculature in trying to escape the farmer's hatchet). We saw earlier that the red colorings of the slow twitch muscle fiber is predominantly due to increased vascularization and blood supply to these fibers. The classification of a particular muscle fiber, based on twitch characteristics, is determined upon stimulation. If, upon receiving a nervous impulse, the muscle fiber responds fast, then it is classified as a fast twitch muscle fiber. If, instead, a longer, slower muscle twitch results, then this is a slow twitch fiber.

Metabolic Classification of Muscle Fibers

Another classification system for muscle fibers is typing them according to their biochemical properties. The metabolic profile of the fiber considers whether that muscle fiber is primarily suited for **aerobic** (longer term, oxygen-present), or **anaerobic** (in the absence

Figure 3.5 A Continuum of Muscle Fiber Types in Human Skeletal Muscles. To the left on the continuum are the slow oxidative (SO) fibers, and on the far right are the fast glycolytic (FG) fibers. Falling in between on the continuum are the fast oxidative-glycolytic (FOG) type. Statements relating to twitch speeds, size, fatigability, and color are *generalizations* regarding skeletal muscles.

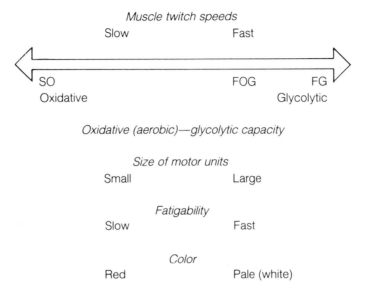

Muscle twitch speeds

Slow   Fast

SO   FOG   FG
Oxidative   Glycolytic

Oxidative (aerobic)—glycolytic capacity

Size of motor units

Small   Large

Fatigability

Slow   Fast

Color

Red   Pale (white)

of free oxygen) physical activity. This classification system considers whether the particular muscle cell is used for very powerful, fast, strength-type muscle contractions, or for slower, longer-lasting muscle contractions of less force. When looking at this particular classification scheme, scientists have broken down this metabolic profile into three areas. The first is the slow twitch **oxidative** fiber. This will be identified by the symbol "SO," standing for slow oxidative metabolic profile. A second category, according to the biochemical or metabolic property of the muscle fiber, is the fast twitch **oxidative-glycolytic** fiber. This category is identified by the initials "FOG," standing for fast twitch, oxidative *and* glycolytic. The third and final category under this biochemical system of classifying muscle fibers is the fast twitch **glycolytic** fiber. This will be identified by the initials "FG." It is important to realize that there may be some overlapping within these different classifications. When looking at a continuum of fiber types, as shown in figure 3.5, the slow oxidative fibers are at one end of the biochemical/metabolic spectrum, while the fast twitch glycolytic fibers are at the other end. The FOG fibers are somewhat in the middle of this continuum, but leaning slightly to the right—toward the FG category. Many of the older systems of classification were based on just two or three individual categories of fiber types. Now we realize that there may be many gradations. Earlier work in this area of investigation was conducted on small animals. Subsequent work on humans has shown that the fiber typing of animal muscle fibers is somewhat different from that of humans. There are differences between species in the number and types of muscle fibers (Edington & Edgerton, 1976; Holloszy, 1982).

Table 3.1 Muscle Fiber Type Classification System (Metabolic and Contractile)

Characteristic	Fiber type terminology		
	SO	FOG	FG
Color	Red	Pink	White
Name	I	II A	II B
Speed	Slow	Fast	Fast
Metabolism	High—oxidative	High—oxidative	Low—oxidative
Fatigue	Fatigue resistant	—	Fast fatiguing
Mitochondria	Many, large	Many	Few, small
Blood supply	Great	Moderate	Small
Speed & metabolism	SO	FOG	FG
Myoglobin	High	Moderate	Low
Neuromuscular junction	Small, simple	Large, complex	Large, complex
Glycogen	Low	High	High
ATPase activity	Low	High	High
Fatty acid use	High	Moderately high	Low

Sources: Edington, D. W., and V. R. Edgerton. 1976. *The biology of physical activity.* Boston: Houghton Mifflin; deVries, H. A. 1980. *Physiology of exercise.* 3d ed. Dubuque, IA: Wm. C. Brown.

So far, we have classified skeletal muscle fiber according to anatomical appearance, muscle function, and biochemical properties. A fourth classification system is based on the enzyme profile of the muscle fiber. Very briefly, this final system involves staining muscle fibers with a particular dye that reacts to certain metabolic properties within the muscle fiber. A summary of the classifications and characteristics of human skeletal muscle fiber types is listed in table 3.1. Table 3.2 displays another classification system using subtypes of muscle fibers for the slow and fast twitch muscle fibers.

Muscle Energy Metabolism

Another way of analyzing human muscular contraction is to consider the ability of the athlete to generate energy. Since superior athletic performance is largely determined by the athlete's capacity to generate energy, a minimal understanding of basic energy generation and energy metabolism can help to explain superior muscle performance. In studying energy metabolism it is important to realize that energy can be generated via two major pathways. The first major pathway is aerobic metabolism, in which the burning of fats and glucose is the major energy production system during rest. A little over 50 percent of the energy necessary for resting metabolism is supplied through fat metabolism, however, as the athlete goes from the resting state into vigorous all-out muscular performance, the energy supply system switches from burning mostly fat to burning mostly carbohydrates.

Table 3.2 Characteristics of Human Muscle Fiber Types

Muscle fiber characteristics	Muscle fiber type	
	Slow twitch	Fast twitch
Morphological		
Mitochondria	Large, many	Small, few
Neuromuscular junction	Small, simple	Large, complex
Sarcoplasmic reticulum	Similar	Similar
Metabolic[a]		
Glycogenesis	↑	↓
Glycogenolysis	↓	↑
Glycolysis	↓	↑
Fatty acid utilization	↑	↓
Krebs cycle and electron transport system	↑	↓
Ketone body oxidation	↑	↓
Protein metabolism	↑	↓
Blood supply	↑	↓
Myoglobin content	↑	↓
Contractile		
Contraction speed	↓	↑
Relaxation time	↑	↓
Force/velocity relationship	Slow/relative load	Fast/relative load
Length/tension relationship	Similar	Similar

Sources: Edington, D. W., and V. R. Edgerton. 1976. *The biology of physical activity.* Boston: Houghton Mifflin, deVries, H. A. 1980. *Physiology of exercise.* 3d ed. Dubuque, IA: Wm. C. Brown.

Note: Findings which are not available from studies using human subjects have been extrapolated from studies using other mammals.

[a] Enzyme activities of the respective metabolic pathways as estimated by histochemical or biochemical analysis have been used as indicators of the capacity of the metabolic characteristics. Arrows indicate higher or lower comparative values.

There are six particular time frames of energy production (Edington & Edgerton, 1976) and three major energy supply systems available to the athlete (fig. 3.6). An immediate energy source system consists of adenine triphosphate (ATP) and creatine phosphate (CP). These substrates are broken down to adenosine diphosphate (ADP). The reaction is then shown:

$$\text{ATP} \xrightarrow{\text{M. Contraction}} \text{ADP} + \text{P (Phosphate)} + \text{approx. 8000 kcal of energy.}$$

This energy system furnishes an immediate source of energy for the contractile mechanism. An intermediate energy source is called into play if the athlete continues vigorous exercise for a period of thirty seconds to two minutes. At this point, the major fuel for this continued muscular contraction is glycogen. Most glycogen is stored in skeletal muscle,

Figure 3.6 Energy Supply Systems Available to Athletes. The sources of immediate energy are ATP and CP *(a)*. Secondary energy *(b)* is obtained from glycogen, or non-oxidative sources. Sources of long-term energy are blood-borne glucose and free fatty acids *(c)*.

Adapted from Edington, D. W., and V. R. Edgerton. 1976. *The biology of physical activity.* Boston: Houghton Mifflin. Reprinted with permission.

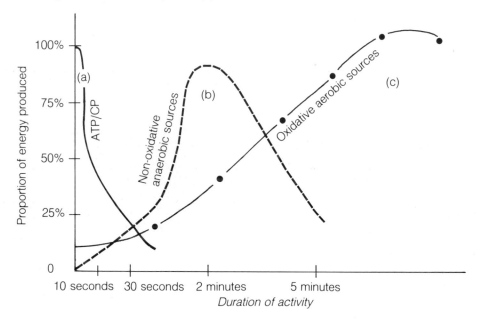

but some is also available in the liver. When the sport calls for long term endurance-type activity, the athlete must turn to the long term energy supply sources of free fatty acids (FFA) and glucose (see fig. 3.6). These energy substrates are circulating in the blood and are brought to the skeletal muscle via the circulation. In events that require continuous motion (a sustained athletic event lasting five minutes or longer), this long term energy source becomes most important. In very long term running events (over five kilometers), this long term energy supply system must be extremely well developed. Table 3.3 shows these various energy source systems together with transition phases that may occur between each of the major energy source phases.

Energy Metabolism Related to Training

Muscle energy metabolism is important to the understanding of training and conditioning. One of the cardinal principles of training and conditioning is specificity of effort—to be successful in an athletic activity, an individual must train specifically for that activity. To give a concrete example, if an athlete hopes to achieve optimum times in the mile run, then training and conditioning must be specific for that particular athletic event. Since the

Table 3.3 Aerobic/Anaerobic Metabolism of Energy Sources

Energy source	Duration of activity	% Aerobic	% Anaerobic
ATP, CP	up to 2 seconds	—	100
ATP, CP	2 to 10 seconds	1–5	95–99
Transition	10 to 30 seconds	5–10	90–95
Glycogen	30 seconds to 2 minutes	10–20	80 90
Transition	2 to 5 minutes	20–30	70–80
FFA & glucose	over 5 minutes	55–65	35–45

Sources: Edington, D. W., and V. R. Edgerton. 1976. *The biology of physical activity.* Boston: Houghton Mifflin; deVries, H. A. *Physiology of exercise.* 3d ed. Dubuque, IA: Wm. C. Brown.

Table 3.4 Aerobic/Anaerobic Energy Source Requirements for Swimming and Track Events

Track event	Swimming event	% Speed/strength ATP/CP	% Anaerobic	% Aerobic
100 m	25 m	98–99	1–2	_____
200 m	50 m	95–98	2–5	_____
400 m	100 m	70–80	20–30	2–5
800 m	200 m	25–30	60–70	5–10
1500 m	400 m	10–20	30–40	55–65
5000 m	1600 m	5–10	20–30	65–75
19,000 m	_____	1–5	15–20	75–85
Marathon	Channel, ocean swims	_____	2–5	95–98

Source: Morris, A. F. 1978. Comparing and contrasting two similar individual sports: swimming and track. *The Journal of Sports Medicine and Physical Fitness.* 18: 409–415.

goal of the mile runner on a world class level would be to achieve a time of well under four minutes, repeated efforts of one to four minutes in duration must be sustained in certain training cycles. The duration of effort indicates that the mile run is primarily an aerobic event, however, there is a significant proportion of anaerobic components to it. Table 3.4 shows that approximately 55–65 percent of the effort of running the mile will come from aerobic sources; the other percentage will come from anaerobic sources. This indicates that the miler should spend approximately this same percentage of training time working on developing the aerobic system. However, since a significant proportion of the event may be anaerobic, this phase of the miler's development must also be attended to in proportion. The intelligent athlete training for this distance should be concerned with practicing speed and short term bursts of activity, as well as longer term aerobic conditioning.

Often, early season training for the mile runner will consist of longer, slower aerobic efforts, while late season or peak training will involve shorter, more intensive anaerobic workouts. This breakdown of aerobic and anaerobic proportions is listed for various individual continuous events in table 3.4.

Comparisons of Sports

Swimming and Running

This scheme of classifying muscle function according to exercise metabolism can also be used quite well to compare and contrast various sports. Morris (1978, 1981) has done this in several published reports. Comparisons made in these writings show certain parallels between different sport activities. For example, the swimmer will complete an event of approximately four hundred meters to the runner's fifteen hundred meters (table 3.4). This tells the exercise physiologist, the coach, the athletic trainer, and the athlete that the same approximate amount of effort is generated over the same time span within these two activities. The ratio of swimming distance to running distance is 1:4.

Cross-Country Skiing and Long-Distance Running

Another sport comparison which can be made is cross-country skiing to long-distance running by looking at the record times that individual athletes have set over the distances of each of these sports. A common event in both cross-country skiing and long-distance running is the ten kilometer race. World class athletes in both sports cover these distances in from twenty-seven to thirty-two minutes, depending on terrain, weather, and environmental conditions. So the sport scientist or coach can compare these two activities on a one-to-one ratio. The maximum distance that has been covered by an athlete in one day in either sport is approximately 168 miles. Whenever such extremely long distances are involved, the terrain and weather conditions play a vital part. The wetness and condition of the snow are of utmost importance to the long-distance skier. Temperature and terrain are vital concerns to the long-distance runner. A hilly rolling course may not be covered within the same period of time as a relatively flat course with a fairly strong favorable wind. In many extremely long-term endurance events, world records are not recognized due to the extreme variety in terrain and environmental conditions.

Speed Skating and Running

With this basic knowledge of muscle energy metabolism, other sporting activities can be compared and contrasted. This has been done in a paper involving speed skating (Morris, 1981). An individual performance by a speed skater over a certain time period is compared with an individual performance by a track athlete during a certain track event. This assumes that both individuals will give maximal effort in their performance over that particular time frame so various events can be compared in terms of energy metabolism. The ratio of skating distance to running distance is 2:1 in events of more than ten thousand meters.

46

Cycling and Cross-Country Skiing

Among the several other sports that may be contrasted here are cycling and cross-country skiing. These two individual sports can be compared and contrasted since they are individual sports and are measured by a ratio of distance/time. This is the best way to compare two different events—events that start at a given time and continue uninterrupted for whatever period is needed to cover a pre-determined distance.

When contrasting cycling with skiing, one can observe that a good skier should be able to cover ten miles in one hour. In that hour of all-out effort a good cyclist should cover approximately twenty-two to thirty-three miles. This demonstrates a relationship developing between these two sports. To compare a cycling workout with a skiing workout, the distance ratios would be approximately three to one. The cyclist covering ten miles would get the same approximate workout as the skier covering three to four miles. ■

Summary

The purpose of this chapter is to introduce the components of human skeletal muscle. There are three types of muscle found in the human body. The first type is smooth and is found mostly in blood vessels and throughout the walls of certain organs of the body; the second type, cardiac muscle, is a special type of muscle found only in the heart; the final type, striated skeletal muscle, is the voluntary type of muscle found in the human body. Since this text is concerned with human movement, a detailed discussion of the structure of human skeletal muscle is given. The components of the striated muscle cell are listed: the cell membrane, mitochondria, and other organisms within the muscle cell. Blood supply for skeletal muscle is covered. Neuromuscular considerations, including the motor unit, patterns of proprioception, and elements of the reflex arc are covered.

Another major section covers the relationship of individual muscle fiber types to human skeletal muscle function. It is pointed out that there are two major fiber types as classified by twitch contraction times. A further breakdown of the classification of muscle fiber types is by muscle metabolism. It is shown that, according to this classification scheme, there are at least three different categories of classification of muscle fibers based on metabolic properties.

In a later section, muscle energy metabolism is given as a means to compare and contrast several different sports. Swimming and running can be compared in an approximate four to one ratio. A swimmer takes approximately four times longer to cover the same distance as a runner. For example, it takes a runner about four minutes to do fifteen hundred meters, or one mile, while in the swimming pool, an experienced swimmer would cover approximately four hundred meters. The importance of anaerobic and aerobic energy metabolism as related to training is also covered in this chapter. The energy sources and time periods of energy utilization for different anaerobic/aerobic events are listed. In short, all-out, intense exercise, the anaerobic system is used primarily. In longer term events (continuous events of five minutes or longer), mostly aerobic mechanisms are called into play. This information is later integrated with various sports comparisons, as indicated earlier, such as swimming and running, cross-country skiing and long-distance running, speed skating and running, etc.

References

deVries, H. A. 1980. *Physiology of exercise.* 3d ed. Dubuque, IA: Wm. C. Brown.

Edington, D. W., and V. R. Edgerton. 1976. *The biology of physical activity.* Boston: Houghton Mifflin.

Fox, E. 1979. *Sports physiology.* Philadelphia: W. B. Saunders.

Ho, K. W., et al. 1980. Skeletal muscle fiber splitting with weight-lifting exercise in rats. *American Journal of Anatomy.* 157: 433–40.

Holloszy, J. O. 1982. Muscle metabolism during exercise. Archives of *Physical Medicine and Rehabilitation.* 63: 231.

Morris, A. F. 1978. Comparing and contrasting two similar individual events: swimming and track. *The Journal of Sports Medicine and Physical Fitness.* 18: 409–415.

Morris, A. F. 1981. A scientific explanation for Eric Heiden's unique olympic performance. *The Journal of Sports Medicine and Physical Fitness.* 21: 156–59.

Strauss, R. H. ed. 1979. *Sports medicine and physiology.* Philadelphia: W. B. Saunders.

Athletic Training and Conditioning for Sports

Part 3

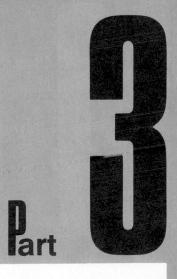

Training Principles and Overtraining

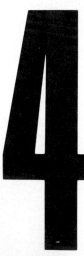

Introduction

In this third part, composed of four chapters, in-depth preparation for sports competition is examined. This section covers **strength, endurance,** and **flexibility** training. Other sections deal with myotatic strength training and the athlete's heart.

If proper training and conditioning programs are followed, the athlete is more likely to encounter success in a chosen sport. Some studies have shown a reduction of injuries in well-conditioned athletes. With all our scientific knowledge, however, much of the training of the athlete remains an art. This is because the athlete is, first and foremost, an individual with all the intricacies and problems that are inherent in human life. The athletic coach or trainer tries to control for all these variables in the athlete's life during the preparation for competition, but many of them cannot be pre-programmed. However, by employing the scientific principles noted in these chapters, the coach can insure that the most modern and advanced training techniques available are used in preparing the athlete.

Almost all authors of textbooks on training include a list of cardinal, universal, or guiding rules of training. These are the general, overriding principles upon which all athletic training and conditioning should be based. In fact, the principles which are listed in this chapter are considered necessary for any athletes who hope to attain improvement in their performance. This section emphasizes that, in order for the athletes to improve their performance, these general principles must be followed intelligently. Comparing the list of principles in this book with those found in other similar books is likely to reveal much overlap because most experts are in agreement concerning many of these training principles. Although some texts on sports training and conditioning may list as many as twelve or more principles, the purpose of this chapter is to emphasize eight major principles which should be of concern to all coaches, athletic trainers, and sports medicine specialists. These principles are also crucial to the athletes themselves. Athletes must consider these training principles during each training session if they are striving to improve their overall performance. Many times all of these principles are not followed in any one workout, however, athletes who continue to neglect or ignore these training principles cannot expect *improvement* in their athletic activity. The eight essential training principles for intelligent athletic conditioning, along with a brief discussion of each, are listed as follows.

Principle One: *The Principle of Overload/Stress*

The first principle of training to be emphasized is that of *overload* or *stress*. Exercise stress occurs in a workout session in which the body is overloaded to the extent that the cardiovascular and musculoskeletal systems are maximally stressed. This overload/stress concept relates specifically to the intensity of effort. A simple way to measure intensity of effort is to have the athletes monitor their pulse rates as they go through the workout session. We know that young athletes can achieve maximal heart rates of about 179–190 or more beats per minute. If the athlete is stressing the body in athletic workouts, then the maximal heart rate will approach these upper limits at least for some periods of time during the training session. In discussing this first training principle, we are equating stress or overload with intensity of effort. For example, in a strength workout, overload/stress would be the attempt to do a slightly greater number of repetitions lifting more weight.

Principle Two: *The Principle of Specificity of Training*

The specificity of training principle states that training must be specific to the sport and to the particular requirements and strategies of that sport. An athlete who wishes to become a better tennis player must practice and participate in the sport of tennis. An athlete who wishes to become a better basketball player should play basketball. To become a better runner, an athlete must run. However, there may be additional strategies that these

The athlete monitors the radial pulse to find out the intensity of effort of the preceding exercise stress.

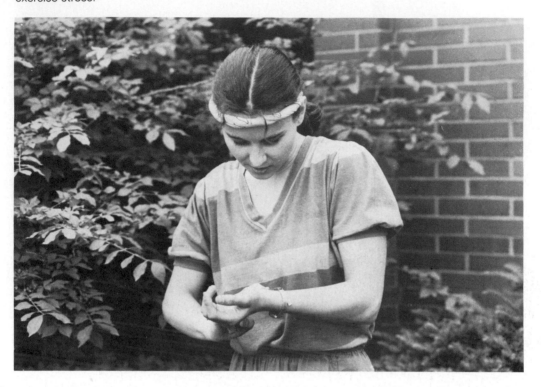

athletes must follow. For example, the tennis player must work on such components of the tennis game as the serve, the volley, or the backhand. Specificity indicates that the training, conditioning, and practice sessions should emphasize drill in the components, as well as practice of the entire sport. Also, specificity of training implies that the athlete continue to work in training and conditioning sessions of the same approximate time period as the actual event. For example, if a high school basketball player is exposed to thirty-two minutes of continuous basketball-type action, then the training and practice sessions must be structured along these lines. The college athlete can be expected to participate for forty minutes, therefore, training and conditioning practices must take into account continuous performance for this length of time. Also, it must be realized that, in basketball, there are breaks in the action for foul-shooting, time-outs, and substitutions. These types of delays may be scheduled into practice and training sessions. The basketball player may need to improve jumping ability, and hand, arm, and shoulder strength. Therefore, conditioning activities, before and during the season, should emphasize jumping drills, as well as hand, arm, and total body flexibility and strength.

Principle Three: *The Training Principle of Progression*

The training principle of progression emphasizes that the athlete must progressively extend the duration of effort in the overall training program over the first few weeks, months, and perhaps even years, of preparation for a sport activity. The first training principle states that overload/stress is related to *intensity of effort*. This principle emphasizes the *progression of effort*. According to the progression principle, the athlete, who is accustomed to running at 65–75 percent effort for a period of twenty to thirty minutes, should try to extend the duration of effort to fifty to seventy-five minutes at the same intensity (65–75 percent) of effort, with the hope of increasing overall performance. Again, using the runner as an example, the progression principle would suggest that the runner increase the total distance run in each single run.

Principle Four: *The Principle of Regularity of Sports Participation*

The principle of regularity of participation implies that the athlete must be willing to work on an almost daily basis to improve athletic performance. One extreme example of regularity in a training program involves the extraordinary British marathoner, Ron Hill, who has attained over six thousand *consecutive days* of training and conditioning. Though not all of these training days have been intense or very stressful efforts, interspersed in this training period have been days when Ron has competed in various marathons, including Olympic marathons. Also during this long, continuous string of activity, there have been days when he has been mildly injured and still continues to work out. One positive factor that this regularity of participation promotes in the athlete is that of a certain discipline, a mental toughness, a commitment to continue training toward an overall goal. Not all athletes—young and old, male and female—must have such obstinate regularity in their training programs, but, in order for any program of training to be intelligent, progressive, and lead to increases in performance, *regularity* must be a component. In certain aspects of training, especially endurance training and some other aspects of skill sports (basketball and tennis), several consecutive days of complete inactivity may intrude on the overall performance. This is why it is extremely important that a running athlete, who sustains an injury to a weight-bearing joint (a joint of the foot, knee, or hip), try to continue endurance training or cardiovascular conditioning through another aerobic activity, such as swimming, other water training, bicycle ergometer exercise, or other type of similar work, to maintain good cardiovascular conditioning.

Principle Five: *The Principle of Recovery/Rest*

The principle of recovery after a severe workout is included with the principle of stress by many authors. It is listed as a separate principle here to emphasize its importance. Many highly successful coaches and trainers feel that, if sufficient recuperation periods are not included in the overall training program, the athlete will become stale and performance will deteriorate. Most coaches will schedule hard workouts only every other day, or even put two light days between very heavy workouts. When the athlete or coach continues to push training to a very severe degree for several consecutive days, staleness or over-training may result. In a later section of this chapter various signs and symptoms of overstress or overtraining will be listed.

Principle Six: *The Principle of Diminishing Returns*

The principle of diminishing returns indicates that an athlete who begins a training program will see modest to good improvement initially, however, as the athlete continues to train beyond a period of weeks and months, and perhaps even years, they will be getting closer to their maximum performance and the rate of improvement tends to level off. The average high school or college student who begins a training program will see a steady increase in performance over the first few days, weeks, and months. Strength may increase to almost twice what it was at the outset; endurance and flexibility capacity could improve greatly. Some authors and scientists report that almost anyone beginning a training program can expect to improve performance by 20–30 percent. Figure 4.1 shows that, as the athlete nears the point of maximum potential in a chosen sport, much more of an effort must be exerted in terms of training and conditioning to gain even slight improvements in performance. As more and more time and effort are devoted to improving performance to a very high level, the risk of overuse injury may become more and more of a problem. A discussion of overuse type injuries will follow in a later section.

Principle Seven: *The Principle of Seasons*

The principle of seasonal efforts means that the athlete does a lot of lower-level pre-season and early season training followed by one to two weeks of much more intensive and stressful training immediately before the championship event. Although some authorities on

Figure 4.1 The Principle of Diminishing Returns. From a baseline condition the athlete may make marked improvements during the first several months of training until a plateau is reached. After this point, only intelligent training will cause the athlete to continue to improve—at a much slower rate.

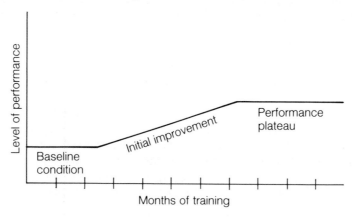

training will combine this principle with their overall scheme of stress and recovery, it is our attempt here to emphasize it by not combining it with another. Many training experts bring their athletes' conditioning to a peak for a particular championship event, and then they allow the athletes to relax for several days before resuming training for the next seasonal effort. Track coaches refer to this pre-season conditioning as baseline training or "putting money in the bank."

Principle Eight: *Training Principle of Individuality*

The training principle of individuality means that, although a group of athletes may receive the same athletic conditioning program, the athletes' *rate of improvement and development may be dissimilar.* A coach may start with a homogeneous group of young athletes, and give them the same intelligent, progressive pre-season training program, but not all of them will develop at the same rate. One of the several reasons for this is the individual genetic makeup of each athlete. We have seen in an earlier section that each athlete brings a different set of fiber types and psychological makeup to a particular sport. Because of this, some athletes may be more successful in speed or strength-type activities and others may be more successful in endurance-type activities. Body build is unique to each individual. The principle of individuality in a training program is also caused by the fact that no coach can control the life of an athlete twenty-four hours a day. For example, although it is known that diet, nutrition, and rest are key components of successful athletic competition, most coaches do not have direct control over these variables. The wise coach and athlete realize the variability of human characteristics and try to tailor training programs to suit each individual for maximum results.

Conclusions Regarding Training Principles

The athlete who hopes to improve and increase athletic performance must pay attention to these eight principles. Although these are not the only major training principles, it is believed that these eight are the most important, and are necessary as part of the athlete's total conditioning program. The athlete who follows these eight general training principles can expect reasonable improvement in sports activities. In fact, any intelligent training program will consist of at least the training principles that have been outlined in this section. Other people have pointed out additional training principles which involve individual motivation, environmental factors, or other training considerations. Certainly, these other principles may be important, but it is believed that the above eight training principles are crucial to an intelligent training program for all athletics. Whether the athlete is trying to improve performance in a strength, speed, skill, endurance, or flexibility activity, all of the training principles must be considered: overload, specificity, progression, regularity, recovery, diminishing returns, seasonality, and individuality. Wise athletes use these eight principles in planning their training programs according to their individuality.

Problems of Overtraining and Overstress

If an athlete is excessively eager or unwise in training and approaches the point of overstress, then certain body signs (outward, objective bits of evidence) and symptoms (reported, subjective feelings, like pain or discomfort) will manifest themselves. These overstresses may fall into one of several categories:

1. *Work Stress.* Job- or school-related; physical, or exercise-induced; doing too much too intensely without sufficient rest.
2. *Emotional Stress.* Due to anxiety, fear (real or imagined), depression, boredom, etc.
3. *Dietary Stress.* Too much, too little, or the wrong kinds of foods.
4. *Social Stress.* Alienation; isolation; peer pressure; overcrowding, etc.
5. *Specific Health Stress.* Illness; injury; accident (not sport related); infection, etc.
6. *Environmental Stress.* Air pollution; excessive cigarette, cigar, or pipe smoke in environment; job noise or air pollution; excessive heat, cold, etc.
7. *Rest Stress.* Inadequate recovery from hard work; sleep deprivation, etc.

All of these problems of overtraining and *overstress,* either individually, or in concert, can draw on the adaptive reserves of the athlete. When the drain becomes too severe, certain mild symptoms may present themselves. If these warning signs are ignored by the athlete, then severe breakdowns (illness such as mononucleosis) could occur.

Warning Signs and Symptoms of Overtraining or Overstress

Some specific symptoms which commonly develop in the athlete who is close to overtraining follow.

1. A six to twelve beats per minute elevation in the morning, at-rest heart rate. This is perhaps the most common, easily-recorded warning that the body has not totally recovered from the previous day's stresses.
2. An elevation in the normal body temperature of a degree or two. Again, this physiological parameter is relatively easy to monitor, and it informs the individual of the resting state of the body.
3. A low-level, but persistent, stiffness and soreness in the muscles, tendons, and joints.
4. Frequent minor sore throats and colds, or development of cold sores in the mouth.
5. Excessive nervousness, irritability, headaches, depression, anxiety with no apparent cause.
6. Inability to sleep, rest, or relax normally.
7. Nagging fatigue and general sluggishness that continues for several days.

8. Unexplained, noticeable drops in performance.
9. Disinterest in normally exciting and stimulating activities.
10. Diarrhea or constipation.
11. Aching stomach or feeling of uneasiness in the abdomen.
12. Loss of appetite and body weight.
13. Elevated readings for monocytes (white blood cells) and atypical lymphocytes (lymph cells) in the blood count.

A very basic concept in this whole area of training and overtraining is reflected by the coaching adage, "train, don't strain." Unfortunately, this is extremely difficult to do because the athlete must continue to push more and more to increase performance, yet plan enough rest and relaxation breaks so that the body can recuperate for another stressful workout. This balance is what coaches mean when they say that athletes must know themselves, listen to their bodies, and try to determine the fine line of optimal stress, combined with proper rest and recovery. The athlete who wishes to excel must push the body to extremes, yet allow for adequate rest and recovery. The athlete who risks these training extremes is pushing toward greatness, but must also be willing to expect some staleness, overtraining, or overstress that may result from these high-level training sessions.

The best athletic performer on any single occasion is the performer who is able to approach the very pinnacle of training and achievement without suffering a breakdown. It must be realized that, for every competitor in the finals of an event, there may be countless others on the sidelines watching because of a training or overuse injury. Such is the nature of top-flight athletic competition. It is the price all athletes pay in preparing to do their absolute best. To strive for greatness is to risk injury. More of this complex interrelationship will be covered in the section on athletic injuries. ∎

Summary

This chapter delineates eight major principles that all athletes must follow in the training and conditioning process. The principle of overload, the principle of specificity of training, the principle of progression, the principle of regularity, the principle of recovery, the principle of diminishing returns, the principle of seasons, and finally, the principle of individuality are listed, defined, and described in some detail. All athletes must pay attention to these training principles in order to improve their performance in sport activity. Also included in this chapter is a section on problems of overtraining and overstress. Since these are common concerns for many athletes, several problems are listed that accompany overtraining or overstress. Specific symptoms and signs of overtraining, such as elevation of resting pulse rate or body temperature, or other nagging ailments, such as low-level pain and soreness, headache, irritability, disturbance in sleeping and eating habits are listed in this chapter. Athletes preparing themselves for top flight athletic competition continually examine the training program that they have set out for themselves, seeing that it conforms to the principles of training which are listed in this chapter, while avoiding the strains and stresses of overtraining.

References

Appenzeller, O., & R. Atkinson. 1981. *Sports medicine.* Baltimore, MD: Urban & Schwarzenberg.

deVries, H. A. 1980. *Physiology of exercise.* 3d ed. Dubuque, IA: Wm. C. Brown.

Fox, E. 1979. *Sports physiology.* Philadelphia: W. B. Saunders.

Mirkin, G., & M. Hoffman. 1978. *The sports medicine book.* Boston: Little, Brown.

Morris, A. F. 1983. Training for the elite athlete. Invited address to the 1st International Symposium on Sports Medicine, San Sebastian, Spain.

O'Shea, J. P. 1976. *Scientific principles and methods of strength training.* 2d ed. Reading, MA: Addison-Wesley.

Sheehan, G. 1980. *This running life.* New York: Simon & Schuster.

Strength Training Programs

Introduction

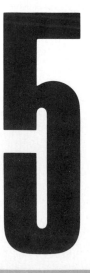

This chapter concerns strength training programs for sports. Strength is important in many athletic activities. In some sports such as weightlifting, the strength component is the most significant factor. In many other sports such as football and lacrosse, athletes must be quite big and strong. Generally, the bigger, stronger athlete will do better in any sport that has a strength component.

This chapter details some of the ways to build strength. Before a discussion of strength training programs is given, the concepts of **isotonic, isometric,** and **isokinetic** muscular strength are listed. Isotonic strength programs involve lifting loose weights a certain number of times. Isometric strength activities require the individual to make a maximal muscular contraction against an immovable resistance. In isokinetic type muscle contractions, an outside device that regulates the speed of contraction is used. All three methods of muscular contraction—isotonic, isometric, and isokinetic—result in increases in strength. However, all training is highly specific as was noted in chapter 4. For the athlete to improve isotonic strength, mostly isotonic conditioning programs must be followed. This is the case with isometric and isokinetic strength training programs as well. Details of these three types of programs and the advantages and disadvantages of each are listed in this chapter.

Muscular strength is operationally defined as the force or tension exerted by a person in a *single maximum muscular contraction,* as measured with a calibrated instrument, or by the single lift of a specified weight or resistance. Strength is important in our everyday lives. The toddler at one to two years of age needs basic strength to pull himself up along furniture so as to learn to walk unaided. A college student needs strength to ride her new motorcycle, especially if she is unfortunate enough to let the bike go down, and has to right it herself. Basic strength is necessary for the older grandparent struggling to open the jar of peanut butter at breakfast. In all these instances and in other innumerable everyday activities, every person needs a basic level of strength to function and lead a successful life.

Athletes especially need strength. For some sports participants, such as weight lifters, their entire events are examples of an expression of strength. In other sports the need for strength may be minimal. In long-distance running, for example, as proficiency increases, leg strength and power may actually decrease (Costill, 1979). However, in most sport activities athletes do need strength. A wise team sport coach once said that, other things being equal, the good, big person (stronger, larger individual) would always have the advantage over the smaller, weaker one, except in crawling through an eighteen-inch pipe.

Isotonic, Isometric, and Isokinetic Strength Programs

There arc many strength training programs in use today both in athletic conditioning programs and in rehabilitation medicine. All of these programs use isotonic, isometric, or isokinetic type muscle contractions. In order to fully understand each of these strength building programs, an in-depth look at the specific types of human muscle contraction in these different human motions is necessary.

Isotonic Muscular Contractions

Isotonic muscular contractions are by far the most common type of human muscular contractions. Simple bending of the elbow joint, as in curling a weight, is an example of an isotonic contraction. Other typical isotonic actions are walking, dressing, and eating movements. Speed of movement in these muscular contractions is irregular and unstable. In certain parts of the range-of-motion (ROM), the speed of movement is faster than in other parts of that same movement. Most sport scientists feel that the reason that the speed of movement is irregular in isotonic contractions is that a muscle or muscle group is stronger at one particular point in the ROM (Morris, 1974). The unchanging aspect of isotonic contraction is the resistance factor (fig. 5.1). The weight or resistance remains stable as one

Figure 5.1 Isotonic Contraction. An unchanging weight or resistance *(a)* is lifted throughout a full joint flexion motion. *Speed is variable.*

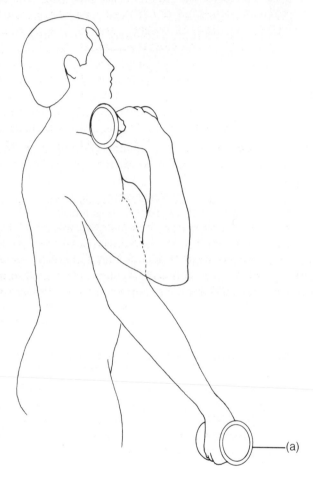

moves isotonically in the curling action cited previously. Likewise, any resistance manipulated by the hands and arms in dressing and eating remains constant through the full ROM. Most isotonic movements may be made throughout the full ROM. This is a very important factor in isotonic exercise (O'Shea, 1976).

In summary, isotonic movements are generally full range-of-motion activities in which the speed may change, but *resistance remains the same.* A specific example of an isotonic movement is simple arm curling with a small dumbbell.

Programs to Improve Isotonic Strength

In order for an athlete to gain muscular strength, the overload and resistance principle needs to be used. This means that the athlete must work with near maximal loads if strength and muscle hypertrophy are to develop. Two physicians (DeLorme & Watkins, 1948), working with veterans who had been injured in World War II, devised a system of progressive resistance exercise (PRE) which is still used today in isotonic strength development.

This system was based on the single repetition maximum (1 RM). A resistance was determined as the maximal weight that an individual could lift one time through the full range-of-motion (ROM). To find the individual's 1 RM was a tedious procedure which involved a trial and error process. However, the 1 RM level had to be determined before the individual proceeded to plan a strength workout. Once the 1 RM was found, the individual could take approximately 70 percent of the 1 RM and try to do 10 repetitions. This was labeled the 10 RM or one exercise set. Therefore, one set in the DeLorme System came to be equal to ten repetitions of a movement.

The DeLorme System of Strength Building

The DeLorme System, as it became known, is based on doing three sets of ten repetitions each in a single workout. The protocol for a basic isotonic workout is as follows: (DeLorme & Watkins, 1948).

DeLorme System
Load-Resisting Exercises
First set of ten repetitions—Use 50% of 10 RM
Second set of ten repetitions—Use 75% of 10 RM
Third set of ten repetitions—Use 100% of 10 RM

As can be seen, in the DeLorme System the athlete makes thirty contractions with each muscle or muscle group. This amount was determined after many studies which manipulated the number of repetitions per set, as well as the number of sets per workout. Another outstanding feature of the DeLorme System is that the muscle is "warmed-up" by doing ten repetitions at 50% of the total of 10 RM maximum in the first set. Then, after a second set at 75% of the 10 RM max, the person is ready to exert a maximum effort in the final set of 10 RM.

Variations of the DeLorme System

Dr. Richard Berger, of Temple University, one of the most knowledgeable and prolific researchers on isotonic strength development (Berger, 1962, 1963; Berger & Hardage, 1967), also experimented with varying the number of sets and number of repetitions and essentially, corroborated the findings of other scientists. Berger (1962) noted that between 5 RM and 9 RM may be more effective than 10 RM. When the number of repetitions is lowered to two to four per set, the performer can increase the resistance lifted and also increase the number of sets per session from three to four, or even five sets per workout.

There have been variations on the basic DeLorme System. In a system called the Oxford System, British researchers reported strength gains using the reverse of the DeLorme System. This is portrayed below:

Oxford System
First set of ten repetitions—Use 100% of 10 RM
Second set of ten repetitions—Use 75% of 10 RM
Third set of ten repetitions—Use 50% of 10 RM

Other variations can be tried and are limited only to the imagination of the athlete, coach, or trainer. Berger & Hardage (1967) had subjects do one set of ten repetitions, but each repetition required a maximum or near maximum effort. By reducing the resistance (weight lifted) with each trial, the experimenter aimed to adjust each repetition commensurate to the subject's strength and fatigue. This system, sometimes referred to as an *exhaustion set,* was more beneficial in terms of strength gained when compared with the typical 10 RM of DeLorme. Berger's method (1967) could be reversed by starting with a light weight and progressively working to a heavier resistance, trying to do at least four or six repetitions (deVries, 1980).

Other variables to consider in an isotonic strength program are (1) number of days per week to hold workouts (every other day seems to be best), (2) initial level of strength that the athlete brings to the sport, and (3) the particular strength requirements of the sport. Quite frankly, it is more important for the football player to be strong than it is for the coxswain in crew. Each particular sport has its own specific strength and fitness requirements.

Early in strength training programs, people improve at a fast rate, however, as near maximal strength is gained, improvements in amount of resistance moved become less. An untrained person can generally improve approximately 30 percent in strength in eight to twelve weeks of strength training.

Strength Building in the Athlete

Most world class weight lifters and Olympic competitors use free weights, as contrasted to machines (Universal® and Nautilus®) to improve strength. These gifted athletes employ heavy resistance training using three to five sets of 2–6 RM during a particular phase of their season.

For hypertrophy, (building bulk) and for body-building, the athlete lifts against lower resistance, but the number of repetitions per set is increased to approximately 8–20 RM. The athlete still tries for three sets of these increased repetitions. See the work of Dr. Michael H. Stone, at the National Strength Research Center in Alabama, for excellent research and references regarding strength building (Stone, O'Bryant & Garhammer, 1981). An excellent journal on strength training is *The National Strength and Conditioning Association Journal*.

Isometric Contractions

Isometric muscle contractions may also be used to improve strength. These types of muscular contractions, however, are vastly different from isotonic contractions. With isometric muscle contractions, the muscle attempts to shorten, but there is *no movement* because resistance is too great to overcome. Since there is no movement, there can be no speed of movement. A performer may try to flex at the elbow joint, but there is no movement because an unyielding resistance is preventing the lower arm from moving (fig. 5.2). In this case the resistance is simply too great to overcome and, although the person strains and attempts to contract the elbow flexors, no movement occurs.

There are many examples of isometric contractions in our daily lives, but they are not as common as isotonic muscle contractions. The grandparent straining to open the peanut butter container gives us an example of isometric effort. As long as the person strains in an attempt to remove the container lid, *and* that lid won't move, that straining muscular contraction is of an isometric nature. Other examples are the spring housecleaner forcibly attempting to open a stuck window, or the person pushing a stalled car. There are some muscular efforts in sports (gymnastics, wrestling, downhill skiing, and water skiing) which are examples of types of isometric muscle contractions. Can a person be trained to become stronger isometrically? The following section will describe how this can be accomplished.

Figure 5.2 Isometric Contraction. The athlete makes a maximum muscular effort but, since the resistance is too great to overcome, *no movement occurs.*

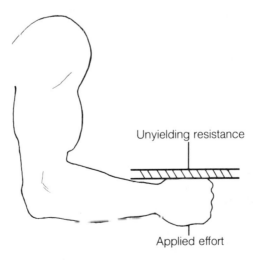

Unyielding resistance

Applied effort

Programs to Improve Isometric Strength

In attempts to improve isometric strength by means of isometric training programs, the individual makes *maximal or near maximal* isometric voluntary contractions (MVC). This simply means that the athlete contracts the muscle with as much force or intensity as possible. Although an effort is being made, the resistance is too great to overcome. Strength gained through isometric exercise is highly specific to a specific angle in the range-of-motion (ROM) of the joint.

Once these variables of joint angle and percent MVC are realized, the athlete or coach can begin to manipulate them in a training or conditioning program. The variables to consider in isometric strength programs are (1) joint angle at which the person exerts the force, (2) number of repetitions, (3) intensity of each effort (e.g., 50% MVC or 75% MVC), (4) duration of the isometric contraction, and (5) the intercontraction rest interval. A person who is at full MVC can only hold this maximum contraction for a short period of time. If a person contracts a muscle group maximally in an isometric fashion for ten to thirty seconds, the percent of MVC begins to decline. It is believed that local muscular blood flow is interrupted in these maximal isometric contractions and, therefore, strength falls, due to local muscular fatigue. Early researchers believed that maximal strength gains could be achieved with a single 75% MVC held for only about six seconds. In later, more refined work, it was discovered that athletes must make six to ten contractions with each contraction at near maximal intensity, and hold each for six to ten seconds. The main consideration with this type of training involves specificity. Strength gains will be essentially isometric in nature, and will relate mostly to the specific joint angle being used. For better utilization of isometric training the athlete should exercise at least three widely separate points in the full ROM. For example, the athlete should make isometric contractions at 45°, 90°, and 135° of elbow flexion to fully develop strength of the elbow flexors.

A final consideration that must be kept uppermost in mind regarding isometric contractions is the rapid elevation in heart rate and blood pressure (both systolic and diastolic) that occurs with isometric exercise (Bove, 1979). In an older individual, or in a person with a compromised cardiovascular system, these sudden rises in both heart rate and blood pressure could be very harmful. If a sedentary person, who is unused to isometric contractions, were to suddenly make a near-maximal effort for a given length of time, cardiac problems or a heart attack could be a result. This point will be amplified in a later section on aerobic endurance muscle activity. It is not all that bad, however, because there are some definite benefits to isometric exercise programs. These will be listed later in this section.

Isokinetic Contractions

From the mid-1960s and into the 1970s, a new type of muscle contraction was studied. This type of muscle contraction is called isokinetic contraction (Hislop & Perrine, 1967). In this type of movement the subject works against a piece of equipment or apparatus (fig. 5.3). A piece of equipment or apparatus designed specifically to regulate the speed of

Figure 5.3 Isokinetic Contraction. An apparatus is needed which can apply accommodating or matching resistance to the applied effort of the contracting muscle. Since resistance equals applied effort, *speed* of contraction *is controlled.*

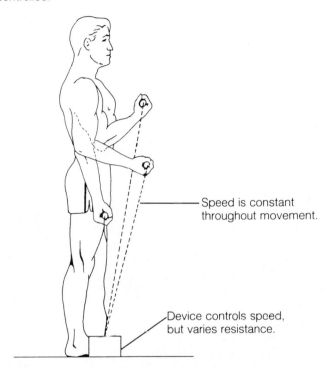

Speed is constant throughout movement.

Device controls speed, but varies resistance.

movement is needed to exercise in an isokinetic fashion. What changes in isokinetic contractions is the resistance. Since resistance varies in these contractions, the devices that the athlete uses in these workouts are often called *accommodating* or *variable resistance devices.* The theory underlying this important development in strength measurement and development is that, since the human being is stronger in certain points in the joint ROM, it would be wise to have a device capable of taxing the individual muscle or muscle group most severely at the muscle's strongest point. These devices employ levers (Universal®) and/or hydraulic arrangements (Nautilus®), or are constructed to provide varying resistance at any speed. The Cybex® is the most accurate isokinetic device used for measuring force and for rehabilitation, since it can provide an accurate stripchart (write-out) of force expressed over time in a single **flexion** and **extension** movement. The other main advantage of a Cybex device is that the researcher/therapist can very accurately set the speed of movement (fig. 5.4).

Figure 5.4 Cybex® Isokinetic Dynamometer. With this device preset at a certain speed, the athlete makes a rapid maximal contraction in both extension and flexion and the resultant force of the contracting muscle group is printed out graphically.

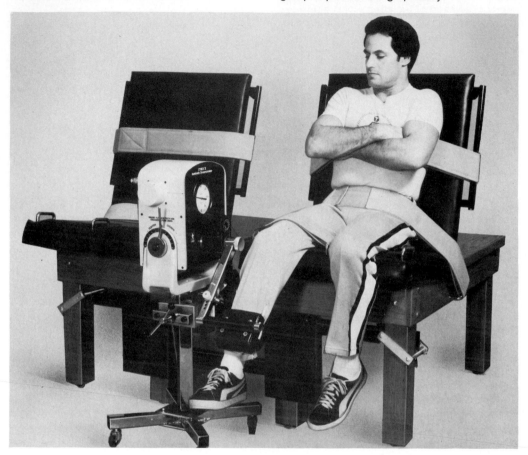

While, in theory, these machines should prove more effective in developing maximum strength, keep in mind the principle of *specificity of training.* Since most human muscle movements in daily life or sports require isotonic movements (accelerated and decelerated movements) as opposed to isokinetic movements (constant speed actions), isotonic training may be more beneficial to the athlete in training. In fact, most top strength athletes use free weights or isotonic training in their fitness programs.

Like many competing theories in science, these various types of muscle contraction training programs all have advantages and disadvantages, and it may well be that athletes who incorporate all three muscle actions (isotonic, isometric, and isokinetic) in their training programs may be employing an intelligent conditioning scheme.

Programs to Improve Isokinetic Strength

Isokinetic training sessions should follow the procedures used in isotonic programs in that repetitions and sets are varied in a similar manner. Some earlier studies have claimed superiority of isokinetic programs over isotonic programs (Pipes & Wilmore, 1975), however, in a later statement Wilmore (1979) notes that earlier reported research may have contained major inconsistencies, so that one system (isotonic or isokinetic) may not, in fact, be superior to the other. In the end, the most important criteria may be the aim or goal of training. If the athlete needs specific isotonic strength in his/her sport, then isotonic muscle strength must be developed. If some sport requirements are of an isometric nature (wrestling), then some isometric strength training would be wise.

Comparisons of Training Programs

There have been studies which have attempted to compare and contrast these various strength training methods. Much of this research is unequal, since there are many variables to control such as type of subjects (age, sex, trained or untrained, etc.), intensity, frequency and duration of workouts, number of repetitions and sets, as well as motivation of the subjects (Ikai & Steinhaus, 1961). Even the methods used to measure human strength are variable.

Nevertheless, some general concepts relating to strength training have emerged. These include the following: (1) Strength training is specific—to improve isometric strength, one must train in an isometric fashion, (2) a performer must work with near maximal loads to improve in strength, (3) exercising every other day to every third day seems to be best, (4) gradual progression must be attempted (an attempt must be made periodically to lift maximal weights), (5) isometric strength is highly specific to joint angle, (6) many repetitions completed in a set develops muscle endurance—fewer repetitions develop strength, and (7) as one approaches maximal strength level after months of workouts, one has to work much harder to see any gain (law of diminishing returns).

Advantages and Disadvantages of Different Strength Systems

Each system of improving strength has advantages and disadvantages. The major advantages and disadvantages of the three different types of strength training follow:

Isotonic Strength Training Advantages

1. Isotonic movements are more natural types of human motions.
2. The athlete can actually see work being done as the lifted weight or resistance moves.
3. The athlete retains full range-of-motion (ROM), if the exercise is made through entire ROM.

4. Maximum strength gains may be made, if the overload principle is followed.
5. Rest period between sets might be good to offset local muscular fatigue.
6. Free weights may be the only way to lift great amounts of resistance for elite athletes beyond the limits of a particular machine.
7. The athlete and coach can devise home-made weights (cement in cans and pipes, etc.).
8. Free weight movements are not limited to machine's movements, as Nautilus® and Universal® weight lifting.
9. Isotonics may be used to build muscular endurance by increasing the number of repetitions in weight lifting.
10. Many repeated sets can increase bulk (hypertrophy) for muscle definition.

Isotonic Strength Training Disadvantages

1. May be unsafe—athlete needs spotters to make certain no injury occurs.
2. May be costly in equipment, especially if very heavy weights are used.
3. May be inefficient in time consumed changing weights.
4. Hard to do isolated neck movements (flexion, extension, rotation, etc.) and other specific movements.
5. Athlete may do an isometric contraction on bar with hand grip as weight is lifted.
6. "Stick point" (point where it is hardest to begin moving the weight) is a disadvantage in isotonics.

Isometric Strength Training Advantages

1. Isometric exercises can be done at any time.
2. Little or no space is required for isometrics.
3. Inexpensive equipment often can be made at local level.
4. Athletes can work in pairs or alone (one athlete may provide resistance for another).
5. There is a therapeutic value in isometric exercise for an athlete restricted by a cast.
6. Isometrics can be done in restricted spaces (e.g., astronauts).

Isometric Strength Training Disadvantages

1. Isometrics may produce rapid increases in heart rate.
2. Isometrics may produce rapid increase in systolic blood pressure.
3. Isometrics may produce rapid increase in diastolic blood pressure.
4. Strength is only gained at certain points in ROM where athlete practices the particular isometric contraction.
5. Isometric exercises are mostly for strength, not endurance.
6. Isometric exercises may produce more bulk than strength.

Isokinetic Strength Training Advantages

1. Isokinetic devices are generally safer—weights should not drop on the performer.
2. Variable resistance may be provided throughout the full range of movement.
3. Athlete saves time in workout (doesn't take much time to change weights or levels of resistance).
4. Athlete can do unusual movements (neck machine work-outs on specific isokinetic devices).
5. Athlete can change resistance without changing body position (e.g., bench press).
6. Weight moves so athlete can see work being done.
7. Athlete can use isokinetic workouts for strength or endurance by alternating resistance level or number of repetitions.

Isokinetic Strength Training Disadvantages

1. Isokinetic movement is not a completely natural human movement.
2. Weights on machine are limited to certain resistances, or certain levels.
3. The athlete is limited to the machine's movements and size.
4. The isokinetic device may take up large amounts of space.
5. Isokinetic equipment is very costly as an initial investment (sometimes up to $4,000).
6. Weights move along a channel and might stick, if device is not lubricated properly.
7. One machine is manufactured to fit all body sizes, even though humans come in different sizes (from the tiny female gymnast or dancer, to the heavyweight football lineman).
8. The athlete may only do one set of twelve repetitions (suggested by manufacturer). ■

Summary

This chapter points out the importance of strength training for sports. Many sports, such as football and basketball require great strength. Generally, the bigger, stronger athlete is the better athlete. It covers three types of programs to increase strength—isotonic, isometric, and isokinetic strength training programs—and gives a definition for each, paying special attention to the speed of movement, the resistance to movement, and the type of movement. Strength training is highly specific. That is, if one trains in an isotonio fashion with loose weights, increases in strength will mostly be isotonic gains. The advantages and the disadvantages of each of the strength training programs are listed.

References

Berger, R. A. 1962. Comparison of static and dynamic stretch increases. *Research Quarterly*. 33: 329–33.

Berger, R. A. 1963. Comparison between static training and various dynamic training programs. *Research Quarterly*. 34: 131–35.

Berger, R. A., & B. Hardage. 1967. Effect of maximum loads for each of ten repetitions on strength improvement. *Research Quarterly*. 38: 715–18.

Bove, A. A. 1979. Heart and circulatory function in exercise. In Lowenthal, D. T., et al. eds. *Therapeutics through exercise*. New York: Grune & Stratton.

Costill, D. L. 1979. *A scientific approach to distance running*. Los Altos, CA: Track & Field News Press.

DeLorme, T. L., & A. L. Watkins. 1948. Techniques of progressive resistance exercise. *Archives of Physical Education*. 29: 263–81.

deVries, H. A. 1980. *Physiology of exercise*. 3d ed. Dubuque, IA: Wm. C. Brown.

Hislop, H. J., & J. J. Perrine. 1967. The isokinetic concept of exercise. *Physical Therapy*. 47: 114–17.

Ikai, M., & A. H. Steinhaus. 1961. Some factors modifying the expression of human strength. *Journal of Applied Physiology*. 16: 157–63.

Morris, A. F. 1974. Myotatic reflex effects on bilateral reciprocal leg strength. *American Corrective Therapy Journal*. 28: 24–29.

O'Shea, J. P. 1976. *Scientific principles and methods of strength training*. 2d ed. Reading, MA: Addison-Wesley.

Pipes, T. V., & J. H. Wilmore. 1975. Isokinetic vs. isotonic strength training in adult men. *Medicine and Science in Sports*. 7: 262–74.

Stone, M. H., H. O'Bryant, & J. Garhammer. 1981. A hypothetical model for strength training. *The Journal of Sports Medicine and Physical Fitness*. 21: 342–51.

Wilmore, J. H. 1979. Letter to the editor on isokinetic exercise. *Medicine and Science in Sports*. 11: iii.

Myotatic Strength Training and Power Development

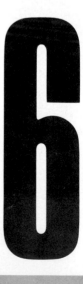

Outline

Introduction

Chapter 6 is a further refinement of strength training. Specifically, **myotatic** (muscle stretch) **strength training** is covered. Various researchers in physical medicine and rehabilitation have noted that, if a slight stretch is applied to a muscle before contraction, the resulting strength from that muscle contraction is greater than if the muscle was not stretched prior to contraction. To do this with human muscle contractions, elaborate precautions must be made to safeguard the muscle and joint being tested. Lagasse (1974), Morris (1974), and Smith (1970) all have shown in studies with humans that, if a muscle is stretched prior to contraction, the resulting strength contraction is greater. However, in all of these experimental studies it was noted that extreme procedures guarding the safety of the subjects had to be instituted. If, in training, the subject can simulate the research condition exposed by the above listed scientists, then muscular strength training should be increased. Another discussion in this chapter is on power. Power is the rate at which work is accomplished. That is, if a very strong individual can do much work within a very brief period of time, this individual is considered to be very powerful. Many sports, football probably being the best example, utilize powerful participants. Specific strength training programs in which the athlete works out with lighter weights, moving them very rapidly through the range-of-motion, are used to develop power. In some activities, such as body building, it is important to build muscle bulk. For this purpose, one moves the muscle slowly through the range-of-motion lifting heavy resistance. Again, the number of total contractions is emphasized and the athlete must get a large number of repetitions completed through each training session.

esearchers and rehabilitation workers have constantly explored new ways in which muscle strength may be facilitated (Knott & Voss, 1968; Beasley, 1956). For several decades, proprioceptive neuromuscular techniques have been used by therapists to aid muscular contraction in weak or partially paralyzed muscles. Proprioceptive neuromuscular technique, in this sense, refers to the awareness of posture, movement, changes in equilibrium, and the knowledge of position, weight, and resistance of objects in relation to the body. However, it is only recently that scientists have examined proprioceptive neuromuscular facilitation techniques in normal subjects. Specifically, Morris (1974) and others (Lagasse, 1974; Smith, 1970) have shown that if a muscle stretches slightly as it is contracting, that same muscle or muscle group may be capable of a supramaximal contraction.

This type of muscle contraction is termed myotatic contraction—derived from myo (muscle) and tatic (stretch). The mechanism at work here is the muscle spindle. These muscle spindles are located in all skeletal muscle and they are sensitive to any change in the length in the muscle. When the muscle spindles are stretched, they signal a reflex contraction of that same muscle. The common knee-jerk response to the patella tendon tap is the most common example of this reflexive muscle stretch response (see chapter 3). The muscle stretch reflex response is designed as a protective response.

Another mechanism which might be involved here is inherent muscle elasticity, which is present in all skeletal muscles. Some researchers who have studied muscle stretching in healthy individuals note that after a muscle stretches, it may contract with more force than it was previously capable of producing. This may happen in muscles which are stretched from previous actions, like jumping from a height.

Several researchers have studied the acute response of muscle stretch in human subjects by forcibly stretching the quadricep muscles during a muscle contraction (Morris, 1974; Lagasse, 1974). This author, in a 1974 study, found an increase of about 25 percent in expressed force of the quadriceps muscle group when these muscles were exposed to myotatic procedures. Lagasse (1974) also reported significant increases in strength (over maximum) when he used a superimposed muscle stretch.

These muscle stretch studies corroborated earlier studies by Smith (1970) and Moore (1966). The studies by Smith and Moore were long-term training studies, but they also reported increments of 25–30 percent in muscle strength (Moore, 1966) in subjects who had been exposed to two months of "active resistive stretch" training. Smith (1970) trained subjects for forty-two consecutive days using myotatic training vs. conventional isometric training and reported that the muscle stretch group increased strength by 23 percent compared to a 13 percent gain in strength in the isometric training group. Smith also reported significant contralateral transfer of strength to the opposite leg (which was not stretched) during the experimental period.

In carefully controlled laboratory studies, muscle force was augmented when human musculature was stretched during an active contraction. In several long-term training studies, the chronic strength improvement was greater in subjects who had experienced myotatic training. From these studies it appears that the ultimate way to train for muscle strength may be to provide a stretch stimulus to an already contracting muscle.

Some top class weight-lifters may actually be providing a stretch stimulus during their competitive lifting when they attempt to *bounce* the weights to a small degree before thrusting the weight overhead in a lift. Innovative coaches, trainers, and athletes, who devise ways to slightly stretch a contracting muscle, may be providing the best single stimulus to enhance strength development.

A word of caution is necessary here. In the earlier stretch studies, these researchers took *all precautions* in their procedures to carefully control the intensity and length of muscle stretch in their experimental studies. This is an absolute must if injury or muscle strain is to be avoided in the athlete who may be using muscle stretch procedures in training.

Building Muscle Bulk

Often, students in my sports medicine classes ask me about specific strength training programs to make one stronger or simply to add muscle definition. This is not an easy subject to address because there is a significant amount of misrepresentation of the facts in this area. To properly understand muscle strength and muscle bulk, one must again revert to the study of the individual muscle and the specific muscle cell.

In chapter 3 it was seen that the basic unit of structure in the skeletal muscle system is the individual muscle cell, or fiber. In striated or skeletal muscle, for all intents and purposes, the muscle fiber equals the muscle cell. In order to make an individual stronger, one must make the individual skeletal muscle cell stronger.

There still exists some controversy in the scientific literature as to whether a skeletal muscle cell becomes larger—*hypertrophy*—with increased overload training, or whether muscle cells can actually split or divide and increase in number—*hyperplasia*—and therefore, also appear to increase total muscle mass. Tending to complicate this issue is the general belief that a larger muscle tends to be a stronger muscle. This is not always the case, since the length of the muscle and other factors also play a role in muscle strength.

Hypertrophy, or muscle enlargement, is generally a by-product of intelligent strength training. Most experts feel that the individual muscle fibers enlarge to produce this increase in girth. How can the athlete set up a training program to effect this increase in skeletal muscle size? For certain athletes, such as body builders, this concept of increasing muscle size or bulk may be more important than increasing muscle strength. The next section will cover programs to increase muscle bulk.

High-caliber body builders typically use high volumes of work in their training. These athletes use more sets (five to ten) or higher repetitions (seven to fifteen) than the person who is interested mainly in strength building. Only two to four sets of fewer repetitions (four to eight) are needed to build strength in a maximal fashion. These differences in training emphasize the specificity of training concept. The person who wants to become stronger must attempt to lift greater and greater amounts of weight. The person whose main goal is muscle definition tries for longer sets and a greater number of lifts per set.

One final aspect in the issue of weightlifter (competitive) versus the body builder is that of symmetry. Competitive weightlifters don't particularly care how they look, only that they are proficient and highly technical in *lifting weights*. On the other hand, the body builder is totally committed to how the body looks. It must be properly developed in all aspects, for the body builder is judged on physical appearance. This is not to say that the body builder is weak. To the contrary, any person who has that much muscle bulk and very little body fat, is most often quite strong. Body builders in top flight competition may only have 3–7 percent body fat (males). Weightlifters may have more body fat than body builders, but these trained athletes still have less body fat than an average non-athletic, age-matched individual.

Power

Before this final section on strength training is completed, a word on power is in order. Power *(P)* may be operationally defined as time—rate at which work is done, or $P = w/t$. Strength is defined as the force exerted by a singular muscle contraction. When we discuss power, we bring in the concept of time or speed of muscle contraction. A powerful person, in the sports sense of the term, is a person who can exert *much force very quickly*.

The javelin throw is an event which requires great power and is an athletic contest that dates back to early human history.

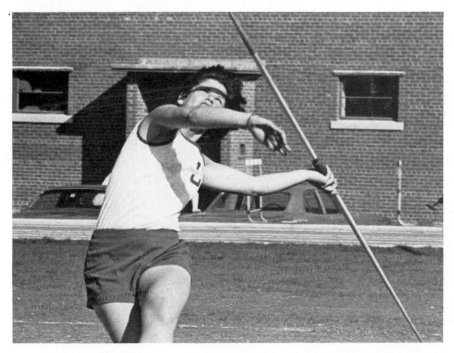

Myotatic Strength Training and Power Development

77

There are certain sport activities in which power is a crucial element of the event. The hammer throw, the discus, and the javelin throw are all events which can be considered power events. To be successful in these events, the athlete must practice power movements in training. Again, the specificity of training principle is emphasized here. Therefore, the power athlete's training sessions involve very high force workouts with very heavy weights. Other workouts involve high speed sessions in which the athlete lifts moderate weights very fast with good technique. Good technique must always be maintained in *all* weight workouts. Both these *high velocity* and *high force* workouts should help to develop the fast twitch fibers noted in the first part of this text.

For more specific information related to strength, power, and body building workouts, consult the *National Strength and Conditioning Association Journal*. This journal, which was started in the late 1970s, is written and edited by experts in the strength training field and offers much valuable information about this important aspect of fitness for certain sports. ■

Summary

In this chapter myotatic strength training and power development are detailed. Essentially, myotatic strength training involves prestretching of the muscle before contraction is made. This is a very difficult type of contraction to make and is done in a highly refined, sophisticated, safe, laboratory condition. If the muscle can be stretched prior to the contraction, several researchers have shown an increase in strength in the contraction following the stretch. If this is done over a period of several training sessions, one investigator has shown an increase in strength over conventional training methods. If the athlete can perform these types of myotatic (muscle stretch) contractions in training, then significant strength gains will be achieved. However, extreme safety precautions must be instituted so that the muscle is not overstretched and there is no joint damage done in the prestretching conditions. Other concerns, such as power development and muscle bulk, are discussed in this chapter. Power involves applying force within a very short period of time. To apply this force, obviously, an individual must be very strong and capable of moving rather heavy weight very quickly. In training to build muscle bulk (as in body building), the athlete attempts to make as many contractions as possible within the given session using the maximal amount of weight. There is a difference between strength training and training for muscle bulk. Essentially, the difference is that the athlete working for muscle bulk continues to work out more days per week, with the emphasis on the total amount of repetitions and resistance used, rather than having an exclusive concern with total weight being used, as does the person who is working for strength development.

References

Beasley, W. C. 1956. Influence of method on estimates of normal knee extension force among normal and post-polio children. *Physical Therapy Review.* 36: 21–41.

Knott, M. & D. E. Voss. 1968. *Proprioceptive neuromuscular facilitation.* 2d ed. New York: Hoeber Medical Division of Harper & Row.

Lagasse, P. P. 1974. Muscle strength: ipsilateral and contralateral effects of superimposed stretch. *Archives of Physical Medicine and Rehabilitation.* 55: 305–10.

Moore, J. C. 1966. Facilitation of a forearm flexor response. *Journal of Applied Physiology.* 21: 649.

Morris, A. F. 1974. Myotatic reflex effects on bilateral reciprocal leg strength. *American Corrective Therapy Journal.* 28: 24–29.

Smith, L. E. 1970. Facilitatory effects of myotatic strength training upon leg strength and contralateral transfer. *American Journal of Physical Medicine.* 49: 132–41.

Endurance Conditioning and the Athlete's Heart

Introduction

This chapter concerns conditioning and training for endurance. The concept of endurance is defined as the ability to continue prolonged performance in a continuous repetitive athletic movement. Endurance involves conditioning of the cardiorespiratory system. In order to condition these systems, practice sessions must consist of long-term, continuous, total body activity involving factors such as duration, intensity, and frequency of the training. Several types of endurance training programs, such as fartlek training, interval training, long slow distance (LSD) training, and circuit training can increase human endurance.

Because endurance conditioning affects the human heart there is a discussion on the Athletic Heart Syndrome in this chapter. The relationship of endurance training to cardiovascular heart disease (CHD), the leading killer in Western society today, and the effects of physical activity of an endurance nature on many of the risk factors of CHD are explained.

The limits of human endurance are constantly being expanded. Following are some recent examples of mind boggling endurance performances which are truly extraordinary human achievements. In the late 1970s a male long distance runner ran a distance of 168 miles on a track in 24 hours. This is an average of 8 min. 35 sec. per mile, or 7 miles per hour for a whole day. A short time later Carlo Sala, a skiing instructor from Italy, skied cross-country over 167 miles in one day. Perhaps the most remarkable human endurance performance takes place annually in Hawaii, in which endurance athletes compete in a triathlon event, consisting of ocean swimming, bicycle racing, and marathon running, all in a single day. A long distance swimmer who won the competition in early 1980, swam the 2.4 mile ocean course in about 51 minutes. Following a change of clothes, he took off on his bike for a 112 mile ride around the island of Oahu. This hilly trek, accomplished in about 5 hours, brought him to the marathon run portion of the event. After competing in nearly 6 hours of exhaustive activity, this gifted athlete covered the popular Hawaiian marathon course in approximately 3.5 hours. This superbly fit athlete had performed for nearly 9 hours and 24 minutes in three exhaustive endurance sports, setting a new world record for the event. To show how rapidly world records are falling in distance events, in the previous year, the record was 11 hours and 15 minutes.

An enterprising young man in Utah has organized an endurance pentathlon which covers 5 consecutive days. A 50 kilometer orienteering event is the first day; the second day, a 10 kilometer swim; the third day, a 25 kilometer kayak race; the fourth day, a 180 kilometer bike race, the fifth day, a marathon (42.2 kilometers) running race.

Another group of outstanding world class endurance athletes who have rapidly improved in performance are the female long distance runners. During the first ten years after they were allowed to enter world competition, they have improved the marathon record by approximately 34 percent. In late 1979, Greta Waitz ran under 2 hrs. and 28 min. for a world record. Somewhat later, Joan Benoit ran it in approximately 2 hrs. and 22 min. for a World and American record. These times would have equalled those of the male winners in many Olympic marathons and other major marathon events until the 1950s, showing the tremendous strides that these women have made in endurance performances when proper training or conditioning is applied. A women's marathon event is now included in the Olympic Games.

Endurance Defined

Endurance may be defined as the ability to repeatedly contract skeletal muscles in an ongoing physical activity. Most physiologists further divide human endurance into muscular endurance and cardiovascular endurance. Muscular endurance may be defined as the capacity of the body to make repeated contractions with a single isolated muscle or muscle group. Lifting weights for twenty to thirty repetitions is an example of muscular endurance. Muscular endurance may also refer to a sustained isometric muscular contraction held for a period of time. Cardiovascular endurance, the fitness of the heart and vascular system, is required in long-term activity involving major muscle groups in alternating rhythmical isotonic activities. These endurance sporting events typically last from five minutes to several hours.

Muscular Endurance

In the discussion of strength building activities it was pointed out that the muscle must work at near maximum loads in order for a training effect to accrue. In muscular endurance activities, a performer must exercise with resistance values of 25–65 percent of maximum resistance for twenty or more repetitions in contractions such as elbow flexion or knee extension. Much of the early work in muscular endurance was done by medical researchers (DeLorme & Watkins, 1948) who found, in general, that increasing muscular endurance requires more repetitions with lower resistance. As the athlete increases the resistance and lowers the total number of repetitions used in training, then the athlete is working primarily to develop muscle strength. Muscular endurance is very important in many sport activities. However, of even more importance is the development of cardiovascular endurance. Sports such as soccer, lacrosse, basketball, field hockey, and, of course, long-distance running, are examples of activities in which the athlete must develop cardiovascular endurance.

Cardiovascular Endurance

Cardiovascular (CV) endurance involves the development of the heart and vascular system. Typically, a person who can complete a marathon race is considered to have excellent cardiovascular conditioning. Training to improve CV endurance involves sustained, rhythmical, isotonic contractions of large body muscles. Common activities for improving CV endurance include walking, running, cycling, swimming, cross-country skiing, skating, rope-jumping, and rowing. All these activities are *timed* events, as they are contested in sports competition. Also, all these events are isotonic in nature and involve large muscle groups or total body activities.

Cardiovascular Conditioning for Sports

This discussion of the intensity, duration, and frequency of workouts pertains to athletes who are training to develop or improve cardiovascular conditioning. All these factors must be intelligently planned for in organizing any cardiovascular conditioning program. It must be emphasized that endurance conditioning activities are generally: (1) large muscle in nature, (2) isotonic, and (3) often consist of walking/running, cycling, skating, cross-country skiing, rowing, or rope-jumping activities.

Intensity of Activity

As an athlete increases effort in physical activity, oxygen consumption also increases. This physiological parameter is very difficult to measure in a field or gymnasium situation, but it represents the best indicator of endurance fitness. Sometimes the coach or athlete will monitor the heart rate during or immediately after exercise. It has been shown that heart

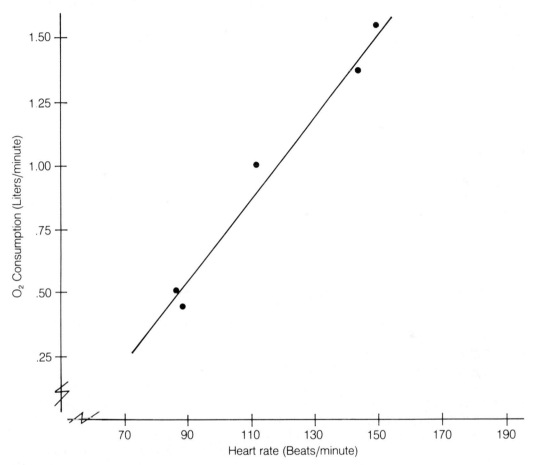

Figure 7.1 Linear Relationship Between Oxygen Uptake and Heart Rate.
Source: deVries, H. A. 1980. *Physiology of exercise*. 3d ed. Dubuque, IA: Wm. C. Brown.

rate increases in a nearly linear fashion with increasing oxygen consumption (Astrand & Rodahl, 1977). This relationship between oxygen consumption and heart rate can be seen in figure 7.1. Knowing this relationship, the athlete or coach can judge how hard the exercise session has been by monitoring the heart rate as the athlete exercises. The athlete may do this for himself by checking the radial or carotid pulse for a six second period and then multiplying by ten to get the minute rate for heart action. It is best to use the tips of the fingers to palpate the pulsating artery because they are the most sensitive area of the hand. The athlete must check the pulse rate *immediately* upon stopping exercise, since heart rate falls precipitously upon cessation of activity.

Intensity of Exercise

Several investigators have indicated that there is an endurance **training threshold** above which an athlete must train to receive full cardiovascular benefit from a conditioning program. Karvonen (1959) suggested that this training threshold is at approximately 60 percent of the difference between the resting and maximal heart rate. Let us take a twenty-year-old college male and calculate his training threshold for endurance conditioning. A general rule of thumb is to use 220 as a constant (determined in repeated laboratory studies) and subtract the individual's age from this value to calculate the maximal predicted heart rate. The maximal predicted heart rate (HR) for this person would be:

$$220 - 20 \text{ (age)} = 200 \text{ (maximal predicted HR)}.$$

If this person had a resting heart rate of 70 beats per minute, further calculation would yield:

$$200 \text{ (maximal predicted HR)} - 70 \text{ (resting HR)} = 130 \text{ (HR difference)}.$$

Now take 60 percent of this HR difference:

$$60 \text{ percent of } 130 = 78.$$

Add this 60 percent of HR difference or 78 beats to the resting level:

$$78 + 70 \text{ (resting HR)} = 148 \text{ (training threshold)}.$$

This pulse rate of 148 is the calculated training threshold heart rate value for this twenty-year-old college male who had a resting heart rate of 70.

Other investigators have proposed a short cut for finding the training threshold. These researchers suggest that this same person exercise at about 75 percent of maximal heart rate for a desired period of time. When these values are used, then the calculations of the training threshold would be 75 percent of 200 or 150 beats per minute. These formulas are nearly equivalent in attempting to predict the training threshold. In the Karvonen formula, the calculated training heart rate is 148 beats per minute while the second method of calculation equals 150 beats per minute. This training threshold represents the level above which the athlete must elevate the heart rate during training activity to achieve a CV benefit.

Aging and Training Threshold

Dr. Herbert deVries (1980), of Southern California, has determined that older individuals may exercise at lower work loads, perhaps 50–65 percent of their maximal heart rates, and that this intensity level may provide a training stimulus to their cardiovascular systems. This may be the case since it is known that the maximal predicted heart rate falls as a person ages (see table 7.1).

Table 7.1 Training Threshold Heart Rates (HR) for Adults

Age of athlete (years)	Maximum predicted HR (beats/min.)	Training threshold HR (beats/min.)
20	200	140.0[a]
25	195	136.5[a]
30	190	133.0[a]
35	185	129.5[a]
40	180	126.0[a]
45	175	122.5[a]
50	170	119.0[a]
55	165	107.3[b]
60	160	104.0[b]
65	155	100.8[b]
70	150	90.0[c]
75	145	87.0[c]
80	140	84.0[c]

Source: Morris, A. F. 1983. Training for the elite athlete. Invited address to the *1st International Symposium on Sports Medicine,* San Sebastian, Spain, March.

[a] Training threshold calculated at 70 percent of maximum heart rate

[b] Training threshold calculated at 65 percent of maximum heart rate

[c] Training threshold calculated at 60 percent of maximum heart rate

The preceding sections point out that a person must work at a near-maximal heart rate level to increase endurance fitness. In reality, paying attention to exercise intensity only will not enable a person to become endurance conditioned. The duration or length of the exercise session must be considered as well. Here again, the concern is with continuous, large muscle isotonic activity, such as walking, swimming, running, or cycling.

Duration of Activity

The American College of Sports Medicine (ACSM) has established a position paper on the quantity and quality of exercise necessary in endurance training. (Appendix #3.) The research in this area suggests that a person should engage in twenty to sixty minutes of continuous activity. The minimum level should be about twenty to thirty minutes of uninterrupted activity. As exercise intensity increases, the resultant trade-off will be a decrease in duration of that activity. The person aiming for an endurance workout would be well-advised to start slowly and with less intensity, but to try to continue working out for twenty to thirty minutes during a single session.

Although there are other considerations, the most important factor in endurance training activity may be the initial fitness level of the beginning exerciser. If the fitness level is low, then initial intensity and duration of workouts must necessarily be kept low. Short amounts of jogging may be interspersed between walking exercise. As the individual becomes more fit, faster running or more running may be included in workout periods. The exercise principle of progression is emphasized here. For the very fit athlete, the intensity level and duration level may be quite high, possibly 70–85 percent of maximal heart rate for about forty to one hundred minutes of continuous endurance activity.

Frequency of Training

This factor of *daily activity* is a final consideration for endurance fitness training. Many studies have been conducted regarding the frequency of training for endurance fitness. The general consensus is that a person needs to work out about three to five days per week to develop or maintain endurance fitness. Most of these training studies have been on college age males or military conscripts between the ages of eighteen and twenty-six. Recent evidence on females suggests that women adapt to endurance training in the same manner as men. The beginner in endurance training should work out every other day, or three to four times per week. To further improve endurance activity it becomes necessary to work out six or seven days per week. The elite performer in track, swimming, or cycling may do multiple workouts every day (Morris, 1980). It is not uncommon for world class distance runners to run twenty miles per day or 120 to 160 miles per week. This could be divided into a seven to nine mile morning run, followed by a ten to fifteen mile afternoon workout. World class swimmers and other endurance athletes also exercise several times per day to spread their total distance over a longer period of time (Morris, 1983).

Types of Endurance Training Programs

Several specific training programs have been devised to improve cardiovascular endurance. These are discussed and formal training regimes outlined in the following sections. Among the endurance programs discussed are: (1) fartlek training, (2) circuit training, (3) interval training, and (4) long slow distance (LSD) training.

Fartlek Training

This form of endurance training originated in Sweden and represents a loose translation of the Swedish word meaning "speed play." **Fartlek training** was advocated in the 1930s by Swedish coach, Gosta Holmer, who wanted a form of training that took advantage of Scandinavian forest trails and rolling hills. Fartlek running periods can be used to develop speed and endurance, if the run is continuous and long.

The main advantage of fartlek is that the athlete can get into condition in a short period of time. Additionally, the feeling of freedom and self-creation on the run is beneficial. It is suggested that the athlete run for thirty to one hundred minutes over a certain area, including bursts of speed for various short distances. In between these speed efforts, which may be from one hundred to one thousand meters in length, the athlete continues to run or jog at a comfortable pace. An additional advantage of this type of workout is that it enables the athlete to gain speed, as well as endurance benefits, without the structure of a track interval type workout.

One of the major drawbacks to fartlek training is the danger that the athlete will not push hard enough in the speed efforts during the exercise session. One remedy for this would be for the coach to suggest at least three to six "speed bursts" of about four hundred to six hundred meters each during a sixty minute workout. Alternatively, a coach may instruct two or more runners of near equal ability to run together while also suggesting the number, length, and intensity of fartlek efforts during the workout. Of course, the more structured the workout, the less likely it is to resemble the true fartlek training.

Interval Training

A program of endurance conditioning may be built out of **interval training.** This type of program is designed to permit the athlete to get the most work accomplished with a minimum amount of fatigue build up. Fatigue is operationally defined as a decrement in performance as a result of preceding work. A program of interval training considers five major variables. These variables are: (1) intensity of effort (usually time), (2) duration of effort (usually distance), (3) rest interval (time period), (4) number of repetitions, and (5) mode of rest (lying, standing, walking, jogging, etc.). Since interval training involves the manipulation of many variables, it permits much flexibility in the athlete's training schedule. This variability appears to be the major advantage in interval workouts.

Many exercise scientists have explored interval training variables in endurance training, and have noted significant factors for the coach and athlete. A prominent Italian physiologist (Cavagna, 1968), noted that intense running (top speed) for about one hundred meters followed by rest intervals of approximately thirty seconds could be repeated almost indefinitely without significant build up of fatigue by-products. On the other hand, running four hundred to eight hundred meters at top speed and then resting would quickly build up fatigue and less total work could be accomplished in an exercise period. Cavagna (1968) claimed that the trained athlete, who exercised in the manner of short, intense intervals with adequate rest, could accomplish nearly thirty times more work than one who did intervals of four hundred meters or longer.

Fox (1979) compared untrained college students at the Ohio State University on a treadmill set at high power (nineteen runs of thirty seconds at high intensity) versus low power (seven runs of two minutes each at lower intensity). Both groups rested (seated) until heart rates returned to between 120 and 140 beats per minute. His results showed that both groups improved significantly in maximum oxygen uptake and both groups showed similar changes in maximal aerobic and anaerobic metabolism.

A generalization which coaches and athletes have experienced is that as the training season comes to its conclusion, the athlete is better off with shorter, but more intense, work intervals rather than the longer, less intense work schedules that were promoted earlier in the season. A corollary to this is that the athletes should gradually curtail the rest intervals as they sharpen for championship performance. The mode of rest may also be more stressful as the athletes change the mode of rest from a slow jog to a run as they peak for competition.

The major advantage of interval training is the myriad of factors (intensity, duration, number of repetitions, rest intervals, and mode of rest) that can be manipulated during a workout session. The major drawback to interval training is often the rigid adherence to the stopwatch (to timed intervals of work, and rest) and the track or pool that may soon lead to boredom in even the most well-motivated athlete. However, it must be emphasized that most good athletes train by using certain types of interval workouts, since they can definitely produce improvements in human performance.

LSD Training

LSD training stands for **long slow distance** training. There is a dispute as to who actually originated this method of endurance conditioning, however, Dr. Ernst van Aaken (1976) is generally recognized as the founder of this particular type of endurance training. This physician originally wrote in German about a "Pure-Endurance Method" of training in which athletes work at heart rates of about 130 beats per minute for long periods of time. Initially, the athlete might have to start out walking, jogging, or jogging and running, but soon runs for longer periods each day. Van Aaken stresses "run long, run daily, and modest caloric intake." These principles are the cornerstone of his endurance program. Many people have been successful with the van Aaken Method (1976), among them Harold Norporth, former European and world record holder at five kilometers.

The individual who actually named LSD training was a writer for *Runner's World* magazine named Joe Henderson (1969). Henderson contended that endurance training need not be a painful experience in order to produce results. He recommended slow running or jogging at a comfortable pace at which it was possible to carry on a conversation with a running partner. As this training continues for thirty minutes to an hour, the pulse rate and body temperature will rise, and the athlete will achieve endurance training benefit.

Although LSD conditioning pertained to jogging or running when first described, it may be applied to other endurance activities as well. For example, cross-country skiers, cyclists, and rowers could also adopt this LSD strategy for portions of their training schedules. It is an excellent device to utilize in preseason or early season workouts, and may be used during the season to give an athlete a break from the more structured (interval) type workouts.

Circuit Training

This type of training program may be used for strength, endurance, or flexibility conditioning. It is a basic exercise program that involves a number of stations set up around the periphery of an exercise area, such as a gymnasium or field. Starting at a particular point on the circuit, the athlete does a specific activity at each station before going on to another point on the circuit (see fig. 7.2).

In a strength type circuit, certain progressive resistive exercises are included. In a flexibility circuit some flexibility activities are done at each station. In an endurance circuit the object is to do a large number of repetitions of an activity in a certain period of time at each stop. The time or distance between stations can be manipulated to get variety into these workouts. One way to insert more running into this training scheme, particularly when space is limited, is to have the athlete run around the outside of the entire circuit before proceeding on to the next station in the circuit. The major advantages of this exercise program are: (1) the different number of activities and stations included, (2) the amount of time required at each station, (3) the time interval between stations, and (4) the

Figure 7.2 Circuit training. The athlete does a prescribed exercise at each of various stations (1–6) on the circuit which is set up in a gymnasium or around a field. Circuit stations may be designed for strength, flexibility or endurance training activities.
Source: Fox, E. 1979. *Sports physiology.* Philadelphia: W. B. Saunders.

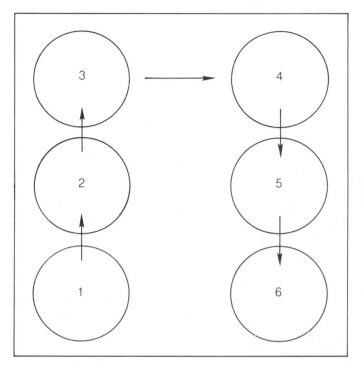

distance between stations. This system can also accommodate many athletes at the same time. Again, it must be stressed that a target heart rate and duration of effort must be maintained throughout the workout, if the athlete is trying to achieve an endurance training effect.

Fatigue in Endurance Activities

The mechanisms underlying human neuromuscular fatigue remain obscure despite extensive efforts to investigate this phenomenon by exercise scientists throughout the world. A monograph on physiological fatigue, written by Simonson (1971), included over two thousand five hundred references on this subject. A major problem in understanding this area is giving an adequate definition to neuromuscular fatigue. Our working definition for fatigue is a transient decrement in work performance due to preceding work activity (Morris, 1977a, 1977b; Simonson, 1971).

Once an operational definition is ascribed to neuromuscular fatigue, another problem that must be confronted is locating the site of neuromuscular fatigue. Many researchers have reported equivocal evidence showing that the fatigue site is predominantly peripheral or of muscular origin, while other scientists point to the brain or central nervous system as the locus of fatigue. Early investigators postulated that there may be several sites of fatigue. Karpovich (1959) noted six different sites for fatigue. However, close scrutiny of his work identifies two basic sites—one muscular and one essentially peripheral in the nervous system. The neuromuscular junction site in the muscle is often considered peripheral.

A unique experiment (Morris, 1977a, 1977b) has been designed to get at possible mechanisms of neuromuscular fatigue in both reaction time (voluntary response to a light stimulus) and reflex time (involuntary response to a tendon tap) actions. Both isometric and isotonic exercise bouts were used to induce fatigue. When fatigue was present, as indicated by a strength decrement of 57 percent following isometric exercise, the involuntary reflex contraction time of the quadriceps muscle was lengthened (Morris, 1977a).

When examining the voluntary reaction time, it was found that both isotonic and isometric exercise inhibited total reaction time. When this total reaction time was analyzed further, it was found that the greatest reaction time change occurred in the muscular component, which suggests that a peripheral site (muscle) is primarily responsible for neuromuscular fatigue.

An important finding that emerges from this type of research is that the type of activity given to a subject to induce fatigue may be crucial. Lind and Petrofsky (1979), pioneer researchers who have examined isometric fatigue at varying levels of maximum voluntary contraction (MVC), note that fatigue may have a different origin at different submaximal tensions. Recently, he proposed that fatigue in sustained, low, isometric tensions contains a component of transmission failure (peripheral fatigue).

Several other factors also enter the picture when attempting to pinpoint an exact site for neuromuscular fatigue. Lind & Petrofsky (1979) noted that blood flow is curtailed in sustained handgrip (isometric) contractions. Kroll (1968) noted that stronger muscles appear to fatigue faster than weaker muscles, and that fatigue curves are related to specific work-rest exercise schedules. Komi and Tesch (1979) recently studied isokinetic exercise and reported that muscle fiber types and motor unit recruitment patterns may play a role in muscle contraction failure. From this brief discussion one may realize that neuromuscular fatigue is an extremely complex process that might be partially explained by a host of competing or complimentary theories.

Neuromuscular fatigue, as presented above, may be represented as a decrement in performance in a muscle or isolated muscle group (handgrip, for example) and may be different from total body fatigue. Total body fatigue, as would occur in distance running, also has many contributing factors. A depletion of foodstuffs (muscle glycogen) and oxygen to the working/skeletal muscle, an increase in lactic acid, a decrease in aerobic enzymes (which changes muscle pH), or extremely high body temperature may all be individual limiting factors to long term endurance performance. Environmental factors, such as high temperature and humidity and altitude, may also limit human performance. The above listing is by no means complete, but merely serves as a guide for the coach and athlete to possible limiting factors in all-out human performance. An excellent reference work by Kuel (1977) discusses many of these limits to physical performance.

Athletic Heart Syndrome

Another concern relative to the whole cardiovascular fitness area is the Athletic Heart Syndrome. This topic was addressed by Simpson and Morris (1979). The Syndrome is characterized by a constellation of findings in the cardiovascular system, which may be suggestive of the presence of pathological changes. The important thing to remember is that these changes (slow, efficient heart rate, additional heart sounds or murmurs, enlarged cardiac muscle due to exercise-induced hypertrophy) are perfectly normal physiological manifestations of intelligent, long-term endurance training. It is important that team physicians, coaches, athletes, and trainers recognize that these changes are normal in endurance training and do not prohibit these athletes from competition. In the past, many people were precluded from sports because they were thought to have heart murmurs or other cardiac problems which would prevent successful participation. Such was the case in the Boston Marathon from 1912 to 1921, when Clarence DeMar was forced to merely watch this race because some ill-advised physician had barred him from competition due to a cardiac "irregularity." DeMar had won the race in 1911 and would win six more championships after resuming racing in 1922. DeMar continued to run the Boston Marathon until age 66 and ran in local races up until his death. When Mr. DeMar died from colon cancer in 1958 at 70 years of age, his heart was examined and found to be extremely large and efficient, as evidenced by his large coronary arteries, which were two to three times normal size.

Coronary Heart Disease (CHD)

If one had to pick the most important area of fitness that has been discussed, without question it would be cardiovascular fitness. This crucial aspect of fitness concerns all individuals, especially young people as they finish their college years. A case could be made that cardiovascular fitness is crucial even to grade school age children. This was learned when scientists examined young soldiers in Korea and Vietnam. It was noted that these young adults had significant atherosclerotic plaques (fatty deposits which obstruct blood flow through vital vessels) at this early adult age. Unless the cardiovascular system is stressed with the endurance type fitness activities mentioned in the previous section, a person is likely to have CHD problems later in life.

Although the CHD death rate is beginning to diminish somewhat, CHD remains the major cause of death and disability in our country and in most other Western societies. CHD gets its name from the coronary arteries that exit from the top of the heart, turn downward, surround, and infiltrate the heart muscle to bring nourishment (oxygen and foodstuffs) to this most important cardiac tissue. With age, the coronary arteries may lose some elasticity and fill with plaquclike fatty materials that begin to shut off or retard blood flow to the important heart muscle. When this happens, a person may experience sharp chest pains (angina) following small blockages in these arteries. Death or loss of function of certain parts of cardiac tissue can result.

Table 7.2 Cardiovascular Disease and Associated Risk Factors

Risk factors	Risk index						Total
Age (years)	10 to 20 1	21 to 30 2	31 to 40 3	41 to 50 4	51 to 60 6	Over 60 8	
Heredity	No known history of heart disease 1	1 relative over 60 with cardiovascular disease 2	2 relatives over 60 with cardiovascular disease 3	1 relative under 60 with cardiovascular disease 4	2 relatives under 60 with cardiovascular disease 6	3 relatives under 60 with cardiovascular disease 7	
Weight	More than 5 lbs. below standard weight 0	− 5 to + 5 lbs from standard weight 1	6 to 20 lbs. overweight 2	21 to 35 lbs. overweight 3	36 to 50 lbs. overweight 5	51 to 65 lbs. overweight 7	
Tobacco smoking	Non-User 0	Cigar and/or pipe 1	10 cigarettes or less per day 2	20 cigarettes per day 4	30 cigarettes per day 6	40 cigarettes per day or more 10	
Exercise habits	Intensive occupational & recreational exertion 1	Moderate occupational & recreational exertion 2	Sedentary work and intense recreational exertion 3	Sedentary occupational and moderate recreational exertion 5	Sedentary work and light recreational exertion 6	Complete lack of all exercise 8	
Cholesterol; fat % in diet	Cholesterol level below 180 mg.; diet contains no animal or solid fats 1	Cholesterol level 181–205 mg.; diet contains 10% animal or solid fats 2	Cholesterol level 206–230 mg.; diet contains 20% animal or solid fats 3	Cholesterol 231–255 mg.; diet contains 30% animal or solid fats 4	Cholesterol level 256–280 mg.; diet contains 40% animal or solid fats 5	Cholesterol level 281–300 mg.; diet contains 50% animal or solid fats 7	
Blood pressure	100 Upper reading 1	120 Upper reading 2	140 Upper reading 3	160 Upper reading 4	180 Upper reading 6	200 or over Upper reading 8	
Sex	Female under 40 1	Female 41 to 50 2	Female over 50 3	Male 5	Stocky male 6	Bald, stocky male 7	

GRAND TOTAL _____

Key To Risk Index Grand Total

6–11 Risk well below average
12–17 Risk below average
18–24 Risk generally average

25–31 Risk moderate
32–40 Risk at a dangerous level
41–62 Danger urgent. See your doctor now.

Source: Edington, D. W., and L. Cunningham. 1975. *Biological Awareness*. Old Tappan, N.J.: Prentice Hall.

When studying CHD in medical terms, one is confronted with CHD as a *multi-factor disease*. This means that there is no single cause responsible for this disease. Physicians and epidemiologists (scientists who study mortality and morbidity in populations) point to some dozen factors which may play a role in CHD. Table 7.2 (Edington & Cunningham, 1975) shows how multiple risk factors can combine to indicate a general, overall *risk index* for CHD.

To fully understand the interplay of the eight risk factors indicated in Table 7.2, a risk index may be computed. Naturally, a young, college-age student is likely to score low (indicating a below average risk), since age is a risk factor in the chart. However, try to determine the risk index for an older aunt, uncle, friend, or parent to see how the risk index may be dangerously high in a person who has high blood pressure and is sedentary, elderly, overweight, a smoker, or follows a poor dietary regime.

Crucial CHD Risk Factors

Many physicians who work in the area of CHD have identified three crucial risk factors: (1) high blood fats and cholesterol, (2) high blood pressure (uncontrolled), and (3) cigarette smoking (one to two packs per day). Other physicians have noted additional risk factors that are not listed in table 7.2: (1) glucose tolerance or onset of diabetes in adulthood, (2) stress and tension on the job or at home, (3) electrocardiographic (ECG) stress test abnormality, (4) personality type which is overly aggressive, time-oriented, and hassled (Type A personality), and (5) high percentage of body fat.

All these factors are certainly involved, to some extent, in this problem, though some are obviously more important than others. The next section makes a case for modifying physical activity as a risk factor and shows that, as a person manipulates this particular risk factor, other risk factors may also be changed.

The risk factors which can be modified are identified as physical activity, tobacco smoking, body weight, blood pressure, and composition of diet. Five out of the eight risk factors noted in the table can be manipulated. Though some may say that the sex factor could be changed, and recent medical advances have noted this capability, this factor will be considered unchangeable for the present discussion.

An increase in physical activity through a planned, intelligent exercise program may lead to several positive trade-offs in the individual. In addition to the well-documented, psychological effects such as increased self-esteem, self-reliance, and feelings of accomplishment, coupled with a decrease in both anxiety and depression, one may favorably affect at least four other physical risk factors by increasing physical activity. Exercise has demonstrated beneficial effects in lowering body weight (especially body fat), blood fats and cholesterol, high blood pressure, and smoking. These positive effects are even more noticeable in individuals who are actively engaged in an endurance training program. Other possible positive transfer effects of endurance conditioning will be listed later relating to stress reduction and control of one's environment through manipulation of physical activity schedules.

Body Weight

Evidence shows that, as physical activity is increased, body weight is reduced—especially if caloric consumption is maintained or reduced. It is important to keep in mind the *long term* effects of physical activity in reducing body weight. For example, a secretary who trades in a manual typewriter for an electric model may experience a five pound weight gain over the course of a year, simply because (all other things being equal) as energy output is lowered body weight increases. Conversely, walking at about 4½ miles per hour for one hour may burn between four and five hundred calories. If this walking program is followed four days per week and if caloric intake is the same, over the long term (one year) a person could lose about twenty to twenty-five pounds. Again, the long term caloric balance must be considered. An increase in physical activity may favorably affect body weight if diet is managed at the same time.

Smoking

The second relationship that will be illuminated involves the risk factors of smoking and physical activity. Many experiments on physically active people note that, as a person increases activity level, smoking is curtailed. In studying long distance runners (Morris, 1980), it has been noted that as weekly mileage figures or months of training increase, consumption of tobacco products is lowered. Indeed, it is easy to see how difficult it is to smoke while playing squash or tennis or while cross-country skiing, so that smoking is curtailed at least during the activity itself.

High Blood Pressure

The evidence indicating a positive effect of physical activity on blood pressure is encouraging. In studies where individuals have increased their physical activity over a period of time, in many cases blood pressure has dropped. Two review articles (Tipton, et al, 1979; Lowenthal & Whiteman, 1979) have shown that an increase in physical activity can have a lowering effect on moderately high blood pressure. For the estimated millions of Americans who have essential untreated hypertension, this relationship between increased exercise and a reduction in blood pressure is a promising discovery.

Blood Fats

Another positive effect of increased energy expenditure is the favorable effect this has on blood cholesterol and blood lipids (fats). Cholesterol is a fat-like substance found in the human vascular system. Again, certain definitive studies have shown that, with increases in weekly exercise, lower serum cholesterol results. Still another positive factor noted in the more recent studies (Hartung, et al, 1981) is that the ratio of beneficial **high-density lipoproteins** increases with increased physical activity. In fact, many scientists now believe that the crucial figures to be concerned with in a cholesterol reading may not be the total blood cholesterol, but the ratio of total blood cholesterol to high-density lipoprotein.

For example, in a person who has a total blood cholesterol reading of 240 mg/% and a high-density lipoprotein reading of 80 mg/%, the ratio would be 240/80, or 3.00. This figure of 3.00 would be a more positive factor when contrasted with another person of the same age and sex having a total cholesterol reading of 240, but a high-density lipoprotein reading of only 40 for a ratio of 6.00. Here, the higher ratio (of high-density lipoprotein to total cholesterol) is indicative of a lower risk index on this particular cardiovascular risk factor. Lamb (1980) notes that ratios of 3.27 to 4.44 indicate an average to below average risk, while ratios of 7.05 to 11.04 may show two to three times the average CHD risk. ■

Summary

Endurance, essentially, is the ability to endure and continue to perform sustained, large-muscle, human activities. The factors of intensity of exercise (at about 70–80% of maximum), frequency of exercise (working at endurance activities at least every other day), and the duration of exercise (working for at least 30 minutes at each exercise session) are stressed. There are several endurance training programs such as fartlek training, interval training, long slow distance training, and circuit training. Fartlek training consists of longer running activities, interspersed with sprinting. Interval training combines different programs of timed, higher-intensity runs with recovery intervals. The number of repetitions and the rest periods are manipulated. Long slow distance training is, as the name implies, going out for longer periods of time at a very slow pace, which provides an endurance stimulus to the cardiovascular system. In circuit training, the athlete runs to different stations in a gymnasium or on an athletic field and performs a series of exercises at each station. The intensity with which the athlete works at the particular station, as well as the intensity with which the athlete moves from one station to the next, is kept quite high in order to provide an endurance training stimulus.

The athlete's heart is the major organ of conditioning for endurance training. Changes that occur in this organ involve mostly volume changes. The heart is able to accept and eject a greater volume of blood during high intensity work. Exercise plays an essential role in modifying certain risk factors leading to coronary heart disease.

References

American College of Sports Medicine. 1978. The recommended quantity and quality of exercise for developing and maintaining fitness in healthy adults. *Medicine and Science in Sports.* 10: vii. (See Appendix 3).

Astrand, P. O., & K. Rodahl. 1977. *Textbook of work physiology.* New York: McGraw Hill.

Cavagna, G. A., B. Dusman, & R. Margaria. 1968. Positive work done by a previously stretched muscle. *Journal of Applied Physiology.* 24: 21.

DeLorme, T. L., & A. L. Watkins. 1948. Techniques of progressive resistance exercise. *Archives of Physical Medicine.* 33: 637.

deVries, H. A. 1980. *Physiology of exercise.* 3d ed. Dubuque, IA: Wm. C. Brown.

Edington, D. W., & L. Cunningham. 1975. *Biological awareness.* Old Tappan, NJ: Prentice-Hall.

Fox, E. 1979. *Sports physiology.* Philadelphia: W. B. Saunders.

Hartung, G. H., W. G. Squires, & A. M. Gotto Jr. 1981. Effect of exercise training on plasma high-density lipoprotein cholesterol in coronary disease patients. *American Heart Journal.* 101: 181.

Henderson, J. 1969. *The humane way to train.* Mountain View, CA: World Publications.

Karpovich, P. V. 1959. *Physiology of muscular activity.* Philadelphia: W. B. Saunders.

Karvonen, M. J. 1959. Effects of vigorous exercise on the heart. In F. F. Rosenbaum & E. L. Belknap, eds. *Work and the heart.* New York: Paul B. Hoeber, Inc.

Komi, P. V., & P. Tesch. 1979. EMG frequency spectrum, muscle structure, and fatigue during dynamic contractions in man. *European Journal of Applied Physiology.* 42: 41.

Kroll, W. 1968. Isometric fatigue curves under varied intertrial recuperation periods. *Research Quarterly.* 39: 106.

Kuel, J. ed. 1977. *Limiting factors of physical performance.* Stuttgart: Georg Thieme Publications.

Lamb, L. E. 1980. Understanding your cholesterol, triglycerides and other blood fats. *The Health Letter.* 15: 1.

Lind, A. R., & J. S. Petrofsky. 1979. Amplitude of the surface electromyogram during fatiguing isometric contractions. *Muscle and Nerve.* 2: 257.

Lowenthal, D. T., & M. S. Whiteman. 1979. Hypertension and exercise. In D. T. Lowenthal, K. Bharadwaja, & W. Oaks, eds. *Therapeutics through exercise.* New York: Grune & Stratton.

Morris, A. F. 1977a. Effects of fatiguing isometric and isotonic exercise on fractionated patella tendon reflex components. *Research Quarterly.* 48: 121.

Morris, A. F. 1977b. Effects of fatiguing isometric and isotonic exercise on resisted and unresisted reaction time components. *European Journal of Applied Physiology.* 37: 1.

Morris, A. F. 1980. Physiological characteristics of female masters long distance runners. Paper presented to the American Medical Joggers Association, Boston.

Morris, A. F. 1983. Training for the elite athlete. Invited address to the 1st International Symposium on Sports Medicine, San Sebastian, Spain, March.

Simonson, E. 1971. *The physiology of work capacity and fatigue.* Springfield, IL: Charles C. Thomas.

Simpson, A. G., & A. F. Morris. 1979. Athletic heart syndrome: some recent observations. *American Corrective Therapy Journal.* 33: 53.

Tipton, C. M., et al. 1979. Exercise, hypertension and animal models. In D. T. Lowenthal, K. Bharadwaja, & W. Oaks, eds. *Therapeutics through exercise.* New York: Grune & Stratton.

van Aaken, E. 1976. *The van Aaken method.* Mountain View, CA: World Publications.

Flexibility Training and Conditioning

Introduction

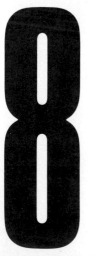

This chapter concerns flexibility, which may be defined as the range of body motion which occurs at a single joint. Flexibility may also be defined as the total range of body movement which can occur at several joints, for example, that flexibility of movement which is permitted between the individual vertebrae of the spine.

There are several devices to measure flexibility, such as the basic, standard **goniometer,** and the Leighton **flexometer.** Also, several researchers have used an electrogoniometer to record human movement occurring at a joint.

The athlete can develop or maintain flexibility through programs of ballistic stretching, static stretching, or by utilizing newer methods of proprioceptive neuromuscular facilitation. These stretching programs should concentrate on specific muscle groups and body parts which need a certain amount of flexibility in order for the athlete to perform well, and include a regular schedule of exercise.

Devices to Measure Flexibility

Several devices are available to measure flexibility. The two most common are the Leighton (1955) flexometer and the standard goniometer.

The Leighton flexometer consists of a compass-type arrangement that is strapped to a particular body segment. When the subject is asked to move the body part, a small weight rotates about an axis point due to gravity, and a needle indicates degrees of movement (fig. 8.1).

A second device to measure flexibility, the simple goniometer, is nothing more than a protractor with two moving segments attached at a pivot point (fig. 8.2). To measure individual joint flexibility with this device, one arm of the goniometer is aligned along one body segment and the second rotating arm of the goniometer along the adjacent body segment. The center axis of the goniometer is carefully placed over the subject's joint center. The subject is asked to move one segment in regard to the other segment and total range of movement (ROM), or the subject's flexibility, is noted at that particular joint. Some investigations have devised elaborate electric goniometers to measure ROM during certain human movements (Morris & Brown, 1976).

In some tasks, such as trunk bending, it is nearly impossible to measure single joint flexibility, so other tests must be devised. One such test for measuring back, hip, and hamstring flexibility is the sit and reach test, in which the performer sits on the floor and, while keeping the knees straight, attempts to touch or reach beyond the toes. This is a good lower body and hip flexibility test, since it is almost impossible to isolate flexibility in different parts of the spine (American Academy, 1965; Humphrey, 1981).

Static and Dynamic Flexibility

In further study of flexibility both **static** and **dynamic flexibility** must be considered. Static flexibility refers to range-of-motion (ROM) at a particular joint when one body segment is manipulated relative to another (deVries, 1962, 1980), as when the forearm is flexed against the upper arm segment in a very slow motion and held in the extreme flexed position. Dynamic, or phasic, flexibility refers to rapid flexibility of movement, as occurs in a hurdler going over the hurdles or a gymnast doing a back flip. These dynamic flexibility movements require rapid, jerking, and often bouncing movements.

How to Increase Flexibility

What type of flexibility exercise movements are best to increase flexibility? This is a difficult question to answer for it may involve a *combination* of static and dynamic flexibility movements in practice or training to achieve maximum improvement. One thing is fairly well established—static stretches lead to larger increases in ROM. This can be tested by flexing the forearm at the elbow as *rapidly* as possible and holding it in the flexed position.

Flexibility Training and Conditioning

Figure 8.1 Leighton Flexometer. Free-moving indicator needle *(a)* is held vertical by counterweight *(b)*. Stationary housing with indicator dial *(c)* is attached to moving body segment by strap *(d)*.

Source: Leighton, J. R. 1955. An instrument and technique for measurement of range of joint motion. *Archives of Physical Medicine and Rehabilitation*. 36:571–75.

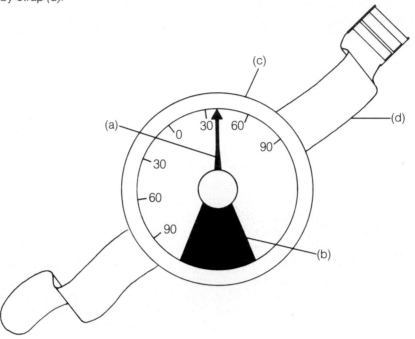

Figure 8.2 Goniometer or Range-of-Motion Device. Center of axis *(a)* is placed over subject's joint center. Segment arm *(b)* is aligned with one human limb. Rotating segment arm *(c)* is aligned with adjacent human limb. An angle of 30° is illustrated.

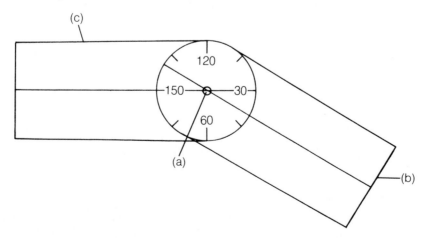

The hand is still several inches from the shoulder. Now, flexing the arm very slowly and gradually, the hand comes much closer to the shoulder than in the rapid flexing movement. The reason for this is the stretch reflex. In the fast flex, the triceps muscle spindles (special muscle sensory receptors) monitor the rapid stretch in this muscle group and, as a protective maneuver, the triceps partially contracts near the end of the rapid flexion movement. The net result is less ROM in the elbow joint. This simple but effective test emphasizes the importance of developing static stretching exercises in training and rehabilitation.

Some authors (Logan & Egstrom, 1961; deVries, 1980) have compared static to dynamic stretching training programs and have found significant increases in ROM with both programs. Although recorded increases were of the same magnitude, there are still some definite benefits to employing slow static stretches. These advantages of static stretches are summarized by deVries (1980) as: (1) less danger of exceeding muscle limits, causing muscle strains and pulls, (2) less energy use in assuming the static stretches, and (3) lesser likelihood of incurring muscle soreness than in fast, phasic stretching. In fact, deVries (1962) has noted that static stretching may actually relieve muscle soreness.

The proper procedure for static stretching is important. Ideally, the athlete should try to hold the final position in the joint ROM of the stretch for ten to thirty seconds. Holding for this period of time, or even longer, allows the muscle fibers to stretch out slowly and remain stretched for this duration, leading to increases in flexibility.

The athlete should go into each stretch slowly and in control. As the maximal stretch is reached, some tension is felt in the stretched muscle. This is natural and it is a good sign that muscle fibers are being stretched. The object is to hold that position for a ten to thirty second period of time. As the performer progresses in holding the stretch from six to twenty seconds, the muscle may be able to stretch out even farther. This is a good indication that the muscle fibers are being elongated. The performer should also return from the stretched position slowly and in control. Breathing should be natural, slow, and controlled during these static flexibility exercises. Some individuals may close their eyes during the exercise to more closely monitor the stretching sensation in the muscles being flexed.

Static stretching is a time-consuming experience and the athlete must have patience to effect a successful flexibility program. The person who practices yoga is often very flexible, since this person often takes the necessary time and effort to practice the various static positions. In most cases, the results of increased flexibility can be demonstrated in their performances.

Important Areas to Stretch

Those body areas that are used most extensively in a particular sport need stretching the most. The runner must stretch the calf group, hamstrings, and lower back. Swimmers and hockey players must concentrate on arm and shoulder flexibility, as well as leg and ankle flexibility. Gymnasts work primarily for hip, back, and total body flexibility. Several flexibility stretching exercises are described in figure 8.3.

Figure 8.3 Flexibility Exercises for Lower Extremities. Some stretching should be performed slowly, with few repetitions, several times a day.

Source: deVries, H. A. 1980. *Physiology of exercise.* Dubuque, IA: Wm. C. Brown.

Hamstrings

Exercise One

1. Spread legs 24″ apart.
2. Bend over (knees stiff).
3. S t r e t c h (do not bounce).
4. Return to upright position.

Exercise Two

1. Cross feet.
2. Bend over to touch floor.
3. S t r e t c h
4. Return to upright position.
5. Change feet and repeat.

Exercise Three

1. Standing on one leg, place opposite heel on table about 30″ high.
2. Bend at waist and touch toes (keep knees stiff).
3. S t r e t c h
4. Return to upright position.
5. Change legs.

Exercise Four

1. Spread feet 24″ apart.
2. Bring arms out at shoulder level.
3. Twist and bend, touching fingers to opposite foot.
4. Return to upright position.
5. Alternate.

Exercise Five

1. Sit on floor with one leg extended, one flexed at side.
2. Grasp toes.
3. Pull body toward toes.
4. Alternate.

Exercise Six

1. Lie flat on back, with hands at side.
2. Roll legs up and over head.
3. Touch floor above head.
4. Return legs to lying position.
5. Repeat.

Quadriceps

Exercise One

1. Lie on front.
2. Reach back and hold ankle.
3. Pull heel to buttocks. Do not jerk!
4. Return to floor.
5. Alternate.

Exercise Two

1. Sit on floor, with one leg extended, one flexed at side.
2. Lie back on floor.
3. Return to upright position.
4. Alternate.

Exercise Three

1. The same as quad exercise one but standing. Many people use this as a quad stretcher, but in this exercise the pelvis moves and you do not get the full stretch. We suggest exercise one instead.

Figure 8.3 (continued)

Heel Cord

Exercise One

1. Stand about 30″ from wall.
2. Lean to wall at arm's length.
3. Push abdomen towards wall, keeping knees stiff.
4. Return and repeat.

Exercise Two

1. Same as exercise one, except swivel pelvis from side to side.
2. Repeat.

Exercise Three

1. Same as exercise one, except flex one knee.
2. Repeat.

Stretching before an athletic event can warm the muscles slightly and serve to prepare the body for more vigorous action.

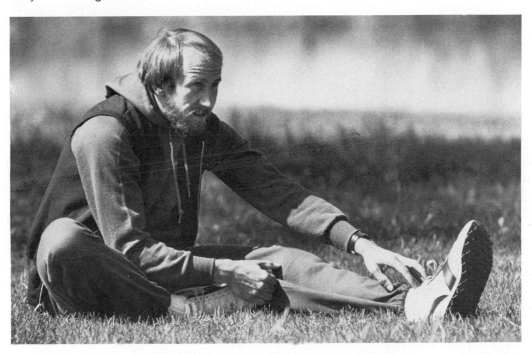

What is the best time to stretch? Ideally, the athlete should stretch before, during, and at the end of a workout session. Flexibility exercises at the beginning of the workout enable the athlete to gradually warmup and prepare the body for action. Stretching during a long and strenuous workout may begin to relieve tight muscles and postpone tightness and cramping in the working muscles. It is most important, however, to stretch after a workout when muscles are often somewhat shortened from repeated contractions caused by the workouts. deVries (1980) has also shown that flexibility exercises after muscular activity may actually relieve some muscle spasm and resultant soreness.

Additional Research on Stretching

Dr. Robert Hutton, of the University of Washington (1979), has noted that when three hamstring muscle stretching conditions were compared, subjects reported that no single stretch condition felt superior to another. In this experiment the subjects were involved in three different conditions. In condition one the subjects used a static stretch. In condition two the subjects contracted the hamstrings, then went into a static stretch. In condition three the subjects contracted the hamstrings, then relaxed the hamstrings, then contracted the opposite hip flexor muscle group in an attempt to further stretch the hamstrings. Results indicated greater ROM for condition three, but also greater discomfort. It was concluded that if comfort and training time are major factors for the athlete, then the static condition may be the most desirable technique to use in flexibility training, since this condition produces favorable results in ROM in a brief period of time with minimal discomfort. ▄

Summary

Flexibility is the range of body motion which occurs at a single joint. Flexibility may also be described as the total range of body movement within a series of joints, such as occurs in the human spine.

There are devices to measure flexibility such as the Leighton flexometer and the goniometer. Joint measurement is recorded in degrees of movement. Generally, the person who has a larger number of degrees of movement at a particular joint, or in a series of joints, is more flexible.

Programs to improve flexibility are either dynamic or static. Dynamic refers to rapidly moving body segments, while static movements are slow, prolonged, muscle stretches. Static stretching is more efficient because it does not conflict with the stretch reflex. Important areas of the body in which to maintain flexibility include the calf muscle group, the muscle groups in the upper thighs (hamstrings and quadriceps), as well as muscles in the groin region. Also, flexibility in the back is important for many types of athletes, such as gymnasts, pole vaulters, and golfers.

References

American Academy of Orthopaedic Surgeons. 1965. *Joint motion.* Chicago, IL.

deVries, H. A. 1962. Evaluation of static stretching procedures for improvement of flexibility. *Research Quarterly.* 33: 222.

deVries, H. A. 1980. *Physiology of exercise.* Dubuque, IA: Wm. C. Brown.

Humphrey, L. D. 1981. Flexibility. *Journal of Physical Education, Recreation, and Dance.* 52: 41.

Hutton, R. 1979. Personal communication. Fall.

Leighton, J. R. 1955. An instrument and technique for measurement of range of joint motion. *Archives of Physical Medicine and Rehabilitation.* 36: 571.

Logan, G., & G. H. Egstrom. 1961. The effects of slow and fast stretching on the sacrofemoral angle. *Journal of the Association for Physical and Mental Rehabilitation.* 15: 85.

Morris, A. F., & M. Brown. 1976. Electronic training devices for hand rehabilitation. *American Journal of Occupational Therapy.* 30: 376.

Injuries in Sports Medicine

Part 4

Introduction to Athletic Injuries

Outline

Introduction

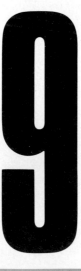

The subject of sports medicine injuries occupies a very large part of the discipline of sports medicine. There are many clinical people involved in the area of sports medicine as outlined in chapter 1 in this text. Physicians occupy approximately 40% of all the personnel within the sports medicine field. At the high school level, coaches, athletic trainers, and school nurses, in addition to the team physician, are involved in the care of young athletes. On other levels (club or YMCA), the youth sports league coaches, therapists, or parents who may become concerned with their youngsters, ultimately become involved in training, conditioning, and the injury aspect of sports. This chapter defines sports medicine injuries, noting the severity of the different types of injuries. The NAIRS (National Athletic Injury/Illness Reporting System) is covered.

Although there are many reasons why injuries occur in sports, essentially, the contact nature of sport and the athlete striving for excellence produce most of them. Classification systems for sports injuries make it easier to understand the means of treatment and prevention.

Methods of Defining Athletic Injuries

By Participation Time Lost in Sport Activity

In most cases, an athletic injury is defined as some physical damage or insult to the body that occurs during athletic practice or competition, causing *a resultant loss of capacity or impairing performance.* Many athletic trainers and coaches categorize the severity of the injury by the period of time for which it prevents the athlete from participating. If the athlete must miss a day or two of practice due to insult incurred in sports participation, then the problem may be considered as an athletic injury. This description of athletic injuries depends on the *time away from the activity.* Obviously, a more severe athletic injury is going to require more missed practice time, more time away from training, possibly missing a competitive event, or even an entire season.

By Necessity for Visiting a Professional

Another definition of athletic injury is the number of visits that the athlete makes to a professional person, seeking treatment for the injury. For example, if the athlete reports the damage or injury to the coach, athletic trainer, school nurse, or team physician, this would be considered an injury. Or, if the injury necessitates a visit to the athletic training room, this may count as one report of an athletic injury. More serious athletic injuries are indicated by the necessity to consult a trained specialist.

National Athletic Injury/Illness Reporting System (NAIRS)

NAIRS, or the **National Athletic Injury/Illness Reporting System** (1978) is founded on functional definitions which attempt to ensure a uniformity of criteria for reportable injuries. These *reportable* injuries are:

a) Any *brain concussion* causing cessation of the athlete's participation for observation before return to play is permitted is reportable.
b) Any *dental injury* which *should* receive professional attention is reportable.
c) Any injury/illness which causes cessation of an athlete's customary participation throughout the *participation-day following day of onset* is reportable.
d) Any injury/illness which requires *substantive professional* attention before the athlete's return to participation is permitted is reportable (i.e., *without such attention, the athlete would not have been permitted to return to participation the next participation-day).*

NOTE: Any program has the privilege of reporting any injury/illness under liberal interpretation of this definition. Further, it is noted that this NAIRS guide also emphasizes the loss of participation (item c) and the visit to professionals (item d).

The risk of injury is inherent in sport. Because football involves many large players and vicious contact, it may produce many athletic injuries.

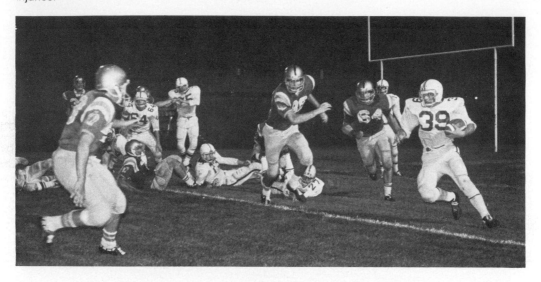

Relationship of Injuries and Sports

Special Considerations of Specific Sports

The number of participants and type of sport involvement determine, in many instances, the number and severity of injuries in that sport. For example, football requires large numbers of participants. The game is often played by two teams with eleven players on each. Most teams have specialty units—offensive teams, defensive teams, kicking teams, and so on. Because of the large number of participants, and also the contact nature of the sport, many injuries occur in football. It is estimated that, during a single season, one out of two football players will miss some practice or game time, due to an injury (Vinger & Hoerner, 1981).

Non-contact sports, like tennis, may not have the severity of the injury or the numbers and types of injuries that football may have. Most of the injuries in those sports involve overuse or improper training techniques. Tennis elbow, problems of irritations occurring at the shoulder, and other types of injuries are examples that are commonly found in tennis. Most of these injuries are overuse or chronic (long-term) type of injuries which may often be prevented if the athlete, the coach, and the trainer are using proper training principles, as outlined in an earlier chapter.

It must be emphasized that the total number of participants involved in a given sport activity often increases the injury potential. Since bicycling is such a popular activity, there may be more total injuries related to bicycling than other sports. This relationship between sport/recreational equipment and frequency of injuries may be seen in table 9.1.

110

Table 9.1 Ranking of Frequency of Injuries Related to Sports and Recreational Equipment

Sports and Recreational Equipment	Number of injuries
1. Bicycling and bicycling equipment	17,411
2. Football and related equipment	12,591
3. Basketball and related equipment	9,492
4. Baseball and related equipment	8,983
5. Sports ball, not specified	3,207
6. Swings	2,788
7. Snow skiing and related equipment	1,887
8. Hockey equipment	1,640
9. Fishing equipment	1,569
10. Swimming pools and related equipment	1,415

Source: Vinger, P. F., & E. G. Hoerner, eds. 1981. *Sports injuries*. Littleton, MA: PSG Publishing Co.

Because it was compiled in the early to mid–1970s—before the great jogging explosion—most running related injuries were absent from this list. If enough people participate in a sport activity, or if the sport activity is particularly risky (like football), then a greater possibility of injury may be associated with participation in that sport activity. Other factors that come to intervene on a particular sport that also affect injury rate are detailed below.

Reasons Why Injuries Occur in Sport Activities

Most authors, when discussing this general area of sports injuries, omit a full rationale of why injuries are apt to happen in sports. This situation is remedied in this section in a detailed examination of *why* injuries may occur. Many injuries in sports can be avoided. By eliminating the contact nature in certain sporting activities, obviously, many of the traumatic injuries would be reduced or sharply curtailed. Reducing the all-out nature, or the drive to excel in sports, would eliminate many of the overuse or overstress syndromes. However, it is the nature of the athlete, the nature of the human being, to attempt to excel in various aspects of human performance. One of the few areas in which participants can assert their own unique selves into an activity is participation in sports. Humans, by nature, are competitive and aggressive and will always seek to perform in such activities as contact sports even though such participation may result in traumatic injuries. In individual sports, such as running, swimming, rowing, or skiing, individual competitors striving to excel may risk injury. In this type of situation, injuries are always going to result, due to overuse and overstress. Improper equipment may be a contributing factor to some athletic injuries. Unprepared participants (training unwisely) may also be prone to injuries. Finally, improper coaching and supervision could lead to injury.

Athletes Strive for Excellence in Sport

Perhaps the main reason why injuries occur in sports is that highly competitive athletes generally do not settle for second best. The very nature of athletic competition implies an all-out striving for excellence by the athlete, pushing the body to the absolute limit. This all-out nature of sports, coupled with the intense drive and motivation of top athletes, often leads to injuries.

Let me provide a little insight here. Walker (1980) has said that a player enters the world of sport as a challenge, accepting the risks and the uncertainty in accordance with his/her own design. Sport and competition at its best, he continues, may be the greatest of the performing arts. When winning is the object of the competition, then all competitors should strive to win. In this all-out striving, in this intense desire to excel, one necessarily exposes oneself to the risk of injuries. Several examples may help to clarify this picture. World-class marathoners, preparing to compete in an Olympic marathon, continue to push themselves through intense two-per-day workouts, vigorous interval training sessions, and longer and longer mileage. As these athletes attempt to peak for this one performance, as they drive themselves to the limit of human endurance, they come closer and closer to the point of injury—the overuse injury. If the athletes, during this intensive period of training, begin to back off somewhat to provide themselves with more rest, then they move away from the overuse or overstress type of injury. But because most athletes on this level are always attempting to improve their past performances, to seek a personal best, they are continually exposing themselves to the possibility of an overuse injury. It is because of this intense, overwhelming desire to excel, to continually push themselves to the limits of performance, that many competitors, especially those in individual sports—gymnastics, swimming, track and field, and cross-country skiing—are more prone to overuse injuries. If athletes, in general, were content to go through the actions of their sport in slow motion, there may be fewer injuries. This, however, is simply not the case.

Physical Contact in Sports

A second reason for the incidence of injuries in many popular sports is physical *contact*. Boxing is an obvious example. Other contact sports are football, hockey, lacrosse, rugby, soccer—the list could go on and on. In all of these games and activities one of the objects is to tackle, to check, or to try to deprive the opponent of the opportunity to win the game. Very large individuals participate in these sports. Football players often weigh in excess of 250 pounds, and are able to bench press their body weight. If contact results between these large, strong players, one may expect some damage or injury. With repeated contact, the risks of injury increase.

Improper Equipment and Apparatus

A third factor as to why injuries occur in sports is the equipment and apparatus used in sport activities. Certain athletic events involve throwing balls, shooting hockey pucks, and so on. Due to the speed which the athletes can impart to these missiles, there may be resulting injuries. In certain activities (hockey and lacrosse) the participants are also wielding sticks. In most cases, there exist strict rules and regulations as to the use of these sticks, but in an attempt to check the opposing player, very often the stick hits the other individual and, obviously, could cause an injury.

Many sports require the use of elaborate protective equipment and padding. In football, for example, the inividual is fitted with head, neck, shoulder, torso and extremity pads. In hockey and lacrosse, many of the participants wear similar equipment. The reason for this entire body covering is the intense contact that takes place in these sports. Also, *if the equipment is not fitted properly, the athlete may be exposed to the risk of injury.* An example is an improperly fitted helmet in hockey, lacrosse, and football. Other examples might be improperly fitted face masks and mouth pieces. Many injuries to the head, face, mouth, and teeth occur when the player is either not wearing the proper equipment, or the piece of equipment is not properly fitted for maximum protection. To excessively pad the individual to the degree where there is the greatest amount of protection, risks losing some of the function of that individual. There is a trade-off between the protection and fit of the equipment and the function that is allowed to the individual wearing the equipment. The athlete, the coach, and the team physician should come to full agreement as to what types and amounts of equipment the athlete should wear for maximum protection without unduly impeding function and performance.

Unprepared Participants

One of the reasons many physicians and athletic trainers list as a prime factor in injuries is the unprepared state of some athletic participants. Early in the season, when conditioning is poor, or in unskilled individuals, the injury rate tends to be higher. If coaches institute adequate pre-season conditioning programs and prepare participants in all aspects of conditioning for their sport, many of these injuries can be prevented. In fact, the unprepared participant and the all-out nature of sports may contribute to most of the non-contact injuries found in athletics.

Poor Coaching and Injuries

It has been reported (Estwanik & Rovere, 1983) that poor coaching practices may contribute to sport injuries. The coach has many responsibilities in this area. Only properly screened (by a physician) athletes should be allowed to try out for the sport. The coach must continually monitor the field or practice environment for safety. The coach must suggest proper guidelines for training and conditioning. If the coach is diligent in all the above mentioned areas, some athletic injuries may be avoided.

Classification Scheme for Injuries

Various authors list several schemoo for classifying injuries. Athletic injuries may be classified by analomical location, or by sport. Some physicians and athletic trainers categorize athletic injury according to the particular participant group, such as women, young children, or older athletes. Still another classification scheme uses the terms ''acute'' and ''chronic.'' Acute injuries are generally very sudden, traumatic, major injuries. Chronic injuries occur over a longer period of time, and are a form of overuse or overstress injuries.

Another system to classify athletic injuries is by the type of tissue which is involved, such as the muscle tissue. Other sections within this classification scheme may cover injuries to ligaments, cartilage, and tendons—soft tissue injuries. Finally, some other classification systems may be by the severity of the athletic injury or be based on the mechanism of the injury. Table 9.2 shows several different methods of classification of athletic injuries listed by various authors. The first one listed, Morris, is the athletic injury classification scheme used in this book—by muscle tissue and by bone tissue. Many sports medicine authors use an anatomical regional approach to athletic injuries. They list a number or series of injuries which can occur to the anatomical part involved: foot and ankle injuries; lower leg, knee and thigh injuries; hip and back injuries; injuries to the trunk, abdomen and pelvis; injuries to the upper extremity, including the hand, elbow, wrist, and shoulder; injuries to the head, face, and neck (Klafs & Arnheim, 1981; O'Donoghue, 1976). Some authors refer to the specific joint involved in the injury. Many physicians favor this particular scheme for reporting athletic injuries.

Table 9.2 Methods of Classification of Athletic Injuries (with sample texts).

Author	Reference	Athletic injury classification method
1. Morris, A. F.	*Sports Medicine* (1984)	Tissue involved; i.e., muscle, bone, etc.
2. Kraus, H.	*Sports Injuries* (1981)	Acute versus chronic
3. Klein, K. & F. Allman	*The Knee in Sports* (1969)	Anatomical location—knees, shoulder, back, etc.
4. Jesse, J.	*Injury and Running Athletes* (1977)	Sport—Track and field, football, basketball, soccer, lacrosse, gymnastics, etc.
5. Klafs, C. & D. Arnheim	*Modern Principles of Athletic Training* (1981)	Anatomical location
6. Haycock, C. (editor)	*Sports Medicine for the Female Athlete* (1980)	Participant group—children, females, males, oldsters
7. O'Donoghue, D. H.	*Treatment of Injuries to Athletes* (1976)	Anatomical location
8. Reilly, T. (editor)	*Sports Fitness and Sports Injuries* (1981)	Three Types (a) Team game injury, (b) Individual sport injury, (c) Orthopedic
9. Strauss, R. (editor)	*Sports Medicine and Physiology* (1979)	List of injuries—hip pointer, shinsplint, blister, etc.
10. Hlavac, H.	*The Sport Book* (1980)	By physician treating injury (e.g. cardiologist, orthopedist, podiatrist, etc.)
11. Appenzeller, O. & R. Atkinson	*Sports Medicine* (1981)	Combination of above methods, but chiefly by anatomical location

Injury Classification by Sport

Another way to describe athletic injuries is to detail them by sport. For example, an author writing about football injuries would cover the most common type of injuries in the sport of football. Knee injuries would be a major category, since this joint is very often involved in traumatic football injuries. Less severe injuries to the musculoskeletal system would also be categorized due to the contact nature of the sport. Other injuries discussed in the category of football injuries might be those occurring to the feet of athletes playing on artificial surfaces, and various types of burns that they may sustain from friction on the artificial surfaces.

Another example of classification of athletic injuries by sport is swimming injuries. In swimmers, the areas most often involved are the shoulder, hand, and knee. Swimmer's shoulder, however, is vastly different from the type of shoulder injuries that the football player might be exposed to. In swimming, it is the repetitive nature of making thousands of revolutions with the arm at the shoulder joint that causes overuse injuries. The knee of the swimmer who does the breaststroke may be injured because of the particular type of kick involved. The angle at the knee joint is extremely important and may cause an irritation to the swimmer's knee, if a lot of force is exerted in certain aspects of the kick. Many swimmers who injure their knees with an overtraining type of injury syndrome do so because of improper training or by merely doing too much too soon in their swimming activity.

Another sport which has a similar pattern of overuse type injuries is gymnastics. Certain types of injuries occur in male and female gymnasts alike. Gymnasts have a lot of all-out running, jumping, and abrupt landings in their sport. Consequently, many of their injuries are due to the impact of vaulting, twisting, and landings. The gymnast is exposed to many traumatic musculoskeletal problems. An author who discusses injuries by sport will often cover all the specific injuries that occur to the athlete participating in a particular sport.

Injury Classification by Participant Group

Another classification system by which physicians and athletic trainers categorize athletic injury is by noting the particular population segment of the competitors. Recently there has been an increase in participation in youth sports, in sports for women, sports for the physically disabled, and adult or older age group competition. With the increase in the number of these participants in various athletic activities, we also see a concomitant increase in the number of sports injuries. Obviously, the number of sports injuries is related to the number of participants in that sport.

Some authors detail athletic injuries to the specific sport group of youth sports. In youth sports, since the young athlete has a growing skeleton, many of the injuries that occur might be complicated by this growing musculoskeletal system. Specifically, injuries to young, immature athletes might involve the growing centers or growing ends of the bones, which are called epiphyses. If the young athlete sustains an injury, such as a fracture, or irritation to these growth centers of the bone, the youngster must be seen by a trained specialist. In such cases as these, it should be the orthopedic physician. In fact, it may be a very specific type of orthopedic specialist, the pediatric orthopedist.

There may also be specific problems that occur in female athletes. These competitors may have difficulty with menstrual problems and other particular female concerns. Often, gynecologists or even family practitioners specializing in this area become involved with the problems of this particular athletic group.

Physiatrists, physical medicine specialists, and neurologists get involved in classifying spinal cord injuries to determine injury classifications for participants in wheelchair sports.

Finally, as more of the population in this country begins to age and these people enter age group athletics, there are more age related injuries in sports. This older age group tends to compete in individual sports; tennis, track and field, swimming, weightlifting, etc. Many of the injuries in these older participants are due to improper training and overuse. These overuse syndromes and incorrect training procedures result in many, many injuries. The person specializing in treating these injuries to the older person may be a geriatric specialist. Other medical specialists involved in this treatment may be the physiatrist and other rehabilitation specialists. Also, we know that, as the individual ages, they very often become prone to degenerative diseases, such as those occurring in the cardiovascular system. Often, the cardiologist is called upon to examine these people to determine their fitness for athletic competition and also to suggest the types and limits of activity best suited for them.

Other Injury Classification Systems (Acute vs. Chronic)

Another type of injury classification in sports medicine may be to describe the injury as either *acute* or *chronic*. Generally, the definition used for an acute injury is a one-time traumatic injury, such as a simple ankle sprain. The person playing basketball, soccer, or some other vigorous activity may turn sharply on the ankle, resulting in an overstretching of the ligaments and tissues about the joint. In contrast, a chronic injury would be an injury sustained over a period of time or caused by prolonged participation in a given sports activity. Common chronic injuries occur in many individual sports where a person has not followed a graduated training program. Examples of chronic injuries occurring in sports are shin splints, tennis elbow, bone stress fractures, irritations of the shoulder in long distance swimming, and other types of overuse/overstress injuries. When describing athletic injuries according to the category of acute or chronic, one must actually define the length of time involved in incurring these injuries. Many practitioners in this area denote chronic as any injury which lingers for many days, weeks, or even months.

Injury Classification by Type of Tissue Involved

Still another area by which one may classify athletic injuries is to discuss injuries by the type of tissue primarily involved. *Most athletic injuries occur as injuries to the musculoskeletal system, specifically to soft tissues* (Kraus, 1981). Soft tissue injury is any injury to skeletal muscle, nerve, ligament, cartilage, or other such tissue. Bone is considered hard tissue. Most soft tissue injuries are to muscles, tendons, ligaments, and skin. Skeletal muscle tissue injuries are the most common soft tissue injuries and they will be discussed in the next chapter. ■

116

Summary

This chapter deals with injuries in sports medicine. Essentially, an athletic injury is defined as a loss in capacity of the athlete which impairs performance. This generally indicates that the injury or illness will cause the athlete to miss one or more practices, or games. If the injury is severe, the athlete may miss an entire season. The number of practices or games missed often denotes the severity of an athletic injury. Another way to note the severity of an athletic injury is to mark the number of visits to a physician that the athlete needs to make in order to seek treatment for the injury. The NAIRS reporting system, devised at Penn State University, is another way of noting athletic injuries.

There are other considerations that must be noted when discussing sports injuries. The number of participants in the sport will directly affect the number of injuries that will occur. The contact nature of the sport must be considered, particularly in an activity such as football or ice hockey. The all-out nature of the athlete in competition is a main reason for athletic injuries. Contact, improper equipment and apparatus, unprepared participants, and poor coaching can lead to injuries.

A practical scheme for classifying injuries involves consideration of soft tissue injuries (injuries which occur to any soft tissue in the body, such as muscle, tendons, ligaments, or cartilage) versus hard tissue injuries (injuries to the skeletal system). Injuries may also be classified by sport or by participant group (runners). Still other classification systems for injuries include acute versus chronic. Acute injuries are any injuries that occur very suddenly during a single practice or game situation, while chronic injuries are those injuries which develop over time.

References

Appenzeller, O., & R. Atkinson. 1981. *Sports medicine.* Baltimore: Urban & Schwarzenberg.

Estwanik, J. J., & G. D. Rovere. 1983. Wrestling injuries in North Carolina high schools. *The Physician and Sportsmedicine.* 11:100.

Haycock, C., ed. 1980. *Sports medicine for the female athlete.* Oradell, NJ: Medical Economics Co.

Hlavac, H. F. 1980. *The sport book.* Mountain View, CA: World Publications.

Jesse, J. 1977. *Injury and running athletes.* Pasadena, CA: The Athletic Press.

Klafs, C. E., & D. D. Arnheim. 1981. *Modern principles of athletic training.* 5th ed. St. Louis: C. V. Mosby.

Klein, K. K., & F. L. Allman Jr. 1969. *The knee in sports.* Austin, TX: The Pemberton Press.

Kraus, H. 1981. *Sports injuries.* New York: Harper & Row.

O'Donoghue, D. H. 1976. *Treatment of injuries to athletes.* Philadelphia: W. B. Saunders.

Reilly, T., ed. 1981. *Sports fitness and sports injuries.* Great Britain: Faber & Faber Ltd.

Strauss, R. H., ed. 1979. *Sports medicine and physiology.* Philadelphia: W. B. Saunders.

U.S. Consumer Product Safety Commission. 1978. *NAIRS—The National Athletic Injury Reporting System.* Washington, DC.

Vinger, P. F., & E. F. Hoerner. eds. 1981. *Sports injuries.* Littleton, MA: PSG Publishing Co.

Walker, S. H. 1980. *Winning: the psychology of competition.* New York: W. W. Norton & Co.

Muscle Injuries

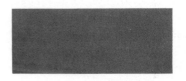

Outline

Introduction

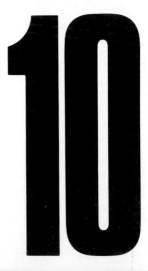

Most sports medicine injuries fall into the category of musculoskeletal injuries. Nearly 80 percent of these injuries are to the skeletal muscle system itself. The purpose of this chapter is to look at muscle injuries in detail.

The immediate treatment for muscle injuries involves the application of rest, ice, compression, elevation, and support to the injured skeletal muscle tissue. There are several common factors that predispose the athlete toward overuse skeletal muscle injuries. This chapter stresses these factors predisposing the athlete to overuse muscle injuries, which athletes neglect in their training and conditioning program. Items such as overtraining and poor training, structural abnormalities, lack of flexibility, muscle imbalances, poor techniques, and factors of growth and maturation are discussed as they relate to the general topic of predisposing factors to muscle injuries.

In the last section of this chapter, specific muscle injuries are covered, such as muscle contusions (blows directly to the skeletal muscle), muscle soreness, muscle cramps, muscle compartment syndromes, and muscle herniations. A detailed description of the different types and severity of muscle strains is also included in this chapter.

Blood Supply to Skeletal Muscle

Nearly 80 percent of all athletic injuries are soft tissue injuries (Kraus, 1981). Of these injuries, perhaps the single tissue which is most often involved is skeletal muscle tissue. Injuries to muscle tissue fall into many categories: muscle strains, muscle contusions, muscle cramps, muscle compartment syndromes, muscle hernias, and excessive muscle soreness. To understand what happens in the muscle injury, it is necessary to review the actual structure of the muscle tissue. Muscle cells are composed of elongated fibers running, in most cases, the entire length of the muscle. In addition, the muscle has much vascularization (it is profusely supplied with blood and blood vessels). Many of these blood vessels are of the very smallest types; the arterioles, capillaries, and venuoles. Any excessive tearing of muscular tissue causes a great deal of bleeding because these small blood vessels are ruptured. Therefore, it is the aim of any initial treatment of soft tissue injuries to attempt to control the bleeding or hemorrhage which will occur in the muscle tissue. In fact, a good guideline to follow with most athletic injuries would be to use a procedure often referred to as RICES.

Immediate Treatment of Muscle Injuries—RICES

Rest

The immediate treatment for muscle injuries always involves rest. Therefore, the first initial in the anacronym RICES, *R,* stands for *rest!* The athlete is immediately removed from further participation and is mandated to a period of enforced rest. This, of course, slows metabolism, and therefore, blood supply to the injured area.

Ice

Secondly, *ice (I)* is applied to the injured area. This ice application may be in the form of an ice massage applied directly to the skin of the injured area, or the ice may be wrapped in a towel, plastic bag, or icebag, which is then applied directly to the area. Sometimes gentle pressure is applied to the area with the ice; sometimes the ice is stroked or mildly massaged on and around the area. This local application of ice should continue for fifteen to thirty minutes out of each hour for the first day. This procedure may be done into the second day of injury. Most medical authorities suggest fifteen to thirty minute applications of ice to the injured area, spaced twenty to thirty minutes apart. This hourly regimen should be continued for at least several hours, and, if possible, throughout the first twenty-four to forty-eight hours after the injury. The ice may be applied over a wrap so as to prevent freezing of the skin. Ice application tends to decrease pain, swelling, metabolism, and spasm in the injured muscle.

Compression

The third initial, *C,* stands for *compression.* In an attempt to limit internal bleeding, a compression bandage is applied to the injured area. Often, the compression bandage is applied directly to the injured site, ice is placed over the first layer of elastic bandage wrap, and more compression elastic wrap is put over the ice. The ice, together with the compression, serves to limit internal bleeding, which is associated with all acute muscle injuries. Compression of the injured area may also aid in squeezing some fluid and debris out of the injury site.

Elevation

The *E* stands for *elevation.* Elevating the injured area limits circulation to that area and, hence, further limits internal bleeding. It is relatively simple to prop up an injured leg or upper extremity so as to limit bleeding. The aim in this immediate first aid step is to get the injured part up over the level of the heart, if possible. This should aid venous return to the heart.

Stabilization/Support

The last letter, *S,* refers to *stabilization* and *support* of the injured area. Movement causes an increase of blood flow to the muscle involved. Since the object is to limit or reduce blood flow to the injured area, it is wise to stabilize the injured area, as well as the joints adjacent to the injury. For example, if the muscle injury is to the calf, one would stabilize and restrict movement to the calf area, as well as to the ankle and knee joints. In this way the injured area is protected and its use limited.

In summary, after an injury to muscle tissue, there will be profuse bleeding due to ruptured blood vessels in the area. The athlete, coach, and trainer all have one immediate objective—to reduce bleeding, swelling, and further insult to the area. RICES (Rest, Ice, Compression, Elevation, Stabilization/Support) should be done immediately. If this procedure is followed, the extent of injury may be reduced and healing should be much quicker. In addition, the athletic coach or trainer should inform the injured athlete regarding possible implications of the injury and refer the athlete to competent medical authorities.

Predisposing Factors to Muscle Injuries

Many of the skeletal muscle injuries that occur to athletes are overuse type injuries. The largest single category of muscle injury is the overuse or overstress injury; the second category is the traumatic contact type injury. Naturally, the number of participants in a sport activity determines the rate of injuries that occur. For example, the highest death rate in any sporting activity is in racing antique airplanes. Although, obviously, there are not many individuals engaged in this activity due to the expense and time involved, it is a very risky activity. There are far more deaths per participant in that activity than in other high-risk activities, such as hang-gliding, mountain climbing, etc.

Many older athletes and weekend athletes, at some time during their lives, experience overuse or overstress injuries. Examples of these types of injuries are shin splints, tennis elbow, sore shoulder, tendinitis, Achilles tendon conditions from excessive or improper running, irritations to the foot, inflammation of the plantar fascia, and others. Gymnasts may develop irritations on the hands and problems in the upper arms due to the excessive arm work that they do. Many factors make an individual more prone to the overuse injury. Some of these factors are outlined below along with a brief description of each.

Overtraining

The athlete who spends too much time at a given activity at one session, or over several consecutive days, is very prone to an overuse or chronic type of injury. This occasionally happens, for instance, after a person has been relatively inactive and then goes out and plays two or three hours of tennis, developing a sore hand, sore elbow, or sore shoulder. They may also have lower extremity problems or even the beginning of shin splints. This is an example of overtraining or overstress occurring within just one session of activity. Occasionally, an individual plays a great deal on Saturday and then goes out again the following day and continues to play, feeling the discomfort of the overtraining later that evening or in the early part of the week. Many other individuals, even trained athletes, may suffer from these overtraining type of injuries. For example, the long distance runner who attempts to increase mileage from one week to the next may be a victim of the overtraining or overstress syndrome. The swimmer who drastically increases the number of meters swum per day, either in one workout or double workouts, may be prone to the overuse type of injury.

Poor Training

The category of poor training deserves a separate discussion in and of itself because it refers to the athlete who increases the intensity and types of workouts at an ever accelerating rate. As an example, the long distance runner may attempt to run at a faster pace in interval work, or to do more hill work, or to do more fast fartlek (speed) type training. The athlete attempts to do too many different types and intensities of training too soon. This results in *poor training.* When this occurs, the athlete is at risk for an overuse type injury.

Structural Abnormality

Many times a trait, either acquired through poor performance or congenital (present at birth), may predispose an athlete to a specific type of injury. Certain abnormalities in anatomical structure, such as high arches, poor posture or a weak spine, excessively flat feet, or a difference in leg lengths, may be a factor in the likelihood of developing an overuse type injury in an intense conditioning activity or program. In conjunction with the coach, athletic trainer, and perhaps the team physician, the athlete must analyze the particular structural deficit and construct an orthotic (a type of aid or assist), which may overcome the structural deficit. Modifications may be made in technique, and, in some cases, the athlete may have to choose an entirely different sport. If a structural abnormality is so severe as to prevent successful participation in one sport, such as in a weight-bearing sport like running, then the athlete may be forced to a non-weight-bearing sport like cycling or swimming.

Lack of Flexibility

An extreme lack of flexibility may serve as a predisposing factor to injury. For example, the athlete who has extremely tight calf muscles may develop problems in the lower legs, such as shin splints, tendinitis, or problems occurring at the ankle and in the foot. Nicholas (1970) has indicated that, in certain athletes, excessive tightness of the soft tissue (muscles, ligaments, and tendons), may be a predisposing factor for that athlete to pull a muscle. There has been a fair amount of data supporting this lack of flexibility as a cause for some athletic injuries.

Muscle Imbalance

A muscle imbalance may also lead to overuse types of injuries. Muscle imbalances could lead to a strain (pull) in the muscle, which may ultimately lead to an inflammation in the muscle. Certain muscle groups in the body have been tested to determine the optimum strength ratio of the muscles at one side of a joint contrasted with those muscles at the other side of a joint. For example, the quadriceps muscle group should be about one and a half times as strong as the hamstring group (Klein & Allman, 1969; Morris, 1974). Some of these ratios have been reported in the literature (Morris, 1974; Lussier, et al., 1983). Another way to express this quadricep-to-hamstring relationship is the hamstrings should be 50 to 60 percent of the strength of the quadriceps. If there is a gross muscular imbalance at one particular joint, that person may be more predisposed to an injury. This has been found to be true in tests of Big Ten track athletes and football players (Morris, unreported data, 1982). Another example of this muscle imbalance, which can occur in the athlete and which may lead to an overuse type of injury, is a muscle imbalance between the left and right side of the body. In most people who are symmetrical in body build, the muscular development on the right side of the body is of the same development as that on the left side. If an individual has excessive muscular development on one side of the body to the detriment of the muscles on the other side, then this individual could be predisposed to injury.

Poor Technique

The athlete who displays poor technique in a sport is prone to injury. An example of this is the tennis player who uses improper stroke mechanics and, consequently, develops tennis elbow. Another example is the swimmer who strokes with improper arm action or kicks with improper leg and knee action and develops knee or shoulder pain. A final example is a runner who has an incorrect foot plant—the point when the runner's foot actually strikes the ground. The runner may have excessive toeing-out (slue-footed) or excessive toeing-in (pigeon-toed). The runner who does not have straight heel-to-toe alignment in the foot plant and toe-off may be more susceptible to the overuse type of injury. There may be other poor techniques which predispose an athlete to unnecessary injury.

122

Body Build

The particular body builds of certain athletes may lead them to injury. We know that, in certain sports, a highly muscular, well-built athlete may be more successful. Sports such as football, lacrosse, and rowing may need a very tall and large muscular individual. In gymnastics, especially women's gymnastics, extra body weight in the form of extra body fat, seems to lead to a decrement in performance. Heath & Carter (1967) have published many works on the relationship between body type and success in athletics. Their findings suggest that athletes of certain body types seem to have more success at some particular sports.

Growth Factor

The growth factor may be another of the factors which contribute to certain types of athletic injuries. We know that maturing young athletes with rapidly growing bones may be susceptible to certain types of injuries. Some authors indicate that young athletes, six to twelve years of age, perhaps should not be competing in long distance running events over 20 kilometers. Others indicate that if the training program is graduated and intelligent in nature to provide for ever-increasing amounts of stress, participation by these youngsters is acceptable. Only time will tell which group is correct. Up until the time of puberty, young athletes have rapidly growing bone centers and bone ends. If injuries occur at these growth centers, the treatment and rehabilitation must be very carefully monitored. Young, growing bones must be set properly in order for the individual to continue to grow correctly. This particular area of athletic injuries is of concern to all involved in the care of young athletes.

Skeletal Muscle Injuries

The largest mass of tissue of concern to the athlete is skeletal muscle tissue. In the male athlete who has conditioned himself with strength and endurance activities, muscle mass comprises 45–50 percent of body weight. In the female athlete who engages in strength training, muscle mass may be 35–45 percent of mass weight. Since many of these muscles are very large in size—often extending up to twelve inches in length—they are often exposed to injury. We will consider *six different categories of injuries to skeletal muscle tissue.* These six categories are: (1) *muscle strains,* (2) *muscle contusions,* (3) *muscle soreness,* (4) *muscle cramps,* (5) *muscle compartment syndromes,* and (6) *muscle herniations.* The following discussion will include a short definition of the particular type of problem, the factors involved in the problem, and procedures for recognition, prevention, and treatment.

Muscle Strains

Perhaps the most common injury is the muscle **strain.** Another term often used by the athlete is *muscle pull.* Skeletal muscles are composed of semi-elastic elements which allow them to stretch and contract. However, if the muscle is stretched while attempting to contract or stretched beyond its normal range of motion due to some outside force, an interruption of the muscle cells will occur. There are various levels or degrees of severity of muscle strains, depending on the degree of the actual muscle tear. Ryan (1969) has offered a classification system using four types of muscle strains. A *grade one muscle tear* is a tear of a few muscle fibers with the fascia (protective covering of the individual muscle fibers) remaining basically intact. There is little loss of function, but some pain may be present. A *grade two muscle tear* occurs when a moderate number of muscle fibers or cells are involved in the tear, and *most* of the fascia remains intact. There will be some localized hematoma (inflammation and rupture of blood vessels), leading to swelling and discoloration in the area. There is loss of function and more pain with a grade two strain. A *grade three muscle tear* is an interruption of many of the muscle fibers and also a partial tearing of the fascia. Diffuse bleeding often accompanies the grade three tear. A grade three muscle strain exhibits much more discoloration and indicates greater internal damage. Pain is often very severe and there is a significant loss of muscle function. A *grade four muscle tear* is often a complete rupture of the muscle *and* the fascia. There is much discoloration and pain with this type of injury. Muscle strength and range of motion may be totally lost at the particular joint involved. Very often, a complete tear (grade four) requires surgical reattachment of the muscle. Figure 10.1 illustrates the types of muscle strains or muscle tears.

The goal in the treatment of the muscle strain is to reestablish the muscle fibers and the continuity of the muscle and muscle tendon junction. Initial treatment of RICES is indicated. This immediate treatment should continue for at least twenty-four to forty-eight hours, perhaps extending to seventy-two hours, depending on swelling.

The above grades of muscle strains indicate the seriousness of the involvement of the individual muscle fibers. With the more severe type strains there is often much pain, discoloration, loss of function, and deformity present in the muscle. We want to emphasize here that often muscle strength and muscle range of motion is greatly reduced and movement is very painful.

There are two schools of thought with regard to the treatment of muscular strains. They were reviewed by the late Dr. Thomas B. Quigley, a former team physician in orthopedics (Strauss, 1979). In his discussion, Quigley noted that one group of physicians feels that the muscle and actual tendon unit should be mildly stretched throughout the entire healing phase so that the muscle does not heal in the shortened position. The second group of physicians contends that the muscle tendon unit should first be allowed to heal for a few days before any activity should be considered. After a few days of complete rest, gradual stretching exercises should be instituted. It may not matter which particular routine is followed, as long as an attempt to increase strength and flexibility is sought. A combination of both programs could be the best course of action by allowing a certain period of time (one to three days) for the muscle to rest followed by light, gentle, stretching exercises to ensure that the muscle will not become contracted and heal in a shortened position. Some physicians have suggested that healing of the muscle tissue may be improved with a steroid injection into the muscle in the area at which it was torn (Birnbaum, 1982). Dr. Patton (1967) has used a very dilute xylocaine (.025 to .05 percent) solution and about five hundred units of hyaluronidase injected directly into the area. He has noted that, especially in quadriceps and hamstring pulls, some chronic problems have been

Figure 10.1 Different Grades of Muscle Strains. A grade one strain *(a)* shows a small tear or interruption of only a few muscle fibers. A grade two strain *(b)* involves damage to a greater number of muscle fibers. A severe strain *(c)* (grade three) involves injury to a majority of the fibers in a muscle, or even a total muscle tear (grade four).

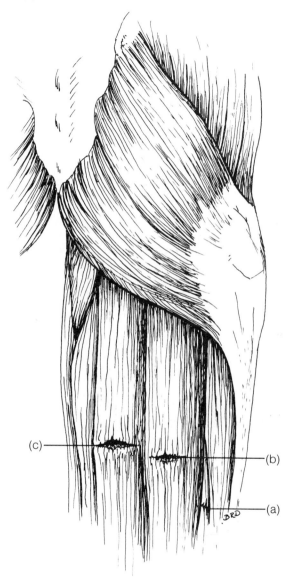

avoided by the injection of these materials into the muscle site. The object of the injection is to reduce the general swelling and hematoma that accompanies the injury. Recently, other physicians have advocated the use of **DMSO** applied to the injured area. At the present time, DMSO is not approved for use in humans for these muscle strain conditions, but some athletes secure DMSO and use it on their muscle pulls. A discussion of the pros and cons of this drug is given in the chapter on drugs and the athlete.

Muscle Contusions

The second major category of muscle injury is the blow to the muscle or contusion. In layman's terms the name for this type of muscle injury is the "charley horse." This term was derived from baseball players who experienced this particular type of athletic injury in the early twentieth century. At that time, the outfield grass of some of the major league ballparks was mowed by horses pulling lawn mowers. At Ebbit's Field in New York, the horse which did this chore was known as "Charley." Charley had a continual limp. When a baseball player was hit in the leg with a ball, or received a blow to the leg muscle sliding into the base, which subsequently caused him to limp, it was said that the baseball player was limping like Charley the horse. Consequently, the muscle blow and contusion to the athlete which caused pain and limping was referred to as a charley horse injury. This term is still quite popular in America today. This injury can occur in any contact sport or in other sports in which missiles and implements are used. It can be a very severely disabling type of injury which may lead to further complications, such as **myositis ossificans.** This occurs when the blow has been so severe as to press the muscle into the bone and an irritation of the muscle or the bone results. Excessive calcium may be released into the injured muscle area and a new bone growth may occur within the muscle mass. There will be extreme pain in the injured area and a lump may be palpated in the muscle. After a period of several days, X-rays might confirm the new growth of bone occurring within the muscle. If the blow to the muscle has been severe enough to cause this condition to develop, the athlete should cease all activity and undergo complete rest. Repeated X-rays could monitor the development of the new abnormally growing bone. If the bone continues to grow and interfere with muscle function, it may have to be surgically excised. Williams and Sperryn (1976) suggest short wave diathermy (heat) with gentle mobility exercises, but caution that the eventual outcome is never certain (Grana & Karnes, 1983). Figure 10.2 shows an occurrence of myositis ossificans.

Muscle Soreness

Many authors include a discussion of muscle soreness under muscle strains (Glick, 1980). For example, all categories of muscle strains include muscle soreness. There are many theories as to what actually happens with muscle soreness; probably the best known is that the muscle has a build-up of the end products of metabolites and these metabolites send out signals of pain and discomfort to the individual. Another theory says that continued hard use of a particular muscle causes minute tears and irritation to some muscle

Figure 10.2 Myositis Ossificans. This muscle/bone injury occurs most often after a severe blow to a muscle which also strikes the bone. A process of new bone growth *(a)* then appears within the muscle belly. It is a painful injury, needing constant medical attention. The example shown is myositis ossificans in the thigh muscles.

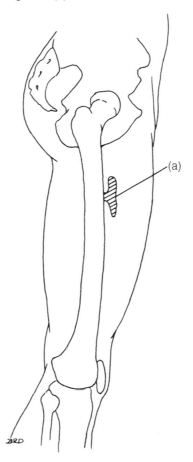

fibers. Much of the muscle soreness the athlete experiences may be due to exposing the muscles to too much work too soon. The pain resulting from muscle soreness may cause a continuous type of contraction or involuntary spasm within the muscle. If this occurs, a cycle may be set up that can only be broken by gradual stretching of the muscle (deVries, 1961). This tends to eliminate involuntary contraction of the individual muscle cells in which some of the blood vessels may go into spasm as a result of the excessive use of the muscle, deVries (1961) has shown that gentle stretching exercises seem to relieve this muscle soreness. In any case, gradual static stretching and range-of-movement activities seem to help.

Muscle Cramps

Another large category of muscle injuries is the muscle cramp in which the muscle goes into uncontrolled spasm or contraction, resulting in severe pain and a restriction or loss of movement. Muscle cramps can occur in any skeletal muscle which is overworked—it may even occur in the breathing muscles. When the cramp occurs in the leg or hand muscles, the athlete may attempt to relieve the spasm or cramp by gradual stretching or massaging of the muscle. Since a muscle cramp is really an uncontrolled spasm or contraction of the muscle, a gradual lengthening or kneading of the muscle may help to lengthen those muscle fibers and relieve the cramp. Other authors have implicated diet or lack of fluids as some of the possible reasons that an individual suffers from muscle cramps. This is discussed further in the chapter on diet and nutrition.

A particular type of muscle cramp that occurs to many individuals, is very disconcerting, and results in a curtailment of athletic activity, is the cramp in the side, which is commonly referred to as the "stitch in the side." What is believed to happen in this instance is that there is a loss of normal function in the breathing muscles—most commonly the diaphragm muscle. Some spasm or uncontrolled contracture of this muscle may be due to either the excitement of the individual in the beginning of the activity, or the failure of the breathing mechanism to adjust to a rhythm in continued long term activity. Causes for the stitch in the side remain largely unknown.

Several remedies have been proposed that may alleviate the stitch in the side. A common treatment is an attempt to stretch this particular muscle or muscle group. The person can stretch this area by bending backwards or bending to either side in an attempt to stretch the muscles of the trunk and the diaphragm muscles. Some coaches and trainers even suggest bending forward from the waist, as in attempting to touch one's toes.

Another alternative is for the individual to forcefully exhale a single breath or several hard breaths through partially closed or pursed lips. This forceful expiration may relieve the cramp in the breathing muscles.

A third recommendation is a technique known as belly breathing in which the person attempts to exhale, again rather forcefully, from deep in the abdominal area through pursed lips, trying to expand the lower abdomen as one inhales and to contract it as one exhales. This is contrary to what one would commonly expect in typical breathing. This deep belly breathing procedure must be practiced to be effective.

A final technique has been reported to help relieve the stitch in the side that is somewhat unique and may be painful. This procedure involves grasping the upper lip between the thumb and forefinger and applying pressure in this area. Obviously, the upper lip is a very sensitive area, and any pinching pressure to this area can cause a great deal of discomfort or pain. The rationale is that a noxious stimulus is applied to one area in an attempt to override another rather noxious stimulus—the stitch in the side or other skeletal muscle cramp.

Another reason put forth for the muscle cramp is poor dietary habits—eating too soon before practice or before a game or contest, or eating foods which are high in gas, or which will produce large amounts of gas. Another reason offered along with the dietary explanation as a cause of the cramp is that the person gets low on body fluids, or particular electrolytes. If, at least three to four hours prior to competition, an athlete eats a well-balanced diet of relatively bland foods, is well hydrated, and has the necessary vitamins and minerals in the diet, diet and nutrients can be eliminated as a cause or as a factor in the different types of muscle cramps. The cramp can still be very disabling and can cause the person to cease activity.

Muscle Compartment Syndrome Injuries

Another type of muscle injury that can occur is a muscle compartment syndrome injury. Perhaps the most well known athlete who has had this condition was Mary Decker, an Olympian and world record holder in the women's mile. For many years, Ms. Decker was plagued with leg cramps and lower leg pain that curtailed her training and competition. After a series of tests to rule out stress fractures, Achilles tendinitis, and other types of shin pain, it was believed that she had a muscle compartment type syndrome. In this type of athletic injury problem, the muscle swells (hypertrophies) with increasing workload (Veith, Matsen & Newell, 1980). More blood and fluid are sent into the area, and this, together with the increase in size of the individual cells during the workout, causes intense pain to the athlete. Tight muscle fascia (connective tissue covering skeletal muscle) may prevent expansion of normal muscle cells. In many cases, the athlete is forced to cut down on workouts. In the example of Ms. Decker, an orthopedic surgeon diagnosed that the fibrous tissue sheaths surrounding the muscles would not give as increased pressure was sent into the muscle, due to the workout. The surgeon then suggested a surgical procedure, involving making incisions in the muscle sheath in several areas. These surgical incisions would eventually repair themselves, accommodating the increased muscle size. Before such an operation is actually begun, the physician may be able to insert a needle deep in the belly of the muscle to get some idea as to the compartment pressure within the muscle. If intramuscular pressure is excessive, an operation may be indicated. Obviously, this surgical procedure is a drastic measure, and should only be used as a last resort. However, it has worked successfully in this particular athlete, and was also performed on the world record holder in the men's mile, John Walker.

Muscle Hernia

A final category of muscle injuries is called muscle herniation. This is not a common injury. Occasionally, the muscle sheath (fascia) will split and allow a portion of the muscle to bulge through the small opening. This condition is known as a muscle hernia. Williams and Sperryn (1976) indicate that there is no conservative treatment for this particular type of muscle injury. Very often a proper rehabilitation program is prescribed to gain strength and flexibility for the injured muscle. The athlete is permitted a gradual return to normal function. ■

Summary

In summary, there are various types of muscle injuries. These types may be categorized into six areas. They are: muscle strains, contusions, muscle soreness due to overwork or overuse, muscle cramps, muscle compartment syndromes, and finally, muscle herniations. In every case the immediate treatment of muscle injuries is the *RICES* technique. After a day or more of this technique, then gradual stretching and strengthening exercises are begun. These exercise routines follow those suggested in an earlier portion of the book on flexibility and strength training. Often the muscle is not injured in isolation; that is, since the muscle is part of the musculotendinous unit, then the tendon may also be injured.

Muscle injuries constitute the major portion of sports medicine injuries. Immediate first aid treatment for any muscle injury is important. The essential, immediate treatment requires the application of RICES (rest, ice, compression, elevation, stabilization). Some of the common factors which predispose the athlete to overuse injuries are over training, poor training, structural abnormalities, lack of flexibility, muscle imbalance, poor technique, body build, and finally, a growth factor. Muscle strains, often called muscle pulls, are a major category of skeletal muscle injuries. The severity of these strains is recorded in terms of one of four degrees. First degree strains would be slight strains, while third and fourth degree strains would be a significant or total rupture of the muscle, requiring surgical repair. Muscle soreness may be due to a buildup of metabolites in the area of the muscle, a spasm of the muscle, slight damage due to over stretching, or minute tears in the muscle as a result of heavy activity. Gradual, gentle training alleviates problems of muscle soreness. Muscle cramps or uncontrolled contractions within the muscle may be relieved through kneading and stretching the muscle, although attention to diet and proper rest and activity cycles are also indicated.

Muscle compartment syndrome injuries occur when muscle fibers (especially groups or bundles of muscle fibers) expand with increasing muscle activity and impinge on blood vessels in the muscle area, leading to pain upon increased physical activity. The athlete with this problem must refer to a sports medicine physician who will determine the pressure built up in the area to see if the fascia should be cut open to alleviate the pressure in this area. A muscle hernia is another type of muscle problem, where a fiber, or portions of several fibers, have protruded through the fascia which surrounds the muscle area.

References

Birnbaum, J. S. 1982. *The musculoskeletal manual.* New York: Academic Press.

deVries, H. A. 1961. Prevention of muscular distress after exercise. *The Research Quarterly.* 32:177.

Glick, J. M. 1980. Muscle strains: prevention and treatment. *The Physician and Sportsmedicine.* 8:73.

Grana, W. A., & E. S. Karnes. 1983. How I manage deep muscle bruises. *The Physician and Sportsmedicine.* 11:123.

Heath, B. H., & J. E. L. Carter. 1967. A modified somatotype method. *American Journal of Physical Anthropology.* 27:57.

Klein, K., & F. Allman. 1969. *The knee in sports.* Austin, TX: The Pemberton Press.

Kraus, K. 1981. *Sports injuries.* New York: Harper & Row.

Lussier, L., et al. 1983. Hamstring/quadriceps strength ratios in collegiate varsity middle distance runners. *The Physician and Sportsmedicine,* in press.

Morris, A. F. 1974. Myotatic reflex effects on bilateral reciprocal leg strength. *The American Corrective Therapy Journal.* 28:24.

Nicholas, J. A. 1970. Injuries to knee ligaments. *The Journal of the American Medical Association.* 212:2236.

Patton, R. 1967. Management of muscle injury. *Journal of the Athletic Trainer's Association.* 2:6.

Ryan, A. J. 1969. Quadriceps strain. *Medicine and Science in Sports.* 1:106.

Strauss, R. H., Ed. 1979. *Sports medicine and physiology.* Philadelphia: W. B. Saunders.

Veith, R. G., F. A. Matsen, & S. G. Newell. 1980. Recurring anterior compartmental syndromes. *The Physician and Sportsmedicine.* 8:80.

Williams, J. G. P., & P. N. Sperryn. 1976. *Sports medicine.* Baltimore: Williams & Wilkins.

Tendon Injuries

Outline

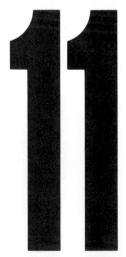

Introduction

Tendon injuries are examined in this chapter. The human tendon is composed of very strong, compact fibers of connective tissue which attach the muscle to the bone. Tendons have less blood supply than muscles, but slightly more blood supply than ligaments. Tendons are often injured along with the muscle they attach to.

Different types of injuries to tendons are listed in this chapter. Essentially, the tendon can become inflamed, resulting in the condition of tendinitis. There can also be a complete rupture or severing of the musculotendinous junction. There may also be degrees of ruptures or partial ruptures of the tendon.

Various treatments for tendon injuries are included. The conservative treatment is a reduction of physical activity, together with warming up of the tendon area before activity, and icing or cooling of the tendon immediately following the physical activity. Sometimes mild oral inflammatory agents are prescribed by the physician.

In all instances where there is suspected injury to the tendon, static stretching and increases in strength in the muscle tendon area is indicated. With this treatment, together with a gradual return to physical activity, the athlete should be able to train and compete without further tendon problems.

Another common soft tissue type of injury that occurs to the athlete is the tendon injury. Often, the muscle tendon may be injured along with the muscle. The skeletal muscle is a collection of single cells that are grouped together to perform a specific function, however, these muscle cells are organized together in a fairly firm fashion and they must work together. These cells are attached together, and they are also attached to a band of fibrous tissue at each end. These fibrous ends are the muscle tendons. Figure 11.1 shows the muscle tendinous junction.

The muscle is not attached to the tendon by a single point of attachment. The muscle fibers taper at their ends and insert into the connective tissue which then forms the tendon. The tendon is a tougher, more fibrous portion of the musculotendinous unit. There is less blood flow and less blood supply to the tendon, as compared with the muscle. The tendon has an appearance of white gristly material when exposed to the human eye. There are several types of injuries which may occur to the tendons.

Types of Tendon Injuries

Most authors note three types of tendon injuries. First, there is the complete tendon rupture. This, of course, is the most severe and indicates that there is a complete interruption of the musculotendinous unit. The second type of tendon injury is a partial tear of the tendon. A third category of tendon injury, the inflammation of the tendon or of the structures surrounding the tendon, is generally classified as tendinitis.

The Complete Tendon Rupture

A complete rupture of a tendon is a very serious athletic injury. A tendon frequently ruptured is the Achilles tendon. This is perhaps the strongest tendon in the body, however, if this particular tendon is subjected to frequent starting and stopping movements, and sudden changes of directions, it may rupture. Sometimes this occurs in middle-aged athletes, who are involved in running, jumping, or quick movement games, like handball or racketball. Williams (1976) notes that there is some disagreement as to whether a rupture can occur in a normal tendon, or whether the rupture occurs at a site of degenerative lesions which make the tendon weak at that particular point. Tendon ruptures also occur in certain arthritic conditions, especially with rheumatoid arthritis.

The complete rupture of the tendon generally provides a straightforward diagnosis, in that range-of-motion and strength are absent because of the obvious loss of anatomical structure.

Figure 11.1 The Muscle Tendon Junction. A site of frequent injury, this is the point where the muscle fibers join the connective tissue portion of the tendon. Each has a slightly different form due to the particular location and function of the specific muscle. Shown are two examples: *(a)* Achilles muscle tendon junction and *(b)* peroneus muscle tendon junction.

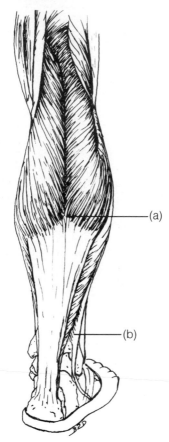

Treatment of Tendon Ruptures

The treatment of a ruptured tendon generally depends on the severity of the lesion and the age of the athlete. Generally, a tendon rupture is treated by surgical repair, although it must be noted that some authorities would urge conservative measures of casting and lack of activity (Williams & Sperryn, 1976).

Partial Rupture of the Tendon

Occasionally, there occur small ruptures of a few fibers of the tendon. This problem may be slight, but still cause swelling in the tendon, and some slight thickening and tenderness over the tendon area. Williams (1976) notes that, with a partial tendon rupture, the symptoms can come on insidiously and that the thickening and swelling in the tendon area is the key point differentiating it from conditions affecting the structures which surround the tendon. In any case, rest is indicated with a partial rupture, and moderate stretching and strengthening activities are indicated.

Tendinitis

Tendinitis is often described as an inflammation of the tendon, or of the sheath (the connective tissue surrounding the tendon). These tendon irritations can occur in almost any tendons of the body which are stressed repeatedly in the athletic activity. Areas often affected are the Achilles tendon, certain tendons about the elbow, and in the shoulder joint. Symptoms of swelling, pain on movement, and some crepitus (a cracking sound produced on movement) occur with tendinitis. Tendinitis is generally easy to observe when evaluating the athlete and often presents as pain on movement. Tendinitis is generally considered an overuse/overstress type of injury, meaning that the athlete has increased the training program in a manner which is not commensurate with the development of the underlying muscle and tendon. It is suggested that one possible way to prevent tendinitis is to insure that there is adequate strength and flexibility in the musculotendinous unit.

Treatment for Tendon Inflammation

There are many controversial remedies (Smart, Taunton & Clement, 1980). Some physicians believe that an injection of a steroid into the area can promote healing. Other physicians report that the repeated injection of steroids into an inflamed tendon may actually cause the tendon to rupture (Ryan, 1978). Still other doctors dispute injecting a substance near the injured tendon for the treatment of tendinitis. The type of steroid or anti-inflammatory agent and the number of dosages that are to be administered is still not certain. Some physicians would suggest oral administration of a non-steroid anti-inflammatory agent. Other physicians believe that a small injection of steroid may be made into the area near the tendon. Still others suggest that an injection of the steroid be made directly into the tendon area. It has been reported that one physician injected one case of tennis elbow eighty times within a three year period (Ryan, 1978). Certainly, this would seem to be an excessive amount of injections at one site for any problem. In fact, it has been suggested that physicians should never repeatedly inject an area. In most cases, after one or two injections, the tendon is weakened. This weakening of the tendon may lead to full rupture of the tendon, if the athlete continues to stress this area.

Aspirin, Ice, Heat

Conservative treatment might include some oral anti-inflammatory agent (aspirin) with rest of the injured tendon. It should be noted that aspirin can irritate the stomach lining and should be taken in buffered form with fluids or food to reduce this possibility. A physician should be consulted before this treatment is followed.

Cold applications, like ice massage, seem to help the injured tendon area in the post-exercise period. After several days, warm applications may be made to the area before exercise and cold treatments after exercise.

There are many conflicting opinions regarding tendon injuries. It may be said that after conservative treatment of seven to ten days of relative inactivity, the athlete can begin to progressively build up strength and flexibility in the injured tendon. This applies to grade one or grade two tendon inflammations. A gradual return to physical activity is always a good routine to follow. Some athletic trainers suggest a small heel lift of twelve to fifteen millimeters in casual and athletic shoes in the treatment of tendinitis in the lower extremities (Smart, Taunton & Clement, 1980). Mild heat before physical activity and icing after activity always seems to help tendon problems. ■

Summary

The tendon is a tough band of connective tissue attaching muscles to bone. The metabolic activity of tendons is quite low. Blood flow to the tendon is much lower than the blood flow occurring in the muscle. Because of this factor, any injuries or inflammation to the tendon results in a longer period of rehabilitation. Tendons may be inflamed, causing a condition called tendinitis. Procedure for treating this condition is a lessening of physical activity, together with a gradual program of strengthening and stretching the musculotendinous area. Sometimes there is a major rupture (a complete tear) of the tendon. In these cases, the athlete would have to be seen by an orthopedist and, probably, be surgically repaired. There may also be degrees of partial rupture of the tendon, which are sometimes treated with rest and oral inflammatory agents. The athlete who has only a mild inflammation in the tendon area may prefer to warm up the area prior to participation in training, and then apply ice in an attempt to cool down the area and resultant inflammation after a period of mild physical activity. Conservative treatment in tendinous injuries involves rest, a mild anti-inflammatory, ice, and heat, with a judicious strengthening and stretching program.

References

Ryan, A. J. 1978. Injection for tendon injuries: cure or cause? *The Physician and Sportsmedicine.* 6:39.

Smart, G. W., J. E. Taunton, & D. B. Clement. 1980. Achilles tendon disorders in runners. *Medicine and Science in Sports and Exercise.* 12:231.

Williams, J. 1976. Soft tissue injuries. *Physiotherapy.* 56:780.

Williams, J. G. P., & P. N. Sperryn. 1976. *Sports medicine.* Baltimore: Williams & Wilkins.

Bone or Hard Tissue Injuries

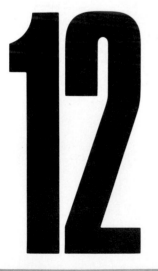

Introduction

Bones are vascular, living, connective tissue, with a high mineral content. Bones are noted for their hardness and power to regenerate after a fracture. A fracture is a break in the bone, which occurs when the bone is exposed to severe stress. Recognition and treatment of bone injuries is of paramount importance. The physician most often involved in these types of injuries is the orthopedic medical doctor.

The most severe type of fracture is the compound fracture, in which there is a break in the bone, as well as a break in the skin, resulting in bleeding, which may also be quite severe. Immediate first aid is to control the bleeding and keep the broken adjacent ends of the bone quiet and splinted. Other types of fractures in addition to the compound fracture are listed in this chapter.

Bone stress fractures are covered in detail because many athletes engaging in individual type sports, such as running, gymnastics, may be exposed to stress fractures. Tests and evaluations for bone fractures such as radiographic examination (X-ray) and newer methods of bone scanning techniques are covered.

Regular Fractures

Another type of injury in athletics is injury to bone. Particularly in contact sports or in sports where there is the use of implements (sticks and missiles), fractures sometimes occur. There can be a complete fracture where the bone is actually broken in half. This type of injury may be compounded when the bone actually breaks through the skin, often causing bleeding. Obviously, in the compound type of fracture with a break in the skin, as well as a break in the bone, there is the possibility of infection. In any case, after a fracture, it is important to seek medical attention as quickly as possible. Bleeding must be controlled at once. Keep the injured athlete quiet. Keep the broken bone and the adjacent bone ends splinted and safe. The physician most often involved is the orthopedist, who resets the bone and casts the area to see that the bone begins to heal itself.

Common Dislocations and Fractures

Some common types of fractures found in contact sports or collision sports are illustrated in figure 12.1. Before a list of these common types of dislocations and fractures are given, some obvious factors are presented so that the athlete, coach, and athletic trainer can recognize and evaluate the different dislocations. A dislocation is the misplacement of two bone ends, generally as a result of some applied stress to the body. Most dislocations in athletes occur to the fingers, and the shoulder joint.

Recognizing Dislocations

There are several ways to recognize a dislocation (Klafs & Arnheim, 1981). Pain is most often present at the area of the dislocation and there may be swelling and point tenderness in the immediate area of the dislocation. Some apparent deformity should be present at the point of dislocation with some loss of limb function as the person attempts to move the bone or joint involved in the dislocation.

Dislocations are severe medical problems and require the aid of a physician. The injured athlete should be splinted and transported to the physician's office with great urgency.

Recognizing Fractures

Some indications of a fracture include:

1. Swelling at the point of the fracture
2. Direct tenderness—point tenderness at the location, even with the slightest touching

Figure 12.1 Various types of Fractures. A *greenstick fracture (a)* is incomplete, and the break occurs on the convex surface of the bend in the bone. A *comminuted fracture (b)* is complete and results in several bony fragments. A *transverse fracture (c)* is complete and the break occurs at a right angle to the axis of the bone. An *oblique fracture (d)* occurs at an angle other than a right angle to the axis of the bone.

From Hole, John W., Jr., Human Anatomy and Physiology, 2d ed. © 1978, 1981 Wm. C. Brown Publishers, Dubuque, Iowa. All Rights Reserved. Reprinted by Permission.

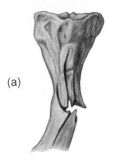 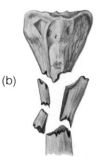 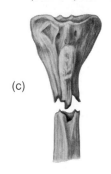 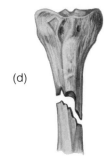

(a)   (b)   (c)   (d)

3. A bony deviation and deformity
4. Crepitus or noise at that particular part, as the athlete tries to move it
5. Discoloration in the area
6. In a compound fracture, the bone may actually protrude through the skin. When this is the case, bleeding must be controlled, with attention to possible infection.

Different Types of Fractures

There is an excellent listing of the different types of fractures by Klafs and Arnheim (1981). Some of the more common types of fractures seen in athletics are covered here.

Perhaps the most common type of fracture seen in athletics is the *longitudinal fracture,* a clean break in one of the long bones of the body. Contact, such as occurs in football, hockey, or lacrosse, generally leads to this kind of injury. A second category is a depressed fracture, which occurs most often in flat bones, such as those of the skull. This may result when the athlete's head hits an immovable object. Any head injury is a most serious injury and must be seen by a physician as soon as possible. A third type of fracture is a comminuted fracture. This consists of a blow to the bone in which it breaks in several pieces (fig. 12.1). Another is the greenstick type of fracture, which occurs in bones that have not yet completely hardened. They occur most frequently to young athletes. A final type of fracture that one sees in athletics is the spontaneous fracture (or stress fracture). Because this last type of fracture is becoming more common in many athletic injuries, especially in running injuries, a detailed section covering the stress fracture is presented next.

Bone Stress Fractures

Any bone which is subjected to repeated stress may begin to wear down and develop slight cracks. In the bones of the lower extremities this may be due to repeated running. It may occur in people who are involved in ski jumping, who are subjected to repeated landings. Stress fractures may occur in hand and arm bones in gymnasts with continual hard exercise on apparatus. It may occur to hikers who suddenly are exposed to long trips with heavy packs, with the pressure of the pack and the strap against the bones of the shoulders. All of these types of stresses can result in a gradual breakdown of the bone, leading to a stress fracture. Other physicians use the terminology of a stress reaction. What they mean is that a stress reaction is set up in the bone when the process of bone repair and growth does not keep pace with the breakdown of the newly forming bone cells.

It has been said that bone layers are often formed in much the same way that an oyster coats the grain of sand to produce the pearl. This continual laying down of new bone is the body's way of changing the shape and size of the bone when new stresses are imposed on it. Just as the skin sloughs off dead cells, the bone continues to replace itself, and changes its size when stress is applied to it. When suddenly exposed to a severe stress, the bone may actually begin to break down, and a stress fracture occurs. Another group of individuals who are prone to stress fractures are military recruits. Because these individuals suddenly have to undergo rigorous physical training without proper prior conditioning, they are more apt to develop stress fractures in the bones of the foot and lower leg.

Evaluating Stress Fractures

How does the athlete recognize a stress fracture? The typical symptom of the stress fracture is pain along the entire length of the bone with a particularly sore spot at the point of the actual bone breakdown. Generally, if one applies fingertip pressure to the spot and there is severe pain, then this is probably the location of the stress fracture. That point on the bone is very tender to the touch, especially if it can be touched or palpated from both sides (Burrows, 1956; Hlavac, 1980).

Radiographic Examination

The only way to accurately determine if there is a stress fracture is radiographic examination. Even with this technique, the simple X-ray examination may not be enough. Serial X-rays are taken once every few days over a period of a week or two. The stress reaction still may not show up under this examination. Then the physician must resort to what is called a radiographic bone scan.

Bone Scan

The **bone scan** is a special type of X-ray test in which a low-dose radioactive substance is injected into the patient. The radioactive particles circulate throughout the body and tend to collect and congregate in an area where the bone is attempting to heal itself. This area is where the particular stress reaction to the bone is occurring. A highly sensitive camera is used to pick up any "hot spots" which correspond to the point of the patient's complaint of the bone pain. The congregation of radioactive particles in the certain area confirms the diagnosis of a stress reaction.

Treatment for Stress Fracture

The treatment for stress fracture is rest. Occasionally, the physician may wish to cast the foot or the leg in an attempt to ensure that the athlete does not place any more stress on the bone. If the athlete were to continue to stress the area of bone reaction, a complete fracture could occur. This has happened to many athletes. In a past world veterans championship a runner was leading in the 50–55 age group in the 400 meter sprint, and snapped the lower leg bone (tibia) as a result of continuing to run on a bone which had a stress reaction in it. After four to eight weeks of very limited activity, the athlete can then begin gentle exercises and some weight bearing (Brody, 1980).

Common Sites for Stress Fractures

There are several common sites where stress fractures appear most frequently. In the running athlete, these are, naturally, in the bones of the lower extremities. The bones of the foot—the metatarsals and the tarsals—are often exposed to stress fractures. The bones of the lower leg—the tibia and the fibula—are also frequent sites of stress fractures. Occasionally, the femur can have some stress reactions to severe weight bearing activities. The most prominent areas of stress fracture on the femur are at the neck and head of the femur. Occasionally, stress fractures have been reported in the pelvis. Any particular location on the skeleton, which is subject to repeated stress, can lead to a stress reaction at that point. In fact, chronic smokers may even have stress type reactions to their ribs caused by continuous vigorous coughing. ■

Summary

We have seen that there are two predominant types of bone injuries. One is the complete fracture of the bone, which is a genuine medical emergency. It is crucial that this person see a physician immediately, especially if a major bone is involved, or there is profuse bleeding. The injured athlete sees a physician to have the bone reset and cast, then goes through a period of rest while the bone attempts to heal. Even though the bone is in the cast, the athlete may continue with some isometric type movements with the hope that only a slight degree of muscle atrophy will set in. Occasionally, some athletes have attempted to exercise the uninjured limb in the hope that some cross-training will take place. The second category of bone fracture is the stress fracture or stress reaction. This is due to repeated bouts of stressful activity at a particular site on the bone. If the buildup of the bone does not keep pace with the tiny irritations that occur as a result of the stress, the bone begins to break down at a faster rate than it is being built up. If continued weight bearing or stress is applied at the site of the bone stress reaction, this may develop into a full fracture with a complete break in the bone. Obviously, moderation, or a very, very gradual buildup of the intensity and duration of the exercise sessions will help to avoid this injury. Bone stress reactions may also occur to the bones of the back—the spine.

References

Brody, D. M. 1980. Running injuries. *Clinical Symposia.* 32:2.

Burrows, H. J. 1956. Fatigue fractures of the tibia. *Journal of Bone and Joint Surgery.* 38b:83.

Hlavac, H. F. 1980. *The foot book.* Mountain View, CA: World Publications.

Klafs, C. E., & D. D. Arnheim. 1981. *Modern principles of athletic training.* 5th ed. St. Louis: C. V. Mosby.

Common Athletic Injuries and Their Treatments

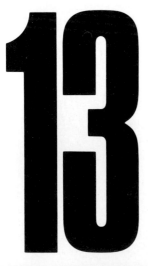

Introduction

    This chapter outlines approximately fifty very specific, but common, athletic injuries along with a brief description of the causes, treatment and prevention scheme for each. These prominent injuries are listed in addition to the more common types of tissue (muscle, tendon and bone) injuries that were noted in the last two chapters.

    This listing starts with athletic injuries to the upper extremities, proceeds to the lower extremities, the back and trunk, and lastly, the head area. These injuries are not presented in order of severity, or importance, but merely by the anatomical location of the particular athletic injury. In the first section, common sports medicine injuries to the shoulder and upper arms are discussed.

Injuries to the Upper Extremities

The Shoulder

Shoulder Separation/Dislocation

Definition and Causes Three bones come together at the shoulder: the scapula (shoulder blade), clavicle (collarbone), and humerus (upper arm bone). These bones and a schematic of the shoulder joint are shown in figure 13.1. The shoulder is the most freely movable joint in the body. There are many muscles and tendons passing over the shoulder joint. A dislocation occurs at the shoulder when the different bones of the shoulder come apart as a result of a blow or a particular movement. This is a severe medical problem and must be seen by a medical doctor immediately. The physician will probably X-ray the area to confirm the diagnosis and then reduce the dislocation (set the bones back in place). The most common shoulder dislocation occurs as a result of a fall on the outstretched hand and arm, causing a jarring up the arm and through the shoulder joint, taking it out of its

Figure 13.1 Shoulder Joint. This complicated joint is often injured in contact sports. Shown are the clavicle *(a)*, scapula *(b)*, humerus *(c)*, and major ligaments *(d)* of the region.

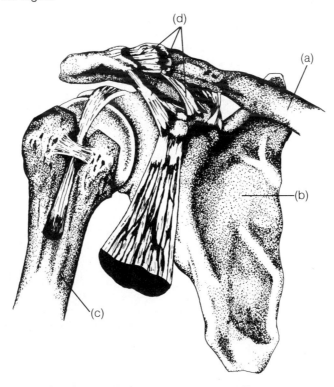

proper place. Another cause of a shoulder separation, or dislocated shoulder, is the trauma of one athlete hitting another, such as occurs in football. The shoulder separation is likely to occur at the acromioclavicular joint (O'Donoghue, 1976).

Treatment Treatment is to immobilize the injured part and adjacent joints by keeping the upper arm close to the body and limiting further movement. Ice and some compression may be used, if it relieves the pain and discomfort of the injured athlete. The injured person must be transported to a physician immediately for further treatment. The physician will generally reset the dislocation and, depending upon the severity, strap the injured arm so that no further harm comes to it. After a period of rest and rehabilitation, the athlete can return to the sport.

Prevention The shoulder separation or dislocation is extremely difficult to prevent when it results from contact. Limiting the contact period in some sports may prevent some shoulder separations and dislocations. Excellent coaching and teaching proper techniques of falling and landing may also help. Finally, both strengthening and stretching exercises for the shoulder area should be helpful in improving the overall integrity of the musculature and tendons of the shoulder.

Fracture of the Collarbone (Clavicle)

Definition and Causes A broken collarbone is defined as a rupture or a break in the clavicle. This is often due to a direct blow or trauma to the area. However, in some instances, a stress fracture may develop in this bone from the pressure of straps of a heavy pack coming over the shoulder or something of that sort. Any continual, severe irritation to this area might result in a stress fracture.

Treatment Immediate first aid should be administered and the person must be taken to a physician. The physician will X-ray the area, stabilize it as much as possible, and prescribe a period of rest, possibly with some medication. Finally, a period of rehabilitation exercises would be recommended for irritated tendons and muscles in the area.

Prevention Avoiding contact, where possible, is the best prevention in certain sports. Another possible preventive aspect is to wear protective padding, such as hockey pads, shoulder pads, etc. Finally, strength and flexibility exercises for the collarbone area insures a very strong, intact shoulder.

Painful Shoulder or Tendinitis at the Shoulder

Definition and Causes A painful shoulder is any irritation of the tendons or muscles surrounding the shoulder area. The cause of the painful shoulder is generally continuous overuse with resultant irritation to the structures of the shoulder. Sports which involve repeated arm movements, like many of the throwing sports (baseball, javelin) or any other sports in which the shoulder is used extensively (swimming) often report painful shoulder. Gymnasts also suffer this athletic injury problem with repeated overuse training.

Treatment The painful shoulder is treated by trying to isolate the specific structure that is involved. Very often, an expert trainer, or physician, can implicate the particular muscle or a tendon which is involved. The physician then prescribes certain exercises and movements to strengthen that particular area. A period of rest is always indicated because, generally, this is an overuse type of injury. Occasionally, some physicians will use a topical injection of hydrocortisone (an anti-inflammatory agent) with some local anesthetic injected into the area. A period of immobilization generally follows such an injection (Williams & Sperryn, 1976).

Prevention The best prevention of this problem is a gradual, intelligent training program. Also, practice of the proper throwing technique or proper stroke mechanics in swimming could avoid this problem. Strengthening and flexibility exercises are indicated.

Fractures of the Shoulder

Definition and Causes Fractures of the shoulder can occur to any one of the three bones (scapula, clavicle, humerus) previously mentioned. A fracture is simply a break in the bone. Generally, this is due to a direct blow to the area.

Treatment Treatment for any fracture occurring at the shoulder is the immediate first aid (RICES) that was listed in the chapter on muscles. Examination by a physician, with X-rays, approximation of the broken ends, and a period of rest and rehabilitation is the sequence of treatment.

Prevention Prevention involves proper padding of the area, avoiding some contact in collision sports, if possible, and strengthening the muscles and other structures at the shoulder joint.

The Upper Arm

Myositis Ossificans

Definition and Causes Whenever a muscle receives a severe, direct blow that compresses the muscle into the bone, there is a great deal of trauma in that area. An irritation to the lining of the bone develops, leading to myositis ossificans. The name myositis ossificans comes from two Latin words—myositis, meaning muscle inflammation, and ossificans, implying a new formation of bone. The definition of this condition is a new growth of bone *within* the muscle (fig. 13.2).

This condition can occur in almost any location, but generally occurs in the long muscles which lay over the long bones. The most common area of occurrence is in the quadriceps muscles, followed by the muscles of the upper arms. This is not a very common condition, but is one that must be watched for whenever the bone and muscle are traumatized as a result of a vicious blow to the area.

Figure 13.2 Myositis Ossificans. This injury is a frequent complication after a new, unnatural bone grows out of the existing bone mass, causing pain and restricted motion. Physical activity should be stopped and a physician must be consulted.

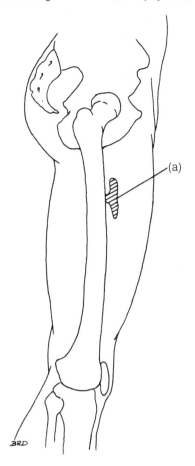

Treatment The treatment for this condition is rest. Further activity would only serve to increase the inflammation of the area, and cause more problems. Resist the temptation to manipulate this area, or to apply heat, which may increase the inflammation. The physician should monitor this problem very carefully, perhaps by taking repeated X-rays to watch the extent of the new bone formation. If the new bone formation continues to grow, surgery to remove the extra piece of bone growth may be necessary.

Prevention Prevention of this condition might be done by padding the area, using proper techniques in blocking and striking an opponent in certain contact sports, and finally, increasing strength and muscle mass.

Tennis Elbow

Definition and Causes **Tennis elbow** is merely an irritation of the extensor tendon of the muscles of the forearm. This is the most common type of tennis elbow problem. It is characterized by pain over the lateral side of the elbow joint. This is an overuse condition brought on by repeated use of the extensor and supinator muscles of the forearm.

Another type of tennis elbow is irritation to the flexor muscle mass. This involves those muscles on the inside upper aspect of the forearm, at just about the location of the elbow joint. Again, this is an overuse condition, generally caused by too much activity too soon in a racket or throwing sport. Elbow injury may also occur in golf and in fishing.

Treatment The immediate treatment for this condition is rest and some ice therapy. The immediate application of cold and compression should help this injury. Some individuals take a local anesthetic, and also a mild anti-inflammatory, such as aspirin. If the condition persists, an injection of hydrocortisone may be helpful. Most physicians avoid repeated injections at the site, since an injection of hydrocortisone almost always causes some weakening in the tendon. The person must reduce activity for at least a short period of time.

Prevention Prevention of this problem involves a gradual buildup and proper training program for the desired sport or activity. Strength training exercises and flexibility exercises to stretch the muscles of this region of the elbow should help. Finally, some participants use strapping in an attempt to hold the tendons of those muscles closer to the bone and provide some support. This may also be used as a treatment modality, but is best if it is used in a preventive nature. Lastly, one cannot overlook the proper mechanics of the sport. Various sports medicine authorities suggest that proper stroke mechanics and proper grip of the racket at the instant the ball is contacted would prevent much of the tennis elbow that occurs in the general population.

Elbow Dislocation

Definition and Causes Elbow dislocation is a somewhat rare occurrence in sports, but it may happen when the athlete falls or takes some vicious contact in a collision type sport.

Treatment As with any dislocation or major joint problem, an orthopedic physician should be sought out and the dislocation reduced.

Prevention Prevention of this injury is proper instruction in the correct techniques of the sport and proper landing after contact.

Thrower's Elbow

Definition and Causes A thrower's elbow is an irritation and strain on the tendons and ligaments of the elbow caused by a round arm (side arm) type of throw. This also occurs in younger athletes and is known as Little League player's elbow. This is an overuse type of syndrome—too much activity too soon, without a gradual buildup of conditioning. Another cause of this problem is poor technique.

Treatment Treatment consists of rest from the activity and normal therapy avenues.

Prevention The prevention of thrower's elbow is the use of correct throwing technique and expert coaching in the proper way of making a throw. It is also advisable, in youth sports, to limit the amount of participation of each athlete. For example, various youth sports oganizations limit the number of innings or the number of throws that the youngster is allowed. This is wise, since the youngster is just developing at this time, and it enforces a limitation on their participation in the activity. For older athletes concerned with thrower's elbow, a strengthening program should be suggested, together with a gradual buildup of physical activity.

The Wrist

Wrist Injuries

Definition and Causes Many wrist injuries occur in sports where the athlete falls on hard surfaces. Examples of these sports are football, rugby, and ice skating. The wrist is a joint composed of the two bones of the lower arm—the radius and ulna—and the eight carpal bones. Many muscle tendons pass over this area. A fall on the outstretched hand can lead to a fracture of either one of the two bones of the lower arm, or any one of the individual carpal bones in the wrist. Most often, one of the smaller carpal bones at the wrist is fractured or broken in a fall.

Treatment The treatment for this type of injury is to visit the physician for X-rays and splinting. Splinting is a stabilization technique. Followup treatment, such as therapeutic exercise (active strengthening and range-of-motion) is indicated.

Prevention The prevention of the wrist fracture is to pad the area well, if possible, and to teach the proper falling technique.

Wrist Sprain

Definition and Causes A wrist sprain is an over-stretching of the tendons at the wrist. It may also be the overuse and resultant inflammation of these tendons. A wrist sprain may occur in racket sports, such as tennis, squash, badminton. It might also occur in rowing, which requires repetitive movements of the wrist. Because there is not much blood directly supplied to this area, the circulation is reduced.

Treatment Treatment is moderate rest, followed by physical therapy modalities.

Prevention The prevention of the wrist sprain can be accomplished by a gradual buildup in the training program for the sport, as well as increasing strength and flexibility to the hand, wrist, and forearm area.

The Hand and Fingers

The Hand and Fingers

Obviously, the most skilled appendage in the human is the hand and fingers. The movements in these joints are very exquisite, and because they are involved in many sport activities, they may be often injured. Fractures, often the result of direct blows, are the most serious injuries that occur to the hand and fingers. Also, in such sports as boxing and karate where the hand is used as a weapon, there is always the danger of a fracture. The fracture is a very serious injury, and must be seen by a physician immediately. After the proper X-rays are taken, the fracture is reduced and set. After a period of time, the bone should heal.

Blisters

Definition and Causes Since the hand and fingers are used extensively in baseball, racket sports, biking, and wheelchair racing, blisters are likely to occur. Blisters are nothing more than points on the skin where friction is allowed to occur, causing a buildup of fluid beneath one or more layers of skin. An important point to remember when considering blisters is that a "hot spot" will always occur *prior* to formation of the blister. In most instances, if the athlete is sensitive to the heat being built up on or under the skin, and stops activity at that point, the blister can be avoided. This is the case whether the blister occurs on the hand or on any other area of the body. If the athlete is monitoring body activity, is aware of the "hot spot" forming, and ceases activity, then the blister may be prevented. However, in certain activities where the athlete is unable to call a time-out, or to stop the activity, obviously, prevention of the blister when the "hot spot" begins is most difficult.

Treatment The treatment for the blister is to use a sterile, sharp instrument to puncture a small hole in the blister. Try to make the hole in the blister in a place where the fluid will drain out. If all of the fluid does not drain from the blister, compression of the outer layers of the skin will force the fluid from the tiny opening made in the skin. It is important not to cut off the entire skin over the blister. This dead, worn skin will protect the tender, underlying skin, which will harden in time. The dead outer layer of skin from the blister will eventually fall off.

Obviously, because there is a break in the skin, the danger of infection is present. The area must be washed well, and kept clean. Some type of padding or adhesive strip over the blister will protect that area during subsequent activity. If it is a very large blister, a piece of padded material in the shape of a doughnut is cut out and placed around the blister, and then padding over the area is applied. Figure 13.3 shows the proper treatment of a blister. New developments, such as "Spenco® 2nd Skin," a new synthetic skin dressing, are designed to relieve pain, prevent infection, and aid healing of skin burns, abrasions, and blisters.

Prevention Obviously, the best prevention method concerning blisters is to avoid their formation. As was indicated earlier, if the athlete can monitor the body for the development of a "hot spot," and then pad the area, many blisters can be prevented. Taping over the fingers and the hand area in certain spots which receive a lot of friction may often prevent

Figure 13.3 Treatment of Blisters. Blisters develop at points where there is excessive friction to the skin. Most often this occurs on the hands and feet of athletes. The site should be covered and protected *(a)* to reduce the possibility of further complications.

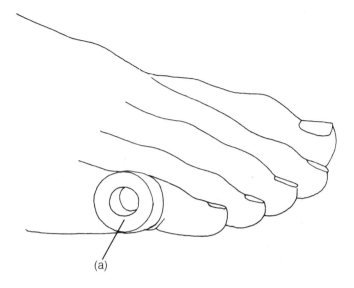

(a)

the blister. In earlier times, many boxers and other athletes who used their hands excessively in their sports, would soak their hands in a salt solution to toughen the outer layers of skin. This can be accomplished just as easily with a gradual buildup of the use of the hands and fingers in the activity, so that the skin will toughen and, consequently, blisters will not form. Wearing gloves or other protective coverings over high friction areas should prevent blisters. Some athletes also use layers of Vaseline® to reduce friction and prevent blisters.

Sore Hands

Definition and Causes Sore hands develop whenever there is repeated pounding and stress placed on the hands and fingers. The sports of handball and wheelchair racing are two common activities where the athlete may develop extremely sore hands. Other sports, such as baseball, where the hand receives repeated blows from catching the baseball, may also cause the hand to become very sore and bruised.

Treatment Treatment for this condition is an obvious, gradual buildup in the activity. Immediately after all the pounding from the session of handball or wheelchair racing, the hand should be soaked in ice water to prevent swelling. Also, it might be possible for the athlete to elevate the hand somewhat to reduce the swelling and minimize trauma in that area.

Prevention Prevention for this condition is to try to pad the hand and fingers as well as possible. Very often, wrapping several layers of tape over the area, wearing gloves with padding in the palm for handball, or padding the hands in some other manner can alleviate some of the problems of sore hands.

Finger Dislocations

Definition and Causes Finger dislocations are common in sports where the hands and fingers are used extensively and exposed to contact. Many times, when the hands and fingers receive direct blows, it is easy for a finger to dislocate. Often the athlete will look down at the misshapen finger and attempt to pull the joint back in place. This is inadvisable. The dislocation should be reduced by the physician after X-rays are taken to see that there is no other injury involved. Broken bone chips can also be seen in the X-rays.

Treatment The treatment is the reduction of the finger dislocation by a physician, and perhaps, some taping and strapping to prevent another occurrence of the injury. Often the finger that was recently dislocated may be splinted to an adjacent, good finger to immobilize it and protect it in future activity.

Prevention The best prevention for the finger dislocation is to use care and good technique in the sports. Protective taping and wrapping can also be used. Other than that, any techniques for prevention of finger dislocations are most difficult.

Mallet Finger

Definition and Causes This injury is a blow to the outstretched finger that causes the tendon to stretch severely, or even rupture, allowing the finger to be bent back in a misshapen form.

Figure 13.4 Mallet finger. This injury often occurs when the outstretched finger is hit on the end by an object (as in catching a baseball). A long tendon or ligament in the region can be snapped or partially ruptured.

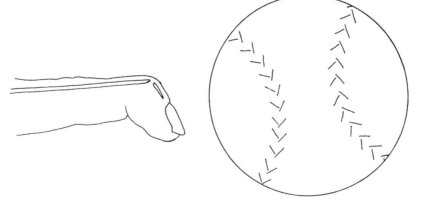

Treatment The treatment of this condition is X-ray to see that there is no other damage present, and immobilization and splinting of the finger to allow the healing process to occur. The physician must determine whether the tendon is actually ruptured and whether surgical repair is necessary.

Prevention The athlete can prevent this type of injury by being alert whenever attempting to catch a ball, such as in baseball or basketball, and try not to injure that outstretched finger. Mallet finger is a very difficult injury to avoid in sports where an athlete is attempting to catch a ball thrown at a very high velocity.

Blood Under the Fingernails (Subungual Hematoma) and Finger Bruises

Definition and Causes Blood under the nail is called **subungual hematoma.** Any direct blow to the fingertip or to the fingernail can cause the accumulation of blood directly beneath the nail. This produces the common purple dislocation which is visible under the nail. This is a minor injury, but it may be very, very painful to the athlete. There may be a blood formation under the toenails as well. This is often due to repeated trauma, such as in running, where the athlete's shoes are continually jarring the front tip of the toes, causing the formation of blood under the nail.

Treatment If there is no pain, the athlete can just disregard this condition. However, if there is pain, and pain is most often found with blood under the fingernails, the athlete must report to a physician or to a trainer who is experienced in handling this problem. The physician or trainer uses a small, sterile instrument, such as a pin or even a small paper clip, to make a small hole through which the blood can escape from beneath the nail. This very simple surgical procedure, performed in a sterile environment, releases the accumulated blood and the accompanying pressure, providing the athlete much relief.

Prevention The prevention of this type of injury is obviously to avoid a blow to the fingernails. To prevent blood forming under the toenails, one should allow ample room between the end of the toes and toenails and the front part of the shoe. Many authorities suggest that one allow at least the width of an index finger, or the width of a thumb, between the end of the toe and the end of the shoe. This will allow free movement of the toe and toenails within the shoe, so that the athlete will not have the problem of blood forming under the toenails.

Injuries to the Back, Thorax, Abdomen, and Pelvis

There are many injuries which can occur to these areas. The purpose of this text is not to go into much detail regarding internal organ injuries. In the area of the thorax and abdomen there are vital organs, such as the spleen, the liver, the kidneys, and, of course, the heart and lungs. It is not the attempt of this review of injuries to cover trauma to these major organs. However, whenever the athlete receives a direct, severe blow to the thorax or abdomen, one might suspect internal injury. If pain is severe, and there are any other obvious signs, such as blood in the urine, rectal bleeding, or coughing blood, there is, obviously, a major problem, which should be seen by a physician immediately.

Low Back Pain (Disk Problems) and Herniated Disk

Definition and Causes Outside of the common cold, the problem for which people seek a physician's advice and guidance most often is low back pain. As athletes get older, many of them develop lower back problems. There are several reasons for this. Poor posture which has been allowed to continue for several years is one reason. Increasing body weight, a problem with many individuals, can also cause back problems. Finally, the lack of proper exercise may contribute to back problems.

A common injury occurring in the spine is the **herniated disk.** The disks are tough, fibrous, connective tissue structures which lie between the bones of the spine (vertebrae). They serve as cushions between the vertebrae and allow movement within the spine. The disk is composed of a soft, inner structure surrounded by a tough, fibrous tissue on the outside. Figure 13.5 is a diagram of the intervertebral disk. In a herniated disk, pressure is brought to bear on some aspect of the disk and a portion of it ruptures. In simple terms, the soft inner part of the disk, which is much like the yolk of an egg, breaks open and is allowed to flow to the outside. The tough outside of the disk then impinges slightly on the nerves running down the spine, causing pain. The pain may be localized in the area of the individual disk which is involved, or if there is pressure on the nerve which runs down the back and into the lower extremities, the pain may be referred down to the lower extremities, or even down to the foot.

Treatment Treatment for the herniated disk is to seek professional advice. The orthopedic physician, after examination, X-rays, and other sophisticated tests, may attempt to isolate the problem in terms of whether a bony structure (the vertebra) is affected or whether the disk, itself, is involved. Initial treatment may consist of remedial exercises,

---

Figure 13.5 Herniated Disk. Inner section, or nucleus pulposus *(a),* occasionally ruptures and flows to the outside, allowing the outer section *(b)* of hardened, cartilaginous material to intrude against the spinal nerves, causing pain and restricted motion.

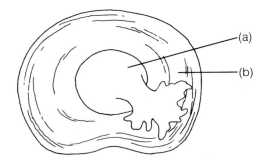

some muscle relaxant drugs, or traction. Also, correct posture will be outlined, and the athlete instructed to practice this correct posture. Occasionally, in severe cases where the disk is ruptured to a large extent, an operation may be necessary. In the operation the herniated or ruptured portion of the disk may be removed, or, in severe cases, the entire disk is removed and the two adjacent vertebrae of the spine may be allowed to fuse together. Obviously, in this drastic procedure, some movement is lost and danger is always present any time the physician opens the spine to do surgery. Most back treatment regimes should be cautious, beginning with low back exercises, a correction of posture, and, perhaps, some traction, wrapping, or back supports and braces.

Prevention The coach, athletic trainer, or therapist should suggest certain exercises in an attempt to relieve the low back pain. Also, correct posture should be presented. Essentially, the postural adjustments to the back are simple—to align the individual bones of the vertebrae, one over the other. Excessive curvature in any area of the spine may exacerbate any problem which may exist in that area. Being overweight can also make the condition worse.

Suggested Exercises in the Prevention of Low Back Pain

The first suggested exercise for low back pain is the bent-knee situp. The individual sits with the feet close to the buttocks, and attempts the situp or the curlup position. This is to isolate the abdominal muscles and, by contracting them in the situp position, to strengthen these muscles. In a second exercise, the individual lies on a padded table or mat and tries to raise both knees up to the chest and hold in this position. Doing this tends to stretch out the lower back lumbar area. A third exercise involves alternately bringing one knee up to the chest while the other leg lies in the extended position on the floor. A final exercise that is suggested is the pelvic tilt exercise. The athlete tries to rotate the pelvis so that the symphysis comes forward and up, and the depression in the lower back is removed. That is, the person tries to press the lower back into the mat. This pelvic tilt position may also be done in the upright position in which the athlete contracts the buttock muscles very tightly and attempts to rotate the symphysis pubis forward and upward.

Some athletic trainers and therapists suggest stretching of the hamstring muscles to relieve a painful lower back condition. If the hamstring muscles are extremely tight and inflexible, they may exaggerate a painful lower back condition.

One final comment about back problems and herniated disks is on treatment by a chiropractor. Very often, skilled chiropractic physicians can manipulate the spine and apply certain traction to the areas of the spine, relieving pressure on the particular disk which is irritated. If all other conservative treatments have failed, a visit to the chiropractic physician might be indicated.

Spondylolysis

Definition and Causes Spondylolysis is a stress fracture of the vertebrae. In this condition, continual stress from landings tends to irritate and wear down the bones of the spine. Tiny cracks develop in the vertebrae and, if continued trauma is applied to the area, may develop into full-blown fractures. Very often, the transverse processes of the verte-brae (the little pieces of bone which extend out to the side of the spine) are slightly frac-tured due to repeated landings. These problems occur in gymnasts, after many dismounts from various apparatus, or in divers, jumpers, pole vaulters, or anyone who is continually landing on a hard surface.

Treatment This condition is treated by having the area X-rayed, or perhaps following the treatment for the stress fracture, which was given in an earlier section on bone injuries. Because of all of the nerves that are running into the spine, a physician must very carefully monitor this condition to see that it does not develop into a severe fracture. Rest, as well as other physiotherapy measures, may be also indicated in the treatment phase of this condition. Proper attention to detail in the technique of the performance of the motor skill is most crucial.

Prevention This condition may be prevented by limiting the types of stress to the back area. This might be done by limiting the number of jumps or falls onto the floor during the athlete's practice routine. Adequate padding or proper placement of floor mats is helpful. A gradual buildup of stresses applied to this area may toughen the spine and the individ-ual to some degree.

Spondylolisthesis

Definition and Causes Spondylolisthesis is a forward slipping of some of the individual vertebrae in the vertebral column. Very often, this involves a single vertebra, but in some cases, may involve two adjacent vertebrae. See figure 13.6 for an illustration of this con-dition. The cause of this condition is repeated, excessive bending, either in flexion or ex-tension of the spine. It occurs often in gymnasts and also in football players, especially interior linemen. When they attempt to block an opposing lineman, the forces generated in the contact bend their own spine in a backward or hyperextended position. It often occurs to younger athletes and may occur in high school football players.

Treatment The treatment for this condition is to reduce the stress to the back. Often-times, strapping or wrapping of the back in a corset-type arrangement will reduce the stresses to this area.

Prevention Prevention of spondylolisthesis involves strengthening the back muscles wherever possible, as well as providing increased flexibility to this area. Correct technique in performing the skills of the particular sport should also be emphasized.

Hip Pointer

Definition and Causes A **hip pointer** is a bruise which occurs to the anterior superior iliac spine, the uppermost front part of the pelvic bone. Because of the several muscle attachments in and around it, and other soft tissue over this area, any blow to this hip point may result in a very tender bruising of this area. A hip pointer most often occurs in

Figure 13.6 Spondylolisthesis in the Lower Back. Sports which cause the athlete to excessively extend the spine place much pressure on the vertebrae, leading to this forward slippage. Pain in the immediate area, as well as radiating down the buttocks and legs, may accompany this injury.

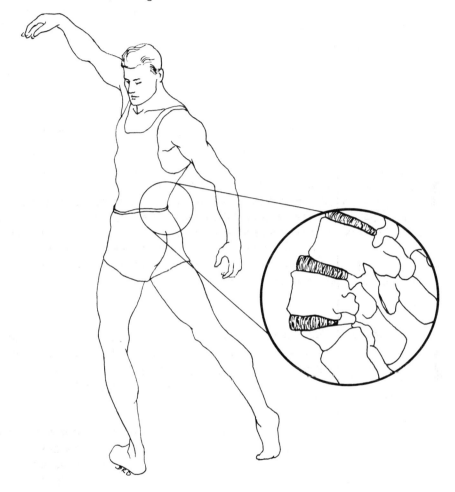

football and other contact sports where a blow to this area overrides the pad or is severe enough to go directly through the padding to irritate the crest of the bone. It is a very severe condition which produces much pain and limits athletic activity.

Treatment The treatment is mostly the same as for any contusion—cold, compression, elevation, and rest, or a cessation of the activity. Some physicians prescribe oral anti-inflammatory medication. The hip pointer can be a disabling condition, and many athletes must rest one to three weeks as a result of receiving this injury. Occasionally, in severe cases of hip pointer, the area is injected with a small amount of cortisone or a related substance, which is diluted in a local anesthetic to diminish the body's reaction to the injury, and also to reduce pain.

Prevention Prevention is to pad the area extremely well so that, when the athlete receives a blow to this area, it is to the pad, and not directly to the soft tissue.

Blow to the Testicles

Definition and Causes Any severe blow which occurs to the lower pelvis in a male is very often damaging to the testicles. The scrotum and immediate area may go into spasm, leading to a very, very painful condition.

Treatment Relief is often brought about by having the athlete lie on his back and alternately bring one knee or both knees up to the chest. A method of treatment suggested by Klafs & Arnheim (1981) is to have the athlete sit with the legs extended at the knee, and have someone come behind him, lift him by the shoulder one to two inches from the playing surface, and let him drop this short distance to the ground. This may relieve some of the spasm to the area.

Prevention Prevention consists of wearing the proper athletic supporter, especially in contact sports. Hard, plastic cup inserts should be supplied to the athlete to prevent vicious contact to this area.

Stress Fractures of the Pelvis

Definition and Causes This is another condition which may occur in the pelvic region. A slight fatigue (or stress) fracture of the pelvis most often occurs in the lower pelvis, right near the symphysis, or occasionally at that part of the pelvis where the thigh bone (femur) comes into the pelvis. Again, a physician would have to conduct certain tests to tell whether a fracture is present.

Treatment The treatment is rest and abstention from the activity until the bone is healed.

Prevention Prevention of the stress fracture of the pelvis is accomplished by a judicious program of gradual exercise. The athlete must build up the running distance or other activity by such a slight degree each day that the bone accommodates and does not begin to break down in a typical stress fracture reaction.

Injuries to the Lower Extremities

The Thigh

Groin Pulls

Definition and Causes A groin pull is a stretching of the muscles in the groin, the area on the inner upper thigh where the large leg muscles come in to attach to the pelvis. The cause for the groin pull is a sudden stretching of that muscle, either due to contraction or overstretching, causing a partial tear or rupture of the muscle.

Treatment The treatment for the groin pull is the same as for any other muscle pull. That is, cold, compression, and relaxation. After this routine is continued for a few days, other aspects of physical therapy are attempted. These other attempts would begin with passive exercise, then active exercise, then the application of heat. There are several ways of wrapping the upper thigh and groin to relieve some of the pressure in this area. See Klafs & Arnheim (1981) for some taping and wrapping suggestions.

Prevention Muscle strengthening in this area and increased flexibility are suggested. It is especially important to stretch and strengthen the adductor muscles. These are the muscles on the upper inner thigh which bring the upper legs together. Resistance should be applied through an externally created means as the athlete attempts to bring the legs together. Also, it is suggested that the athlete work on flexibility in all of the movement that the thigh can make with the pelvis—flexion, extension, abduction and adduction, as well as internal and external rotation. Athletes who have much strength and flexibility in these muscles are less susceptible to groin muscle pulls. Adequate warm-up and lead-up activities to the athletic event should thoroughly warm the area and make muscle contraction in that area easier and less stressful.

Charley Horse

Definition and Causes See chapter 10.

Treatment The treatment is the same as for any muscle contusion.

Prevention The prevention is accomplished by proper padding to lessen the impact of a blow to the muscle area.

Hamstring Pull

Definition and Causes A hamstring pull is overstretching, partial tearing, or rupture of the hamstring muscles. There are three muscles in the hamstring group, the semimembranous, semitendinous, and the biceps femoris. These three large muscles originate at the ischial tuberosity, the point on the pelvis which is most inferior. The muscles run from this point down to the inner and outer aspects, respectively, of the bones of the lower leg. The hamstrings received their names because hogs were hung up by these strong tendinous type muscles as they were slaughtered.

Treatment The treatment for a hamstring pull is the same as that for the other muscle pulls—cold, compression, and rest to try to eliminate hemorrhaging and further irritation to the area. Following this, the treatment is gradual movement and some local applications of heat, followed by stretching and strengthening exercises to this musculature.

Prevention Prevention is avoidance of any activities in which there is a sharp, sudden pull on the muscles without sufficient warm-up and gradual stretching of the area. The best way to get into an activity is to start doing the actual event, but going through the motions at 50 to 75 percent effort, and then gradually increasing to 85 percent, 95 percent, and finally, maximum effort. Also, adequate conditioning, in terms of strengthening and stretching the area, is indicated.

Contusions to the Thigh

Definition and Causes Any athlete who is exposed to a kick, a flying object, such as a ball hitting the thigh, or any implements striking the thigh (baseball bats, hockey sticks, lacrosse sticks) is subject to a contusion of the thigh. This sets up a hematoma (collection of blood in the area) as well as the disruption of muscle tissue. Myositis ossificans, which was noted earlier, might form in the area, since it is caused by a direct blow to the muscle.

Treatment The treatment is to apply ice and compression, and rest the area. Some physicians prescribe some anti-inflammatory medication. Long term treatment is gradual stretching and a gentle increase in activity.

Prevention Prevention would be to pad the area to alleviate any blows to this musculature.

The Knee

Of all of the injuries that occur to the athlete, probably the most serious area of concern is the knee. In contact sports the knee is often injured. In other sports, such as running, skiing, and swimming, the repeated motions made at this joint also cause overuse injuries at the knee. There are many reasons for the large number of injuries to the knee. Some of these reasons and an explanation will be provided in this section. The knee is the biggest joint in the body. It is also a very complicated joint. This can be seen when one looks at the various structures which compose this joint. Another reason for many knee injuries is the very exposed nature of the knee joint. Still another reason for knee injuries is that the knee is a very crucial joint in enabling the athlete to stand and bear weight on the lower extremities. Finally, the knee joint is a very shallow joint, since one bone does not fit very tightly into another bone. This shallowness accounts for still other knee injuries.

The knee is a hinge joint. This means that the prime movements at the knee should be flexing and extending. Flexing is bending the knee, extending is moving the lower leg out in a kicking motion. Many injury problems occur at the knee when athletes try to rotate the knee. In 90° of flexion (the knee is one-half bent) there is some rotation permitted at the knee. However, if the leg is in full extension, because of the very tight musculature of the quadriceps, there is really no rotation permitted at the knee. Some rotation may occur, but that rotation occurs up at the hip joint. The next section provides a brief anatomical description of this area.

Anatomy of the Knee

Ligaments at the Knee There are many ligaments in the knee. Ligaments attach bone to bone. There are two very strong, prominent ligaments that lie on either side of the knee joint. These are the medial collateral ligament, and lateral collateral ligament (fig. 13.7). The medial collateral and lateral collateral ligaments provide stability to the sides of the knee. There are two other very important ligaments at the knee which help provide anterior/posterior (front-to-back) stability. These ligaments are the **anterior** and **posterior** cruciate ligaments. The anterior ligament starts on the front upper portion of the lower leg bone (tibia) and it runs to the back lower portion of the upper leg bone (femur). The posterior cruciate ligament starts at the upper back end of the tibia and it runs forward to the lower front portion of the femur. The other important ligament at the knee is the patella ligament. This structure may also be referred to as the patella tendon.

Figure 13.7 Knee Joint Structure. This is the largest, most exposed, weight-bearing joint of the body. It consists of the tibia *(a)*, fibula *(b)*, femur *(c)*, cruciates *(d)*, collateral ligaments *(e)*, and the meniscus cartilage.

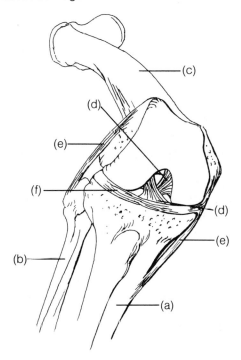

The patella ligament attaches to the lower leg at the tibial tuberosity. This is the large bump on the upper anterior aspect of the tibia (the main bone of the lower leg). Please refer to figure 13.7 for this important landmark. The patella ligament is very strong and serves as the insertion of the quadriceps muscle. The quadriceps is the front part of the thigh. There are many other, smaller ligaments at the knee, but the five mentioned here are the main ligaments at this joint.

Cartilage at the Knee   There are many pieces of cartilage at the knee. It is this cartilage that often causes many problems at this joint. There are two semilunar cartilages (menisci) located within the knee joint. There is one at the medial side of the joint called the medial meniscus, and there is one on the lateral side called the lateral meniscus. These small pieces of cartilage serve as shock absorbers within the knee joint. They also provide stability, to a certain degree, at the joint. It is also important to remember that cartilage covers or encloses all of the bone ends found at the knee. Cartilage covers the bone end of the tibia, and cartilage also lines the bone ends of the femur. This cartilage lining covers the bone ends as they come together at the joint to further protect the ends of the bone, and to provide for efficient movement of the knee joint. In certain sports, this cartilage may be damaged by a direct blow to the joint, or the cartilage may begin to wear away at the joint, as a result of repeated movements.

There is another cartilage on the back side of the patella (knee cap). The patella is a sesmoid bone—a bone lying in the tendon of the quadriceps. This cartilage on the back side of the knee cap may become irritated, leading to another problem, covered later in this chapter.

Dislocated Patella

Definition and Causes   The dislocated patella is a patella which is misplaced from its normal alignment at the knee. Most often, the patella, due to a blow or a very forceful, unnatural contraction, is dislocated to the lateral side. The kneecap moves to the side of the joint. It can be a very painful injury and must be treated immediately.

Treatment   The treatment for this dislocated patella is to reduce the dislocation as quickly as possible. Sometimes the athlete can attempt to straighten the knee. An experienced trainer may be able to slide the patella bone back to the midline of the knee without too much stress. If in doubt about this condition, the dislocated patella must be resolved by a physician.

Prevention   The prevention for the dislocated patella is to try to pad and protect the area. Also, strengthening exercises for the muscles which cross the knee joint tend to put the patella in a very strong position at the knee. Preventive taping and strapping is also used to avoid recurrence of this condition.

Ligament Injuries of the Knee

Definition and Causes There are many ligament injuries that can occur at the knee because of the many ligaments that are involved here. Generally, if a blow is delivered to the side of the knee, as is the case in contact sports, such as football, the medial collateral ligament is injured. When the knee is hit from the outside, it tends to buckle inward, and the medial structures are stretched or torn. The medial collateral ligament is the ligament most commonly injured in a contact blow to the knee. Because the medial collateral ligament is attached to the medial meniscus (the semilunar cartilage at the knee) this cartilage is also often injured in a vigorous blow to the lateral aspect of the knee. There may be other ligament injuries at the knee, depending on the direction of the blow. There are many on-field tests to determine the stability of the knee after it has been hit. Some of these tests involve attempting to move the knee and applying certain stresses in different directions. The physician or trainer may move the lower leg bones forward or backward, or to either side, in an attempt to determine which ligament has been stretched or ruptured as a result of a direct blow. Very often, pain is present in the area; normal movement is not allowed because of the pain; and there is much instability of the joint. Locking of the knee joint may also occur. These are all indications that there is serious ligament damage at the knee.

Treatment The immediate treatment would be RICES. This is followed by X-rays of the joint and an assessment by a physician as to whether the ligament injury should be placed in a cast and treated with further rest, or whether surgical intervention is necessary. If any ligament is torn completely or torn to a large degree, surgical repair may be necessary. There are many diagnostic tools which may be used by the physician to determine the extent of the injury. One such diagnostic tool is the arthrogram.

Prevention The prevention of ligament injuries at the knee is a very difficult task. The more strapping, padding, and wrapping at the knee, the more movement will be limited. Although the athlete may receive some protection from knee pads and knee braces, the trade-off is limited movement of the knee joint.

One thing that the athlete may do for prevention of knee injury is to try to build up the strength of the quadriceps muscles as much as possible. Studies have shown that athletes with very strong quadriceps muscles have very tight, secure knee joints (Nicholas, 1975). Correct application of running technique is also important in preventing ligament injuries. Controlling contact activities in sports is another preventive measure. There are rules which eliminate clipping (hitting from behind) and regulations in some sports which prohibit contact below the waist or any full body contact at the knee joint. Some athletes routinely undergo knee taping to further protect the knee structure, especially the ligaments, as they participate in contact sports. A vigorous conditioning program emphasizing strength activities is probably the best preventive aspect that the athlete can take regarding knee ligament injuries.

Diagnostic Tools for Injured Knee Evaluation

The Arthrogram In this procedure a dye is injected into the knee, and then X-rays are taken as the knee is moved into certain positions. If the ligaments are torn or stretched greatly, abnormal movement will result, and this will be picked up on the X-ray. Arthrograms are studied by radiologists and then orthopedists to determine the exact extent of the injury.

The Arthroscope A newer procedure for detecting knee ligament injuries is use of the arthroscope. This involves the drilling of one to two millimeter holes into the joint and inserting an instrument into the knee joint. This procedure, often done under local anesthesia, allows the physician to insert a very small camera lens into the joint, and actually take a look at the ligaments deep inside the joint. The anterior and posterior cruciate ligaments, as well as the other internal structures, such as cartilage and fluid within the joint, may be seen with the arthroscope. Some physicians are so skilled with this device and this procedure, that they may actually use it to remove small portions of cartilage and other debris which may have built up in the joint as a result of the injury.

Cartilage Injuries of the Knee

Definition and Causes Cartilage injuries at the knee are any tearing, compression, or wearing away of the cartilage of the knee joint. The two major portions of cartilage at the knee are the two menisci. Very often these menisci are injured in contact sports when the athlete takes a direct blow to the knee. This most often occurs in football, hockey, lacrosse, rugby, or other contact sports. Since most athletes are hit on the lateral side of the knee, very often the medial collateral ligament is stretched and torn. Since this medial collateral ligament also attaches to the medial meniscus, this meniscus also is very often injured in a blow from the lateral side of the knee. A very severe injury at the knee is the ''unhappy triad injury,'' when the medial collateral, anterior cruciate, and medial meniscus all are torn. The meniscus can also be injured if the athlete applies a great deal of stress to the knee joint without using proper technique. A common example of this is if, while attempting a deep knee bend (bend at the waist and knee to the extent that the buttocks almost touch the heels), the athlete attempts any turning, lifting movement that places great stresses on the knee. In this situation the cartilage (the meniscus at the knee) may be compressed or torn.

Treatment Treatment includes evaluation of the knee by a trained orthopedic physician or therapist, and then further diagnostic evaluation with the use of X-ray, arthrogram, or the arthroscope.

Prevention The prevention of cartilage injuries at the knee is accomplished by the proper lifting techniques, the proper running techniques, and an excellent program of strength conditioning activities for the knee. It is also important that a gradual long-term program of strengthening exercises be used so as not to apply too much stress to this area early in the sport season.

Knee Pain—Overuse Knee Syndromes

Definition and Causes Knee pain caused by overuse syndromes at the knee is any pain that develops in the knee as a result of repeated movements of that particular portion of the body. Knee pain most often occurs in runners, swimmers, cross-country skiers, crew rowers, cyclists, and other athletes who make repeated bending and flexing movements at the knee. The various structures within the knee—the ligaments, the tendons crossing the knee joints, the cartilage present at the joint, or other loose pieces of cartilage and tissue which may be present in the joint—are irritated by the many repeated movements of the joint.

Treatment Treatment depends upon accurate diagnosis by the orthopedic physician. The physician, with the aid of manipulation, X-rays, and other tests, must determine which particular structure, (ligament, cartilage, or muscle tendon) is the source of the irritation and then prescribe a program of rehabilitation. Very often, a cessation of the workouts is prescribed. Occasionally, anti-inflammatory agents are taken orally, or may even be injected into the joint to help reduce some of the pain caused by the overuse.

Prevention The prevention of this overuse syndrome at the knee is a gradual reduction of activity and a total reevaluation of the training program to determine what particular training stress seems to be causing the problem.

Jumper's Knee

Definition and Causes Jumper's knee is an irritation to the patella tendon or the patella ligament. It occurs in sports, such as the jumps in the field events (long jump, triple jump, and high jump). This condition may occur in any other sport which has a large jumping component, such as volleyball and basketball. Because of the repeated stress to the patella ligament, the ligament becomes irritated and slightly inflamed.

Treatment The treatment for this condition is the application of ice, compression, and rest to the area immediately following the activity. Sometimes rest is the best treatment for this condition. This may be followed with some local anti-inflammatory agent, or oral anti-inflammatory medication.

Prevention The prevention of jumper's knee is to use an intelligent training program. The conditioning process must be very gradual, and involve a great deal of strength and flexibility activities. One final preventive aspect that may be undertaken is to apply a wrap or some type of strapping to the area in an attempt to hold the patella tendon to the bone. This tends to keep heat in the area as the athlete is working out, and also tends to reduce the strain which is placed on that tendon as the athlete jumps.

Osgood-Schlatter's Disease

Definition and Causes This condition is an irritation at the point of insertion of the quadriceps muscle into the tibial bone. This point of insertion is called the tibial tuberosity. In the young, growing athlete, the bone growth and buildup in this area may not be commensurate with stresses that are placed on it. Consequently, repeated flexing and extending of the knee joint, due to vigorous contraction of the quadriceps muscle, places a great deal of stress at the point where this quadriceps muscle inserts into the lower leg bone. This results in a spur growth of the bone and an irritation to this area. Osgood-Schlatter's disease may also be caused by a fall on the knee joint, hitting the upper, front part of the tibia. This also can irritate the bone. A similar condition to this is called housemaid's knee, and sometimes arises when an individual is working on the floors in the kneeling position. The irritation is to the upper front portion of the tibia, resulting in an irritation to the bone at that spot.

Treatment The treatment of this condition is again a gradual buildup in the training program with careful attention to any symptoms of pain or stress that occur in this area. The athlete should engage in some strengthening activities, which may improve the integrity of the quadriceps muscle, as well as the point at which the muscle inserts into the bone.

Prevention Prevention is to carefully regulate and monitor the amount of activity that the young athlete is engaging in. Also, padding and wrapping support may be provided to this area to protect it from the jarring of landing. Careful attention to detail in the athlete's training and conditioning program are very important throughout adolescence.

Chondromalacia

Definition and Causes The definition of **chondromalacia** is an irritation and partial wearing away of some of the cartilage lining the back portion of the patella. This is an overuse type of injury. A direct blow or other single irritation to the knee may start the condition, but in most cases chondromalacia develops because of repeated wear and tear to the structure at the back of the kneecap. This is a condition which is commonly found in runners and other people who use their knees extensively in repeated motions.

Treatment The treatment for chondromalacia is rest. Sometimes physicians administer anti-inflammatory agents to help control some of the irritation and inflammation which is present. Another method of treatment is to analyze the functional alignment of the kneecap with the other structures at the knee and attempt to provide some type of orthotic (an assist placed in the athlete's shoe) to correct alignment of the knee which may help reduce this condition.

Prevention The prevention of chondromalacia involves a very gradual and intelligent buildup of the activity of the athlete. Occasionally, if there is a great deal of misalignment of the kneecap, an orthotic device may be placed in the athlete's shoe to help correct it. Sometimes running on a soft surface or using shoes with extra thickness, support, and padding may minimize this condition.

Ilio-Tibial Band Syndrome

Definition and Causes The ilio-tibial band syndrome is an irritation to the tough, fibrous connective band which lies at the lateral outer aspect of the knee. The ilio-tibial band comes down on the outer aspect of the thigh, and crosses over the femur at the knee joint. It may be irritated when athletes use repeated movements, such as running.

Treatment The treatment for this condition, as suggested by Brody (1980) is a thorough stretching in an attempt to loosen all of the structures in this area. Sometimes it is treated with regular anti-inflammatory agents.

Prevention The prevention of this syndrome would be to modify the activity to such a degree as to allow a gradual buildup and toughening of the structures at the outer aspect of the knee. Stretching exercises which consist of those suggested in the chapter on flexibility seem to help relieve this condition.

Shin Splints

Definition and Causes The term **shin splint** is used to denote pain in the shin or lower leg. The real enigma with this athletic injury is in determining what particular structure in the shin is causing the problem. One of the best articles on this condition was written by Benas and Jokl (1978). They note that the pain of the shin splint injury could be divided into three categories. The first category is pain of a *bony origin,* or some type of irritation or stress fracture to the bones of the lower limb. The second category of pain in the shin is that of *vascular origin,* or pain in any of the blood vessels of the lower limb. The third and final category of pain in the shin area might be due to an irritation of some of the other *soft tissues* in the area, the muscles or the fascia. We will examine each one of these possible causes of pain in a little more detail. In most, if not all cases, the problem of shin splints arises when the athlete attempts to do too much activity too soon. Very often, lots of running on a hard surface, preceded by inactivity, seems to cause the shin splint problem. Shin splints are an overuse type of injury (fig. 13.8).

Treatment The treatment of the shin splint problem involves trying to isolate which particular structure is involved, and then attempting to treat that structure. In order to determine whether there is a bone problem causing the shin splints, X-rays and procedures for diagnosing a stress fracture of the tibia should be followed. Once pain of bony origin is ruled out, one can look at the other possibilities for pain arising in the shin area. The pain may be due to the cutting off of the blood supply to some of the muscles in the area. This is a very difficult area to diagnose and to treat. There are some physicians who will inject a needle into the area to see if there is a buildup of compression and pressure in the muscles of that area, to see if there is an interruption of blood flow due to expansion of the tissue in the area. This topic was presented in a discussion of compartment syndromes. The shin splint problem which causes the most concern to the athlete is pain in the soft tissue—an inflammation of the muscle or the fascia of the lower legs. Included in a discussion of soft tissue injury is a comment on the membrane which connects the two

Figure 13.8 Shin Splints. The interosseous membrane *(a)* in the front of the lower leg becomes inflamed when injured, causing pain in the shin area. There may be other complications.

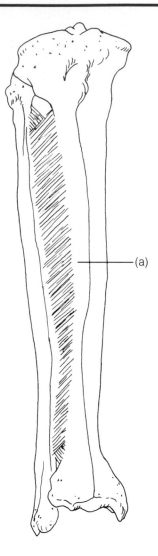

(a)

bones of the lower leg. This is called the interosseous membrane. Very often, the interosseus membrane, which has many blood vessels and serves as attachment for many muscles of the lower leg, becomes inflamed with the repeated running and jarring of the lower limbs. If this is the case, then the athlete must take adequate rest to allow this structure to heal.

Prevention of Shin Splints There are many things that the athlete can do in an attempt to prevent shin splints. The first thing is to have a wise, intelligent, gradual buildup in the training program. Intensity and duration of the training program should be rigidly controlled. Attention must be paid to the type of surface that the athlete is training on. Attention must also be given to footwear. Proper padding and support is necessary in all athletic shoes. Often, inserts can be placed in athletic shoes, which serve to cushion foot-falls. Also, the athlete may wear thick, cushioning socks to absorb some of the forces which are transmitted to the foot by running or by the stresses of starting and stopping on hard surfaces. Other preventive aspects might include some support taping of the structures of the lower limb. This seems to work for some athletes. Stretching and gradual strengthing of all structures of the lower limb may help prevent shin splints. Since shin splints are an overuse type of injury (Benas & Jokl, 1978). By following all of the suggested guidelines presented here, they may be avoided.

The Lower Leg

Achilles Tendinitis

Definition and Causes Achilles tendinitis is a painful inflammation which may be present with or without swelling around the Achilles tendon (Brody, 1980; Williams, 1976). Further discussion of tendon injuries can be found in chapter 11. The Achilles tendon is the larg-est, strongest tendon in the body. However, this tendon is peculiar in that it does not have the true synovial sheath that normally surrounds most tendons. This synovial sheath around tendons is generally a double layered tube through which the tendon passes, and which serves to lubricate the tendon as the tendon moves with muscular activity. Achilles ten-dinitis is an overuse type of injury.

There have been several causes put forth for this condition. Running on hills, wearing very rigid, stiff shoes, and lots of running on very hard pavement have all been identified as possible causes (Brody, 1980). Repeated running on hard surfaces (cement), up or down hills, or on other uneven terrain may inflict small cumulative tears in the tendon that set up the inflammatory process. The athlete may experience a painful, burning sensation early in the run or workout. Many times the pain of Achilles tendinitis subsides as the athlete gets into the workout and blood flow is increased to the area. This masks this injury problem, and it becomes a difficult condition to acknowledge.

Treatment In the acute phase of Achilles tendinitis the symptoms are treated with ice, rest, and elevation. This may be followed some days later by gentle and gradual stretching exercises at the ankle. Occasionally an oral anti-inflammatory medication may be helpful. The injection of steroids into and around the tendon is *not indicated,* because the steroids tend to weaken the tendon and the possibility for rupture of the Achilles tendon is in-creased.

Prevention The athlete can prevent Achilles tendinitis by following a very gradual con-ditioning program. The shoe that the athlete wears for the activity must be very supportive and not too stiff. Attention must be paid to the type of surface and terrain that the athlete is training on, and excessively hilly areas or uneven terrain should be avoided early in the conditioning period. Maintaining strength in the muscles at the front and back of the ankle joint are important as is proper flexibility in this area.

Achilles Tendon Rupture

Definition and Causes The Achilles tendon rupture is a nearly complete or total tear in the Achilles tendon. This is a very painful condition, which needs surgical repair immediately. It is caused by a very rapid contraction of the gastrocnemius muscle group. When this happens, the athlete is totally incapable of any propulsive action with the foot.

Treatment The treatment, as was noted for the rupture, is surgical intervention and repair of the tendon. The foot is then casted and the athlete follows a period of immobilization, followed by further rehabilitation. Strength and flexibility activities are crucial in the rehabilitation process.

Prevention The Achilles tendon rupture is prevented by trying to prepare for the activity in the best possible way. This includes proper warmup and easing gradually into the activity. The athlete should start going through the particular sport motions at 50 to 75 percent intensity, and then *gradually* build up to full intensity. It is important to avoid quick starts and stops on the tendon before adequately warming up. In addition to these suggestions for prevention of this problem, proper strength and flexibility in the area should be maintained throughout the season.

Ankle Sprains

Definition and Causes Ankle sprains are one of the most common types of athletic injuries, occurring to both female and male athletes at all competitive levels. The problem with this particular type of injury is that it is often dismissed as a slight sprain, with improper attention given to it. *Ankle sprains are ligament injuries.* It is important to remember that *sprains* occur to *ligaments,* while *strains* occur to *muscles.* Both, however, involve an overstretching of the particular type tissue. The ankle is basically a hinge joint. The movements of flexion and extension, or dorsiflexion and plantarflexion, are permitted at the joint (see fig. 13.9). There is also some inversion and eversion permitted at the ankle. Inversion is turning the ankle inward so that the big toe comes up toward the knee. Eversion is turning the ankle outward so that the big toe points down and the small toe then comes up toward the outer aspects of the knee. There are only a few degrees of inversion and eversion permitted at the normal ankle joint. The ankle is supported by many small, tough ligaments which are present at the joint. The ankle joint is also reinforced by some of the longer tendons of the muscles of the shank or lower leg.

Most sprains at the ankle occur to those ligaments that are on the lateral, or outside of the ankle. The ligaments of the ankle are named after the two bones that the ligaments connect. Recall that a ligament is a piece of tough, fibrous, connective tissue that attaches bone to bone. One of the most common ligaments injured in an ankle sprain is the calcaneofibular ligament. As the name suggests, this ligament attaches the calcaneus (heel bone) to the fibula (long, slender bone on the outside of the lower leg). Ligament injuries were noted earlier in the section on soft tissue injuries.

Figure 13.9 Ankle Joint. The major bones in the ankle are in the tibia *(a)*, fibula *(b)*, talus *(c)*, and calcaneus *(d)*. The ligaments are named for the two bones they connect, such as the calcaneo-fibular *(e)* ligament. Most injuries (sprains) to these ligaments occur to the lateral (outside) aspect of the ankle.

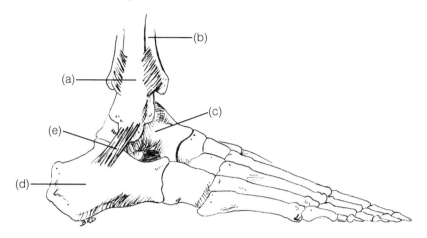

Sprains are described in severity as first, second, or third degree by the amount of stretching or tearing of the ligament. A first degree sprain is a minor sprain, while a total rupture of the ligament is a third degree sprain. Some authors note four degrees of sprains, using the same classification system with a first degree being a minor sprain, and a fourth degree being a total rupture. The causes of the ankle sprain are generally inversion injuries, common in basketball, volleyball, or other running and jumping sports. The ankle "rolls in" under the lower leg and there is a stretching or tearing of the ligaments on the outside of the joint. In severe sprains the joint capsule, that area which surrounds and nourishes the joint with fluid, may also be torn. Inversion-type ankle sprains account for nearly 70 to 85 percent of all of the injuries that occur at the ankle joint.

Treatment The treatment for ankle sprains involves a proper evaluation and diagnosis of which particular ligaments and structures are involved. Often the physician will take several X-rays of the area to help in the diagnosis. Other indications, such as swelling, deformity, discoloration, or restricted motion, may also help the physician get an idea of the extent of damage at the ankle. Of course, immediate treatment is rest, ice, compression, and elevation. Very often, if this is done in the first few seconds following the injury, blood flow into the area is reduced and swelling curtailed. After the first twenty-four to forty-eight hours, a rehabilitation program may begin. Initially, this may be limited movement, with some passive and active stretching at the joint, followed by the application of heat to the joint. Often a whirlpool bath is used. Long term treatment might involve protective taping and strapping of the joint. In severe ankle sprains, where total rupture of a ligament is present, surgical intervention may be required, and it may be necessary to cast the athlete's ankle. The important concept here is to protect the motion and stability which remains at the joint.

Prevention Prevention of the ankle sprain is one of the prime objectives the athlete can have. In sports where there is a lot of jumping, and also some degree of contact, the athlete can protect the ankle by wearing high-topped shoes. Here, again, one trades support and protection for mobility. The athlete may also choose to tape or to wrap the ankles. There are supportive devices on the market which allow the athlete to help protect the ankle. These supports may be reused each time the athlete reports for practice. In addition to these supportive devices and taping, the athlete can make an effort to increase the strength of the area by doing strengthening exercises at the ankle. Also, in conjunction with the strengthening program, the athlete may wish to do certain flexibility exercises at this particular joint.

The Foot

The foot is a very complicated structure. It consists of twenty-six bones, many ligaments, and many small muscles and tendons which contribute to the total function of the foot. The foot also has several arches. There are two arches that run along the longitudinal axis of the foot. In addition, there are several arches which run across the medial aspect, from the outside to the inside portion of the foot. The arches provide support to the body when the person walks or runs. Another function of the foot is propulsion, or propelling the body forward in the walking or running gait. Still another function of the foot is to aid in absorbing the landing of the body whenever the person crosses uneven terrain. There are many types of injuries which can occur at the foot.

Calcaneal Bursitis

Definition and Causes Calcaneal bursitis is defined as an irritation to the bursa, which lies directly beneath the Achilles tendon, and immediately above the calcaneus (heel bone). Generally, this overuse type of injury occurs whenever there is an abrupt change in physical activity and too much stress is placed in too short a time to the foot and to the area of the Achilles tendon.

Treatment Conservative measures which follow the same course as those for treating Achilles tendinitis are also used to treat calcaneal bursitis. This includes the application of cold, rest, and perhaps some oral anti-inflammatory medication. Occasionally, a physician may try some local injection of steroid into this area. However, extreme caution must be used so that the injection of the steroid does not go directly into the Achilles tendon. As has been noted before and is stressed here again, the injection of any steroid into a tendon tends to make that tendon weak and more liable to rupture.

Prevention A method of prevention for this condition is to engage in a very gradual, intelligent, training program, combined with proper footwear, and doing the workouts on a soft, supportive surface, where possible.

Plantar Fasciitis

Definition and Causes The plantar fascia is a tough, fibrous connective tissue that runs along the bottom of the foot and inserts into the heel bone, or calcaneus. Plantar fasciitis is often called "heel spur syndrome." It is a very common cause of heel pain in athletes who do a lot of running. It is an overuse type of syndrome which involves an inflammatory reaction at the point where the plantar fascia inserts into the heel bone. The runner generally experiences pain in this area upon the first few steps taken in the morning (Brody, 1980). The reason for this is that this area of the foot is extremely cold, due to slight circulation at this time. The athlete consequently feels pain. Palpation (touching the area with the fingertips) also brings pain to the area.

Treatment The treatment for this overuse condition is immediate ice, rest, compression, and elevation. Occasionally, other support measures are tried. Plastic heel cups may be used in the running shoes. Occasionally, some taping or strapping of the area is indicated. Sometimes a horseshoe-shaped pad is placed in the heel of the shoe to alleviate the pressure to that area as the athlete stands, walks, or runs.

Prevention Prevention of this condition involves a very gradual buildup of the activity. Again, good supportive shoes which protect the foot, and also allow free movement of the foot, are indicated.

Heel Spur

Definition and Causes The heel spur is an irritation of the bony growth on the underside of the heel bone. This condition is also mentioned simultaneously with plantar fasciitis by many authors. The normal pull of the plantar fascia on the bottom of the foot at this location on the heel bone can cause an irritation of the bone (see fig. 13.10). It must also be remembered that many small nerves cross the area at the side or the bottom of the foot, and possibly some nerve entrapment may occur with this condition. Hlavac (1980) notes that nerve involvement may be a complication in heel spur problems.

Treatment Treatment for heel spur is the same as that for plantar fasciitis. Ice, compression, elevation, and rest are of the first order. Then, the area should be padded, and an examination of the shoes is indicated. Occasionally, the athlete will try to do a low-dye tape support to the foot. This is essentially a method of supporting the plantar fascia so that it (the fascia) does not pull or tear away from the heel bone.

Prevention Prevention of this condition follows the rationale for the prevention of many of the overuse syndromes—a gradual buildup of the training program. Proper shoes and a gradual increase in the amount of work that the athlete can tolerate is suggested. Occasionally, as the athlete feels this type of condition coming on, he or she may report to an orthopedist or podiatrist and have an orthotic made for the foot. An orthotic is a supportive device which, when inserted in the shoe, provides protection to the structures at the bottom of the foot. The orthotic may also help in correcting alignment of the foot, as well as preventing possible injuries which can occur up the leg, at the knee, and at the hip.

Figure 13.10 Plantar Fascia. A tough, fibrous, connective tissue, this fascia *(a)* starts at the calcaneous or heel bone *(b)* and runs forward to the toes, spanning the bottom (plantar) surface of the foot.

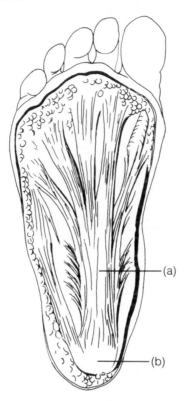

Bone Bruise

Definition and Causes The bone bruise is an irritation to any of the small bones of the lower foot. The cause of this problem is a very hard footfall on a stone or some other small, hard object, which tends to irritate the lining of a small bone of the foot.

Treatment The treatment for this condition is rest and ice, to prevent some of the swelling, pain, and discomfort in the area.

Prevention Prevention of this condition is to wear adequately protective shoes in all phases of the athletic activity. A suggestion for preventing further harm is to pad the area with a felt pad or small rubber covering, or to cut a doughnut-shaped pad to place around the bone bruise to alleviate further pressure on that area. This would also minimize the pain in that area.

Morton's Foot

Definition and Causes Morton's foot is a long, second metatarsal (long bone of the foot). Because of this long second metatarsal, the first metatarsal (one closest to the midline of the body) appears short. With this condition a lot of stress is placed on the first metatarsal. Because of this, the athlete tends to pronate (turn the foot over in an inverted position) to a large degree. This may place a lot of stress on some of the structures on the underside of the foot, and may lead to irritation in these structures. Occasionally, the Morton's foot problem can be so severe as to cause a tiny stress reaction in the metatarsals.

Treatment The treatment of this condition is the prescribing of an orthotic or some proper taping or padding of the arch of the foot.

Prevention The prevention for this condition follows the treatment suggested previously—an orthotic prescribed by a podiatrist or an orthopedist. Other suggestions involve certain preventive tapings and strappings of the foot. The latter preventive mode is difficult because the taping would have to be applied before each workout. Also, it is important for the athlete to wear an athletic shoe which provides ample room for all the toes. A good guide is for the shoe to be at least one finger's width longer than the longest (second) toe.

Intermetatarsal Neuroma

Definition and Causes A neuroma is defined by Hlavac (1980) as a benign nerve tumor. It can occur in the athlete where there is friction or trauma to the foot. The irritation is set up along the protective covering of the nerve. The constant irritation to the nerve sheath causes a reactive thickening to this covering, which produces scar tissue and causes much pain. A common location for this condition is between the first and second metatarsal heads. This is shown in figure 13.11. There may be other nerve injuries to the foot, such as compression or compartment-type nerve injuries. There is always much pain present with these types of nerve injuries.

Treatment The treatment for this condition involves careful examination and evaluation by the physician to understand why there is compression being brought on the nerve. Very often, a simple change to a longer or wider athletic shoe will remove much of the pressure to that area. Often, cushioned insoles which tend to separate the metatarsals, may help (Hlavac, 1980). If these conservative treatments do not work, professional guidance is necessary. The doctor may have to do some surgical removal and scraping of the scar tissue which has built up, or may prescribe some other orthotic, support, or pad to the area.

Prevention Obviously, it is best to look ahead and try to prevent a neuroma or nerve entrapment-type injury. Wearing properly fitted shoes and paying careful attention to the training program may avoid this condition. If the pain in the foot is of a burning type, this suggests a nerve injury and, perhaps, padding of the shoes with insoles or other protective padding may resolve this problem before it develops into a full-blown neuroma.

Figure 13.11 Neuroma. Generally a benign tumor or irritation most often occurring between the metatarsals of the foot due to impact on hard surfaces. Shown is a growth (a) on and around the nerve between the first and second metatarsals. The neuroma causes much pain and irritation in the area.

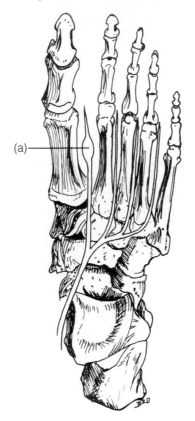

Stress Fracture

Definition and Causes   Stress fractures can occur to any bones in the body. When they occur in the foot, they generally occur to the small, long bones called metatarsals. The repeated pounding of long distance running, or repeated jumping, such as occurs in volleyball or basketball, can cause a gradual stress reaction or breakdown of the bones of the foot.

Treatment   The treatment and discussion of the stress fracture was given earlier in the section on bone injuries. Essentially, the treatment for a stress fracture involves a gradual rest or cessation of the activity. Perhaps padding the inside of the shoe with soft, supportive insole material might help to alleviate some of the jarring that is taking place in this area.

Prevention The prevention of the stress fracture is wearing the best possible shoes that the athlete can find. It might be wise to wear a layer of insole material to further cushion the jarring occurring during jumping and running. Finally, the athlete must use a very gradual, progressive buildup in the training or conditioning program.

Skin and Toenail Problems of the Athlete

Most athletes, sooner or later, are confronted with skin or nail problems in the foot. This section discusses some of the more common problems that happen to the skin and nails of the foot. We talked about blisters when we looked at problems that could occur to the hand. By way of review, blisters are created any time there is an abnormal source of friction, and pressure builds up between the skin and an outside surface. Before the formation of a blister begins, there is always a "hot spot" or burning area, usually on the bottom or side of the foot, before the blister actually forms. If the athlete can stop the activity at that time and remedy the situation, generally a blister will not form. If a blister does form, the area must be cleaned properly and a small puncture made in the blister to allow the fluid to drain. Conservative treatment then follows with the application of an antiseptic and proper covering and bandaging of the area. It is extremely important to avoid infection whenever there is a break in the skin.

Corns and Calluses

Corns and calluses are defined by Hlavac (1980) as local accumulation of thickened skin which forms because of a reaction to stress. Generally, a corn is considered a formation of hard skin on the toes, while a callus often occurs on the bottom of the foot. However, they both consist of the same type of hardened, mostly dead, skin tissue. Generally, corns are deeper and denote a focal point of pressure. Causes of corns and calluses are similar to those of the blister—pressure and friction. Athletes must consider their shoes in eliminating areas of pressure and friction. First, they must allow for the proper length and width. They should also look for any irregularities in the shoe which may be causing pressure points at any particular point on the foot.

The treatment and prevention of the corns and calluses obviously takes into account properly fitting shoes. Occasionally, the athlete may take an emory board or similar abrasive material and attempt to file down the corn or the callus. Special preparations are often sold, which tend to remove some of this hardened dead skin. In extreme cases surgical removal of the corn or callus may be indicated.

Warts

Warts are caused by a *viral infection* and may be mistaken for corns or calluses. The warts may or may not be on a friction or pressure area of the skin. Warts are contagious to certain susceptible people, and many times are found in the adolescent (Hlavac, 1980). Warts, if not treated, may spread and multiply. One should see a podiatrist or a dermatologist to have medication placed on the wart to control this problem. In some cases, surgical removal is indicated.

Hematoma

Hematoma results when blood forms under the toenail because of a blow or constant bruising in that area. The hematoma must be drained, as was suggested with the hematoma of the finger. After drainage, a pressure dressing is applied. Very often, the hematoma can be prevented by wearing properly fitted shoes and gradually building up athletic activity.

Athlete's Foot

The final consideration of the foot is a short discussion of athlete's foot. This is a type of *fungus infection* which affects many athletes during their careers. The most common areas of involvement are the bottoms and sides of the feet, and in the spaces between the toes. The key to treating the fungus infection is to remember that the organisms which cause athlete's foot thrive in hot, dirty, damp, and dark areas. If the area can be kept cool, clean, dry, and well aerated, the athlete will not have a problem with this fungus. Wearing clean, dry socks is a must. Exposing the foot to light occasionally should also help this condition.

Injuries to the Head, Neck, and Face

There are, essentially, two main categories of sports injuries within the entire field of sports medicine. Those two main categories are traumatic-type injuries, and overuse or repeated microtraumatic-type injuries. Most of the recent discussion regarding lower leg, ankle, and foot injuries have involved microtraumatic injuries. These overuse type of injuries are caused by the repeated stressing of the musculoskeletal system. They are contrasted with the severe injuries of a traumatic nature which can occur in the combat sports. These combat sports, in which there are many head injuries, are the sports of boxing, wrestling, judo, and karate. Most of the injuries that occur in these sports are traumatic, single blow type of injuries. Whenever one sustains a traumatic-type injury to the head, neck, or face, a medical emergency is present. The injured athlete must see a physician immediately, and many times various physician specialists must be called in. With any injury to the head, neck, or face, often a neurologist, as well as other medical specialists, such as ophthalmologists, dentists, or others, may be called in. Some of the more common head, neck and face injuries will be discussed briefly in the sections that follow.

The Head

Concussion

Definition and Causes At its simplest definition, a concussion is a sudden loss of consciousness at the moment of injury (Williams & Sperryn, 1976). In most cases in sport, the person who sustains the concussion has only a momentary lapse of consciousness, and full recovery takes place within a few minutes. However, the loss of consciousness, even for such a brief time, is a cause for concern. With the loss of consciousness there is a slowing down of the entire system. The heart rate, breathing, and reflexes of the system are all diminished. The unconsciousness mechanism is a protective measure that the body takes to protect itself from further injury. Anyone who receives a concussion should be seen by proper medical personnel. In no case should the person be allowed to return to the same athletic contest or event after they have received a concussion. No matter what the cause, whether a direct blow to the head, or a fall, this unconsciousness must be viewed as a major emergency.

Concussions are generally described by seriousness as a first, second, or third degree concussion. In a first degree concussion, there may be momentary loss of consciousness, or there may be temporary confusion of mental state. There may also be a slight ringing of the ears, followed by a dull headache (Klafs & Arnheim, 1981). In a second degree concussion, there is considerably more damage and this poses a distinct medical emergency. Finally, there may be a loss of consciousness, perhaps lasting for several minutes, followed by mental confusion, a disturbance of balance, and an inability to remember recent events. In a third degree concussion, which is the most severe, the person reverts to a so-called "knocked-out" state. It implies very serious damage to the brain and the nervous system. In this condition the person must be seen by the physician, preferably a neurologist, and *must abstain from the sport for a certain period of time*.

Treatment The treatment for any severe head injury is to report the incident immediately to a physician, and transport the athlete to a hospital where further examination can be made. The physician will order X-rays of the skull and may take a CAT Scan of the area. The CAT Scan (Computerized Axial Tomography) is a more in-depth picture of what is happening inside the skull by contrasting different areas inside the skull with certain other areas. In the treatment phase, the injured athlete remains under the *direct supervision* of the physician until released to everyday activities. The physician very rigidly controls when that player may return to practice or competition. If the athlete continues to report any of the symptoms of the head injury—headache, dizziness, light-headedness, or balance problems—then the athlete should refrain from further participation in the sport. Head injuries are critical sports medicine problems, and cannot be taken lightly under any circumstances.

Prevention The best way to handle this type of an injury problem is with adequate safeguards. Prevention of the head injury consists of padding the skull in whatever way possible for the athletic event. In boxing, the contestants often wear head gear to prevent concussion-type injuries. In other contact sports, such as football, lacrosse, and hockey, helmets should be worn <u>at all times</u>. In fact, in many leagues and organizations, it is a requirement that all athletes wear protective head gear at all times in these contact sports. Even wearing the head gear does not insure that the athlete will be immune to concussion. Vicious blows to the head may still occasionally result in a loss of consciousness. However, if the athletes are adhering to the rules of the game, and are taking as much precaution as they can, in terms of padding and the wearing of helmets, then this risk of the head injury may be minimized. The importance of *proper fit* of the helmet or head protector cannot be over-emphasized.

Common Athletic Injuries and their Treatments   181

The Neck

Definition and Causes Neck injuries are other genuine medical emergencies, which occasionally occur in sports. Because of the spinal cord and the pairs of spinal nerves which exit from the sides of the spinal cord, any blow to the head, neck, or spine area could cause a very severe paralyzing type of injury. Neck injuries occur whenever there is a violent blow or jarring to the head and neck. Most of the injuries occurring to the neck occur as a result of a forced flexion or hyperextension at the neck. In most cases, before the neck bones fracture, either a partial dislocation or a complete dislocation of the bones of the spine (vertebrae) will usually occur (Klafs & Arnheim, 1981). Whenever there is this violent jarring to the neck, there is always the danger that spinal cord and nerve injury has taken place. Extreme caution must be used in analyzing and diagnosing this type of injury. First aid for this condition is crucial. The athlete must receive medical attention immediately, but utmost care must be taken in moving and transporting the injured athlete to a physician. It is best to always use trained emergency medical technicians to splint and to stabilize the injured athlete before being transported to the hospital emergency room. If the coach or athletic trainer is in doubt as to whether to move an athlete with an injured head or neck, the best advice that can be given is to *not move the athlete* until proper medical aid is on the scene.

Treatment The treatment of a severe neck injury involves further examination with the use of radiographic techniques. Once the physician can pinpoint the exact area of the problem, that portion of the anatomy is splinted and stabilized. It must be emphasized that whenever anyone has a severe neck injury, an orthopedic physician and trained neurologist should both examine the individual to see that there is no further hemorrhaging or damage to the area, and the athlete must receive an adequate period of rest and rehabilitation.

Prevention In some sports, athletes wear special collars made of foam rubber or other padded material to help stabilize and support the neck. This is becoming a more common procedure in American football and in other sports where athletes are likely to receive jarring blows to the head and the neck. In addition to this padded protection, athletes should make certain that they engage in a proper strength conditioning program for all of the musculature which supports the head. These muscles include the neck flexors and extensors, and the muscles which rotate the head and neck. There are several sporting goods manufacturers who presently make specific exercise devices to condition the neck muscles. (Nautilus® is one excellent example of an exercise manufacturer with a device to especially condition the neck muscles.) If the athlete properly builds up the muscles in and around the neck, the likelihood of sustaining a severe injury to this area might be lessened to a degree. However, there is always the danger of the traumatic, sudden blow to the neck area which would cause a severe sports injury to that area.

The Face

Many injuries to the face can occur in contact or combat sports. This section focuses on injuries to the eyes, nose, teeth, and ears. In addition to injuries to these specific parts, the face may also receive blows or contusions. A contusion or a laceration is any blow which results in a tearing of the skin or a local hemmorhage to the area. Obviously, if a blow to the face is severe enough, the person would sustain a concussion in addition to the contusion. These injuries are treated in the same manner as a contusion to any other part of the body—ice, minor compression, and, certainly, rest and avoidance of the activity. With any blow to the face, there is the possibility of concussion, and attention must be paid to possible loss of consciousness, confusion of mental recall, and clarity of vision. A more detailed look at injuries to the particular structures of the face follows.

Eye Injuries

Definition and Causes Serious eye injury is rare in sports, but does occasionally occur in certain contact sports or sports in which balls are used. Perhaps the most common eye injury, other than a bruise or laceration, is the detached retina. In the early 1980s, a World Boxing champion, Sugar Ray Leonard, suffered a detached retina injury. This injury occurs whenever the eye receives a blow which tends to jar the eye in its socket. Detached retinas occur more often in persons from forty to seventy years old.

Treatment The treatment for an eye injury is examination and a proper diagnosis by a trained ophthalmologist, who will examine the eye, perhaps take X-rays of the skull to see if there is any other damage, and use various other diagnostic procedures. Because of the danger of blindness, any eye injury must be seen by a physician and treated immediately.

Prevention Obviously, the best prevention with this type of injury is to wear a protective device which covers the eye and protects it from injury. In contact sports, such as ice hockey, football, and lacrosse, players are advised to wear helmets with face masks to protect the eyes. In other sports, like tennis, handball, racquetball, squash, badminton, and other activities where a ball or projectile may be coming in to injure the eye, there are various types of eyeglasses and goggles which the athlete can wear for eye protection. Protection is the route to go in avoiding eye injuries.

Teeth Injuries

Definition and Causes Teeth injuries are any injuries which occur to the teeth as a result of a direct blow to the jaw or to the teeth themselves. In any case where there is a traumatic blow to this area, the athlete should be seen by a qualified dentist.

Treatment Detailed treatment for injuries to the teeth are outside the scope of this text, but referral to a dentist is mandatory.

Prevention Prevention of teeth and jaw injuries should be of concern to the athlete. In contact sports, face masks and jaw protection should be worn at all times. In addition, most athletes now wear some type of self-molding mouthguard that fits over the teeth very snugly in an attempt to prevent or reduce dental injuries that occur as a result of direct trauma to the teeth. Athletes should be encouraged to wear teeth and mouth guards at all times in contact sports. In many cases, it is wise to have rules which forbid the athlete from participating in a contact sport without wearing a proper mouth guard or teeth guard.

A new device, known as a Temporo Mandibular Jointsplint (TMJ) is suggested to aid certain athletes in the reduction of the number of jaw and teeth injuries. The proponents of this device explain that it also helps the athlete to relax during the competition, and, additionally, may provide more strength to the athlete. Tests to scientifically determine the worth of the TMJ in improving strength have not been performèd as of this date, so these claims remain conjecture at this point. However, the TMJ device may be of value in reducing the trauma which occurs when the athlete is hit in the jaw, teeth, or lower face. Other similar devices are referred to as mandibular orthopedic repositioning appliances (MORA). These are said to be helpful in reducing tension and stress in athletes who report jaw or head pain.

Ear and Nose Injuries

Cauliflower Ear

One type of injury to the ear is the blow or contusion to the area, which generally occurs in combat or contact sports. Boxing and wrestling are two common sports in which the participants are likely to get a "cauliflower" ear. An extreme contusion, friction, or wrenching of the ear leads to this condition of hematoma auris, commonly known as the cauliflower ear (Klafs & Arnheim, 1981). Most of the tissue of the outer ear is of a cartilaginous nature. Repeated trauma to the ear may cause hemorrhaging and fluid accumulation to this area, giving the appearance of the cauliflower ear. Initial treatment should be cold compression of the area. Very often, a physician may attempt to reduce the swelling by withdrawing some of the fluid that has built up in the area. The prevention is to wear properly fitted head gear or other protective device which covers the ears.

Swimmer's Ear

A second type of injury which occurs very often to the ear is ear infection in swimmers. Swimmer's ear results when certain microorganisms get into the ear and set up an infection. The athlete who is in a fatigued state because of severe training is more susceptible to these harmful organisms. If the athlete keeps the ear cleaned and washed properly before and after the workouts, this problem may be avoided.

Nose Injury

Whenever the athlete exposes himself to a combat sport, or a contact sport, there is likelihood of nose trauma. One of the common injuries to the nose is the nasal fracture as a result of a direct blow to the nose. This is most often recognized by deformity, swelling which will soon occur in the area, and, very often, bleeding from the nose itself. Treatment is to stop the bleeding as quickly as possible, and try to splint the nose so that the athlete may be transported to a physician for X-rays and further diagnosis. Applying slight pressure to the nose and tilting the head backwards is often enough to stop bleeding. ■

Summary

Chapter 13 covers specific, common, athletic injury problems and their treatment. Approximately fifty specific athletic injuries are detailed as to their causes, treatment and prevention.

References

Benas, D., & P. Jokl. 1978. Shin splints. *American Corrective Therapy Journal.* 32:53.

Brody, D. M. 1980. Running injuries. *Clinical Symposia.* 32:2.

Hlavac, H. F. 1980. *The foot book.* Mountain View, CA: World Publications.

Klafs, C. E., & D. D. Arnheim. 1981. *Modern principles of athletic training.* 5th ed. St. Louis: C. V. Mosby.

Nicholas, J. A. 1975. Risk factors, sports medicine, and the orthopedic system: an overview. *American Journal of Sports Medicine.* 3:248.

O'Donoghue, D. H. 1976. *Treatment of injuries to athletes.* 3rd ed. Philadelphia: W. B. Saunders Co.

Williams, J. 1976. Soft tissue injuries. *Physiotherapy.* 56:780.

Williams, J. G. P., & P. N. Sperryn. 1976. *Sports medicine.* Baltimore: Williams & Wilkins.

Other Topics Related to Sports Medicine

Part 5

Nutrition for Today's Athlete

Outline

14

Introduction

In top flight athletic competition, the difference between winning and placing may very often be measured in tenths, or even hundredths, of a second. The athlete who is striving for excellence attempts to gain every possible edge over the competition. One vital concern for the athlete interested in improving performance and maintaining a winning edge is the area of nutrition. Nutrition is the science of nourishing the body (Marine Corps, 1977).

This chapter is subdivided into five parts. In the first part, the basic nutrients (fats, proteins, carbohydrates, vitamins, minerals, and water) are discussed. Classes of nutrients, a discussion of foodstuffs, categories of vitamins and minerals, and water are included. In the second part, the current American diet is noted. Finally, a general list of topics dealing with athletic nutrition is covered. These general topics include:

The pre-game meal
Fluids for athletes
CHO loading
Food supplements (vitamins, minerals, iron, etc.)

In the second part of this chapter, the American Diet and the Athlete's Diet are looked at. Weight control and diet are examined next, including recommended body weights for children and adults, and a section on gaining and losing body weight.

The human body, like any other energy system, runs on fuel. The fuel for an automobile engine may be gasoline. In the human body, the fuel is food. Humans are not like plants that can convert sunlight and soil minerals directly into fuel. The human system must get its fuel from plant sources or from animals, who have eaten the plants. Today, humans are considered both herbivorous (plant-eating) and carnivorous (meat-eating). In fact, if one studies human eating habits in the percent of the population that is overweight in Western society one might think people are omnivorous, that is, they eat everything. This is like my friend who is on a seafood diet—he eats all the food that he sees! Actually, it is not bad if people eat food from a large variety of sources, since then they are most likely to include in their diets the nearly forty different nutrients needed to remain healthy. The key factor is to include quality, not necessarily quantity, in the diet.

Some definitions needed to understand this chapter follow.

Nutrition Nutrition is the science of nourishing the body.
Nutrients Nutrients are chemical substances in foods. They function to furnish the body with fuel, to build and repair body tissue, or to protect and regulate body processes.
Diet The diet consists of all food substances regularly consumed in the course of normal living, over a long period of time, aimed at a positive state of health.

In order to nourish the body, the individual must consume various foods which serve the body in several ways. One function of food is to furnish the body with fuel that provides energy for one's daily activities. A second function of food is to build and repair body tissue. Certain cells in our bodies (red blood cells and skin cells) are continually being replaced, while other cells (nerve and muscle) must survive throughout the entire lifetime of the individual. Therefore, the food that a person eats not only goes into building new cells, but into maintaining cells which are not replaced during one's life. A final function of food is to protect and regulate certain body processes. In order for proper metabolism (energy transformations) and other body functions to occur, certain regulators must be present. These substances (vitamins and minerals) are necessary, in small amounts, to all people.

Nutrients are typically divided into six classes. These are shown schematically in figure 14.1. The six classes of nutrients are carbohydrates, fats, proteins, vitamins, minerals, and water. The first three classifications provide the body with calories (energy which the body uses for its internal and external work). A **calorie** (large calorie or kilocalorie) is the amount of heat necessary to raise one kilogram of water one degree centigrade. Calories are units of energy. The final three nutrients do not provide any calories. A brief description of each of these six nutrient classes follows.

190

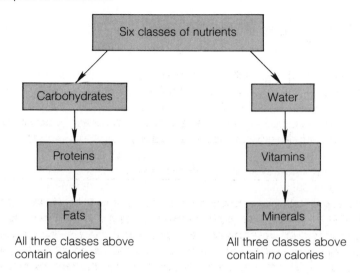

Figure 14.1 Six Classes of Nutrients.
Source: Bogert, L. J., G. M. Briggs, and D. H. Calloway. 1973. *Nutrition and physical fitness.* 9th ed. Philadelphia: W. B. Saunders.

Carbohydrates

These are the starches and sugars found in cereal grains, fruits, and vegetables, and the other sugars added to foods for sweetening. Carbohydrates are a major energy source for the body, especially during intensive exercise. Most unprocessed carbohydrates are rich in food fiber—that structural or fibrous part of plants that is essential to a healthy digestive system.

Fats

This nutrient adds flavor and variety to foods and makes foods taste good. Fats provide high energy (calories)—twice as much energy as proteins and carbohydrates do. Fats are mostly found in oils, fatty meats, butter, and other dairy products.

Proteins

After water and, perhaps fat, protein is the most plentiful substance in the body. Proteins are broken down in digestion to form amino acids, which are used by the body to repair and build body tissue. Major sources of protein are meats, poultry, fish, milk products, and eggs. Whole grain cereal products, beans, and nuts can also be good sources for protein.

The final three major nutrients provide no calories to the body, but they are, nevertheless, crucial to proper body functions.

Vitamins

These are chemical substances needed in small amounts by the body. They serve to regulate body processes.

Minerals

These are a nutrient class of chemical elements essential in small amounts for good health.

Water

This largest body component (about two-thirds or more of the body is water) is absolutely necessary to the body because it serves as a regulating substance in the body by holding other substances in solution in the digestive tract, blood, and tissues. Water, an essential nutrient, aids in regulating body temperature and other body functions.

The three nutrients named above (carbohydrates, fats, and proteins), which contribute calories, are often called foodstuffs. These common foodstuffs are examined in the next section in more detail. Specifically—what are they, what do they do in our bodies, and where can they be found in nature?

Carbohydrates

Carbohydrates may be subdivided into sugars, starches, and cellulose.

Sugars

The human body only uses carbohydrates for energy when they are in the form of simple sugars. Therefore, complex sugars and starches must be broken down by digestion into simple sugars before being used by the body. Some sources of both simple and complex sugars are refined sugars, syrups, fruits, milk, jams, and jellies.

Starches

This carbohydrate is formed by plants and consists mostly of seeds and roots. Before starches can be used by the body, they, too, must be digested into simple sugars. Most starch sources are breads, cereals, macaroni, cakes, pastries, peas, beans, and root vegetables (potatoes, carrots, etc.).

Cellulose

The fibrous, or structural, parts of fruits, vegetables, and whole grains is termed cellulose. This cellulose is undigestible residue which remains after the digestible portions of carbohydrates are absorbed into the system. Technically, cellulose is not a foodstuff, but, nonetheless, it serves a necessary regulatory function in the digestive process. Unprocessed vegetables, fruits, and whole grains are the major sources of cellulose.

There are several carbohydrate-rich foods. Unfortunately, most foods with a high carbohydrate content are refined carbohydrates. These are listed in table 14.1.

The best carbohydrates to eat are fresh
fruits, vegetables, and whole grains.

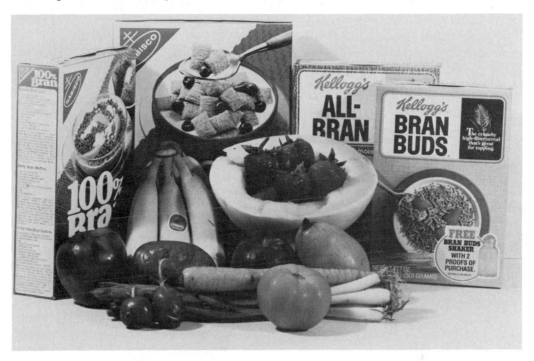

Table 14.1 Foods Rich in Refined Carbohydrates

Food	Percent of Carbohydrate
White table sugar	99+%
Dry cereals	55–75%
Cookies	65–75%
Chocolate cream candies	50–70%
Jams and jellies	71%
Dried fruits (raisins, prunes, apricots)	70%
Plain cake, with icing	62%
White bread	52%
Cooked rice, spaghetti, macaroni, and sweet potatoes	25–30%

Source: Marine Corps Institute. 1977. *Basic nutrition.* Washington, D.C.: Marine Barracks.

Fats

Fats, like carbohydrates, are composed of carbon, hydrogen, and oxygen. However, they contain twice the number of calories as an equal weight of carbohydrates (9 cal. per gram to 4 cal. per gram). Fats are found in the form of solids or liquids (generally oils). Fats are insoluble in and lighter than water. Therefore, cream (a milk fat) will rise to the surface on standing milk.

Fats may be saturated or unsaturated. Saturated fats are mainly animal fats, like butter, fatty meats, yolks of eggs, etc. These are not as easily digested as unsaturated fats.

Unsaturated fats are found mainly in vegetable oils and are liquid at room temperature. Unsaturated fats are generally easier to digest than saturated fats. One should try to include twice as many unsaturated fats as saturated fats in the diet.

Fats serve to provide a concentrated source of fuel in the diet and serve as carriers for fat soluble vitamins.

Some foods high in fats are listed in table 14.2.

Most fats are found in fatty meats, oils, and rich dairy products (cream, high-fat cheese, etc.).

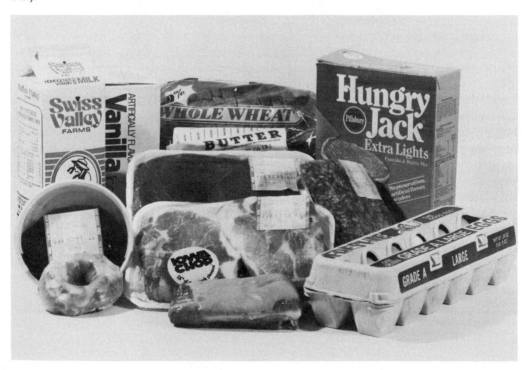

Chapter 14

Table 14.2 Foods Rich in Fats and Oils

Food	Percent of Fat
Lard and vegetable oils	100%
Butter and margarine	81%
Mayonnaise and salad dressing	78%
Walnuts	64%
Unsweetened chocolate	53%
Peanut butter	48%
Pork sausage	45%
American cheese	32%
Ice cream, plain to rich	12–23%
Pastries, doughnuts, cakes, pies, and cookies	6–21%

Source: Marine Corps Institute. 1977. *Basic nutrition.* Washington, D.C.: Marine Barracks.

Table 14.3 Foods Rich in Protein

Food	Percent of protein
Cooked meats and poultry	22–30%
Fried liver	23%
Cooked fish	19–25%
American, cheddar and cottage cheese	19–25%
Nuts	18%
Whole eggs	13%
Dry cereals	11%
Dried or cooked beans and peas	6%
Cooked cereals	2.5%

Source: Marine Corps Institute. 1977. *Basic nutrition.* Washington, D.C.: Marine Barracks.

Proteins

Proteins are larger, more complex molecules than either fats or carbohydrates. Proteins and their constituent parts, the amino acids, are essential to life. There are often twelve to eighteen different amino acids linked together to form protein molecules.

The body can manufacture some necessary proteins called nonessential proteins. However, some other amino acids are only found in certain foods and the body must receive these essential amino acids from good nutrient sources. As a general guide, animal protein, such as is found in meats, eggs, milk, and milk products (cheese, yogurt) will provide adequate (essential) amino acids.

Proteins function to build and nourish tissue growth in the body. They also regulate body processes and may be used as energy sources in rare (starvation) circumstances.

Some protein-rich foods are listed in table 14.3.

Excellent protein sources are low-fat dairy products, bean products, fish and poultry, and enriched pasta products.

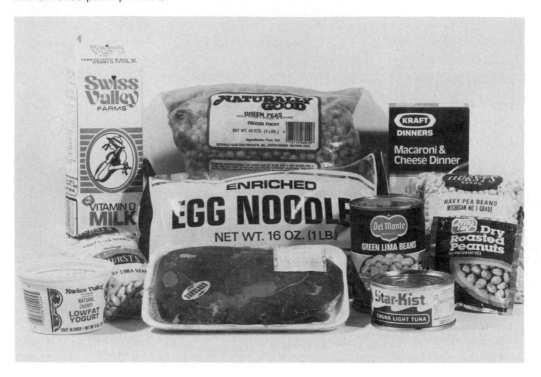

Vitamins

Vitamins are defined as organic compounds (other than the amino acids, fatty acids, or carbohydrates), which are necessary in small amounts in the diet of higher animals for normal growth, maintenance of health, and reproduction (Bogert, Briggs and Calloway, 1973). Thus far, about one dozen or more vitamins have been discovered. All animals may need vitamins, but not every vitamin that has been discovered is needed by all animals (e.g. choline is a vitamin for some animals, although no such need in humans has yet been discovered). A letter of the alphabet was assigned to each vitamin as it was discovered, starting with Vitamin A in 1913. Most vitamins have just recently been discovered and new scientific experiments are still uncovering the exact amounts of these tiny organic compounds which are necessary for proper metabolic functioning. Several additional points are worth noting concerning all vitamins: (1) the cell cannot synthesize these specific substances and, therefore, it must get them from ingested food or through vitamin supplements, and (2) vitamins provide no caloric or energy value to the diet.

Classes and Functions of Vitamins

Vitamins are divided into two classes depending on their solubility. Vitamins A, D, E, and K are the fat soluble vitamins, while the B complex and C vitamins are water soluble. Water soluble vitamins should be consumed daily in wholesome foods, since they are not stored long-term in the body. Fat soluble vitamins are stored in the body fat stores and, therefore, should not be taken in excess, since toxic effects may result if those particular fat soluble vitamins (A, D, E, and K) are allowed to build up in body tissues.

Vitamins perform varied functions in the human body. Many serve as essential links in the metabolic chain within cells. Others provide important regulating aspects to certain body processes, similar to the action of hormones. Each of the thirteen identified vitamins is presented in the next section in outline form. The major function of each vitamin in the body is discussed, followed by where that particular vitamin is found in the food chain. Possible deficiencies are then outlined. If the individual vitamin is crucial to athletic performance, this fact is noted. The recommended dietary allowance (NAS, 1980) for each is also given.

The Fat Soluble Vitamins

Vitamin A

This vitamin can come from two compounds in the diet: (1) animal sources only (liver)—which is Vitamin A, itself, or (2) both plant and animal foods, such as carotene—which can be changed by the body to Vitamin A.

Function. Vitamin A functions in the body to maintain mucous membranes. It also helps to maintain proper vision, especially dim or night vision. Vitamin A is necessary for body growth, teeth development, and general body vigor and stamina.

Sources for Vitamin A. Carotene is found in egg yolk, fish liver oils, butter, carrots, sweet potatoes, cantaloupe, and leafy green vegetables. Beef liver is the single best food source for this vitamin.

Deficiencies. Over time, a lack of vitamin A will lead to a stunting of growth, inability to see in dim light, diseased conditions of skin and body membranes, and abnormalities of teeth development.

RDA. 1000 μg for adult males, 800 μg for adult females and 400–700μg for children. The RDA is sometimes listed in international units (i.u.). Expressed this way, the RDA for men is 5000 i.u., for women, 4000 i.u., and for children 2000 to 3500 i.u.

Overdoses. Overdoses of this vitamin are likely to occur when ten times the normal amount is ingested (e.g. eating one pound of polar bear liver). Overdose symptoms in adults include dry, scaly, coarse skin, loss of hair, and cracked lips. Overdose symptoms in children include appetite loss, failure to grow, and severe itching. Death may result from an overdose of this vitamin.

Vitamin D

Function. This vitamin is required primarily for the body's proper utilization of calcium and phosphorus for making strong bones and teeth.

Sources for Vitamin D. This vitamin occurs in small amounts in many common foods. Liver, butter, eggs, fatty canned fish (tuna, salmon, and herring), and fortified milk are the best sources. Sunlight falling directly on the skin can produce vitamin D in the body.

Deficiencies. The most striking sign of deficiency is poor growth and lack of normal development of the bones and teeth. Rickets (a bone disease) is the most prominent disorder due to a lack of vitamin D.

RDA. 400 i.u.

Overdoses. Overdoses of this vitamin are likely to occur when ten times the normal amount is ingested. Death may result from an overdose.

Vitamin E

Function. This vitamin, discovered in 1922, is still very controversial. It is known that vitamin E is important in the body for its ability to unite with oxygen and thus protect red blood cells from certain blood-destroying agents. This antioxidant property protects other compounds (vitamin A and certain fatty acids) from the negative effects of oxidation. It is also essential for normal reproduction.

Sources for Vitamin E. The main sources for this vitamin are vegetable oils, leafy vegetables, butter and margarine, whole grains, liver, peas, and beans.

Deficiencies. Contrary to much popular literature, there is no convincing scientific evidence that vitamin E deficiency in humans causes reduced athletic performance, heart disease, weakened sex drive, or reduced longevity (Bogert, Briggs and Calloway, 1973). In fact, deficiencies in humans are quite rare because of the great distribution of this vitamin in common good foods. In test animals deprived of vitamin E, there have been reported cases of skeletal muscle weakness, abnormal growth, and reproductive problems in both males and females.

RDA. Not finalized at this time.

Vitamin K

Function. This last fat soluble vitamin was discovered in 1935. It is essential for the proper coagulation of blood, and normal functioning of the liver.

Sources for Vitamin K. The best dietary sources of this vitamin are green leafy vegetables, fruits, cereals, dairy products, and some meats. Some vitamin K can be produced by normal bacteria in the intestines.

Deficiencies. Because of the wide availability of this vitamin, deficiencies are rare. In some individuals who have problems absorbing fat, deficiencies of this vitamin could be manifested. However, since vitamin K can be synthesized in the intestine and is readily available in a variety of foods, deficiencies are not generally known. There is no exact RDA for this vitamin for the above listed reasons.

A final comment on the fat soluble vitamins (A, D, E, K) deserves mention again. They tend to build up in body fat tissues and overdoses of these substances can produce toxic effects, even death. Excessively high dosages of both vitamin A and D have been known to be poisonous to human infants, children, and adults. It is extremely unwise to suggest excessive dosages of these vitamins. While vitamin E and K excesses are not as widely reported as A and D, they are all fat soluble vitamins, so a potential hazard may exist with continued high doses.

The Water Soluble Vitamins

These particular vitamins make up the remaining group of vitamins known to man. They consist of the B complex and C vitamins. Although these vitamins can be stored in the body to some degree, most excesses are usually excreted, thus preventing the possibility of toxicity from overdoses, as with the fat soluble vitamins.

The discussion of water soluble vitamins is divided into two areas, the B complex vitamins and vitamin C. The three major B vitamins are thiamine (B_1), riboflavin (B_2), and niacin (B_3).

Thiamine (B_1)

Function. This first B vitamin is crucial in energy metabolism, especially metabolism of carbohydrates.

Sources. The best sources of thiamine are whole grains, enriched white bread, and rice. It is also found in pork, liver, peas, milk, oranges, and sweet potatoes. Thiamine is unstable in heat, so some of this vitamin may be lost in cooking, due to both the loss to heat and loss to the water.

Deficiencies. Severe deficiencies of thiamine involve the nervous and muscular systems, indicated by a feeling of extreme tiredness. The disease, beriberi, a clinical syndrome of neuritis, muscular weakness, heart problems, and edema, are results of a severe deficiency of thiamine.

RDA. From 1.0 to 1.5 mg.

Riboflavin (B_2)

Function. The function of riboflavin is to promote growth and to aid in proper carbohydrate metabolism.

Sources. Primary sources are milk and milk products. It is also found in liver, eggs, leafy vegetables, lean meats, beans, and peas. This vitamin is generally stable to heating.

Deficiencies. Improper metabolism of carbohydrates, as well as skin abnormalities, cracked and inflamed lips, mouth sores, and inflamed eyelids are all reported with riboflavin deficiencies.

Niacin (B_3)

Function. Like thiamine and riboflavin, niacin functions in carbohydrate metabolism. It also aids fat metabolism and tissue respiration.

Sources. Liver, lean meats, whole grains, nuts, peas, and beans are good sources of niacin. It is often added to enriched breads, rice, and flour.

Deficiencies. A lack of this vitamin may cause pellagra, a condition of skin lesions, inflamed mucous membranes, and faulty digestion.

RDA. 13 to 18 mg.

Lesser B Vitamins

Pyridoxine (B_6)

Function. This vitamin functions in amino acid metabolism.

Sources. Liver, muscle meats, some vegetables, and whole grains.

Deficiencies. Similar to the three main B vitamins, i.e., muscular weakness, nervous disorders, skin inflammation, general depression, and irritability.

RDA. 1.8 to 2.0 mg.

Pantothenic Acid

Function. This vitamin is essential to all metabolism.

Sources. Liver, kidney, meats, whole grains, legumes.

Deficiencies. Rare in humans.

RDA. None established.

Biotin, Folacin

Function. These two B vitamins function in growth and the formation of red blood cells, respectively. Both are essential to human nutrition.

Sources. As listed above for all the B vitamins.

Deficiencies. Since they are needed in the diet in such small amounts, deficiencies are highly unlikely.

Vitamin B₁₂

Function. This vitamin also functions in amino acid and fatty acid metabolism. Additionally, it is linked to the regeneration of folacin.

Sources. Liver, kidneys, muscle meats, cheese, eggs, green leafy vegetables, and whole grains.

Deficiencies. A deficiency may occur after some time in individuals on a strict vegetarian diet devoid of meat, eggs, and dairy products. Pernicious anemia, a blood disease marked by loss of red blood cells leading to muscular weakness, may occur with vitamin B₁₂ deficiency.

Vitamin C (Ascorbic Acid)

Function. This controversial vitamin functions in the body to hold cells together and in other complex, but poorly understood functions. It is believed to be involved in metabolism, leucocyte functions, absorption of iron, and the synthesis of epinephrine and anti-inflammatory steroids by the adrenal gland.

An excellent drink for athletes, orange juice provides vitamin C, vitamin A, some protein, and many important minerals.

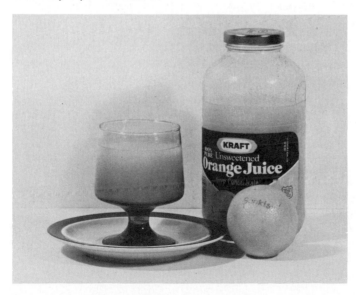

Sources. This vitamin is present in fresh citrus fruits, tomatoes, potatoes, and leafy vegetables. However, vitamin C is unstable in heat and easily destroyed by oxidation.

Deficiencies. A deficiency of vitamin C leads to scurvy, which is characterized by weakness, anemia, bleeding gums, and skin problems.

RDA. The recommended dietary allowances for this vitamin have changed since it was first isolated in 1928. Prior to 1980 the RDA for adults was about 45 mg. Now it has been raised to 60 mg. This may indicate that the American diet is deteriorating and we may need to consume more vitamin C.

Vitamin Supplements and the Athlete's Diet

There are two major classes of vitamins—fat soluble and water soluble. If the individual athlete is eating a variety of good foods, there is no reason to take any vitamin supplement. This assumes that athletes are choosing their foods from the four main food groups, and that they are eating as many unprocessed vegetables, fruits, and whole grains as possible. Extremely large dosages of the fat soluble vitamins may produce a toxicity in the individual, so it is unwise to ingest large amounts of them.

There have been many reports of people taking large doses of ascorbic acid (2 to 6 grams per day, or one hundred times the RDA). These large doses may be unwise due to their negative effects on the body. However, the athlete who is working out for one to two hours a day in hot weather may need additional vitamin C, since vitamin C is heat sensitive and some may be destroyed in the body by the extremely high internal temperatures created by long-term, vigorous exercise (for example, a ten mile run in the heat of summer). Therefore, if the athlete is not taking in large amounts of natural vitamin C, it might be wise to supplement the diet with small amounts (100 to 500 mg. daily) of this vitamin during these high temperature exercise stress periods. In fact, some authors (Bassler and Burger, 1979) note that a runner may take one gram of vitamin C for each six miles run. Since vitamin C is an acid, it may cause some gastric upset, so as a supplement, it should be taken with other food or drink. Any vitamin supplement should be taken with food, since most vitamins serve to increase the efficiency of body metabolism. It might also be wise to spread out the vitamin supplement dose over the course of a day, since large amounts tend to enter and exit the system rapidly. Because the B complex vitamins are so intimately involved in energy metabolism, many athletes take a small supplement of these vitamins during extremely stressful training or competitive schedules.

Minerals

Minerals are basic inorganic elements or compounds found in nature—in the soil, water, plants, and animals. Minerals are also found in our bodies in large amounts and are required in our diets in larger quantities than the "trace elements." Minerals serve several vital body functions: (1) they are essential components of cells, (2) they form parts of nails, bone, and teeth, (3) they regulate body processes, and (4) they play an important role in water metabolism and blood volume. Three major minerals have been identified. They are calcium, phosphorus, and magnesium.

Calcium and Phosphorus

Since calcium and phosphorus are closely associated in the body in the formation and maintenance of bones and teeth, these two minerals are often grouped together. Calcium, the mineral found in humans in the greatest quantity, is present mostly in the skeleton. Calcium is also necessary in the blood, and for normal blood clotting. It is also present in intra- and extra-cellular fluids and in muscle tissue.

Phosphorus, the second most abundant mineral, combines with calcium to form strong bones and teeth. It is also crucial in forming **adenosine triphosphate (ATP)** and **creatine phosphate (CP),** the high energy compounds necessary for muscle contraction. Phosphorus also combines with substances in the blood and aids energy metabolism.

Sources of Calcium and Phosphorus. Main sources include milk and dairy products, liver, fish, poultry, meats, leafy vegetables, eggs, and whole grains.

Deficiencies. A diet lacking in the above minerals leads to poor metabolism, poor nerve and muscle function, stunted growth and development, and poor quality bones and teeth.

Magnesium

This third major body mineral is similar in function to calcium and phosphorus in that it combines with them in bones to insure proper bone function. Magnesium also functions in carbohydrate metabolism and is important in normal neuromuscular functioning.

Sources of magnesium. Whole grains, nuts, beans, and green leafy vegetables.

RDA. The RDA for the three major minerals is from 300–400 mg. per day for magnesium, and 800–1200 mg. per day for calcium and phosphorus.

Trace Elements

There are roughly nine trace elements that have been identified as necessary in proper nutrition. These are labeled trace elements simply because they are necessary in the human diet in trace amounts—less than 100 mg. per day. These include iron, zinc, iodine, copper, manganese, fluorine, chromium, selenium, magnesium, silicon, and molybdenum.

Recently, much attention has been given to the three trace minerals of magnesium, chromium, and selenium. Table 14.4 outlines the minerals, possible functions, food sources where the minerals are found, and possible effects of deficiencies.

Of all the trace minerals, iron is the most important for the athlete, especially the female athlete. Studies (NAS, 1980; Bogert, Briggs and Calloway, 1973) indicate that between 10 and 25 percent of the total population may be iron deficient. Menstruating women seem to be most prominent in this group, since 15 mg. of iron may be lost per period. This

Table 14.4 Guide to Minerals

Mineral	Function	Food sources	Effects of deficiency
Calcium	Gives structure and strength to bones and teeth; assists in blood clotting; allows muscle contraction and relaxation and nerve transmission.	Milk and milk products, meat, fish, eggs, cereal products, beans, fruits, vegetables.	Nerve-muscle excitability; facial spasm; abnormal sensations of lips, tongue, fingers, feet; convulsions.
RDA	1000 mg. for men 800 mg. for women		
Chromium	Necessary for proper glucose metabolism.	Black pepper, calf liver, American cheese, wheat germ, brewer's yeast.	Diabetes (adult onset); atherosclerosis.
Copper	Acts as a component of many vital enzyme systems; assists with iron storage and its release to form red blood cells.	Seafood, meat, eggs, legumes, whole grain cereals, nuts, raisins.	Anemia.
RDA	2 mg. for men and women		
Fluorine	Incorporated in bones and teeth; helps protect against dental cavities; may help protect against osteoporosis, a bone-thinning disorder.	Seafood, tea, drinking water.	Increased dental cavities; possibly increased tendency to osteoporosis.
Iodine	Goes into the making of thyroid gland hormones, which help determine the body's metabolic rate or use of energy.	Seafoods, drinking water, iodized salt.	Thyroid gland enlargements (goiter).
RDA*	150 micrograms for men and women		
Iron	Acts as component of enzyme systems; aids energy utilization; combines with protein to form hemoglobin, the red blood cell pigment that transports oxygen.	Liver, red meat, beans, prunes, figs, dates, raisins, fish, oysters, enriched or whole grain products, and cereals.	Anemia; fatigue.
RDA**	10 mg. for men 18 mg. for women		

Source: The National Academy of Sciences. 1980. Recommended Dietary Allowances. 9th ed. Washington, D.C.

*1,000 micrograms = 1 milligram

**During menses and pregnancy, iron requirements may exceed 18 mg. daily and supplemental iron may be prescribed.

Note: RDAs are listed for only seven minerals by the NAS. The other six may be considered trace minerals.

Mineral	Function	Food sources	Effects of deficiency
Magnesium	Necessary for muscle and nerve function and various enzyme functions.	Black-eyed peas, buckwheat, whole wheat, leafy green vegetables, seafood, nuts, and fruit.	Insomnia; tension and anxiety; muscle twitches and tremors.
RDA	350 mg. for men 300 mg. for women		
Manganese	Enters into normal bone structure; forms part of many essential enzyme systems.	Whole grain cereals, green leafy vegetables.	No human deficiency reported.
Phosphorus	Combines with calcium to give strength to bones and teeth; enters into energy production.	Milk and milk products, meat, poultry, fish, eggs, whole grain cereals, legumes.	No human deficiency reported.
RDA	1200 mg. for men 800 mg. for women		
Potassium	Contributes to muscle contraction, nerve transmission, water and acid base balance in the body.	Whole and skim milk, bananas, prunes, raisins.	Heart rhythm disturbances; muscular weakness; muscle twitching.
Selenium	Aids in controlling blood pressure and associated problems of heart attacks, strokes, aneurysms.	Whole grain breads and flour, egg noodles, rice, seafoods, meats, liver, garlic, mushrooms, beer.	Cancer(?); high blood pressure(?)
Silicon	Maintains cellular structural integrity.	Alfalfa and cereal bran.	Arthritis(?); Poor tissue repair(?)
Zinc	Becomes part of insulin and a great number of enzyme systems involved in many activities in the body, including growth, reproduction, and wound healing.	Meat, liver, eggs, oysters, seafoods, milk, whole grain cereals.	Growth failure; impaired wound healing; skin disturbances; appetite impairment; taste and smell disturbances.
RDA	15 mg. for men and women		

iron loss may be exacerbated in a female athlete who is using an IUD, since menstrual iron loss appears to be greater in these individuals. Iron is necessary to prevent anemia, which is characterized by general fatigue, loss of appetite, and disinterest in training (Nickerson & Tripp, 1983).

Sources of Iron. Major iron sources include liver, vegetables, dried, uncooked fruits, organ meats, egg yolk, and shell fish.

RDA. Children need about 10–15 mg. of iron per day, while adult males need 10–18 mg., and adult females need 18 mg. or more per day. Pregnant or lactating women may need much more.

The other trace elements are furnished in a diet which includes large amounts of unprocessed fruits and vegetables, whole grains, meat, milk, and egg products.

Water and Electrolytes

Water and electrolytes are the other main nutrients to be discussed. Water accounts for 60 to 75 percent of body weight, depending on age and percent of body fat. It provides a medium for many chemical processes in the body. A person needs between six and twelve glasses of water per day, in addition to water obtained in various foods. Athletes who sweat a great deal in their workouts may need more than a dozen glasses of water per day. More about water will be discussed in the dehydration section.

Major Electrolytes: Sodium, Potassium, and Chloride

Sodium and potassium are the major cations (positively charged ions) found in the body. Sodium and potassium electrolytes, so named because they exist in the body as electrically charged particles called ions, are found in the extra-cellular fluid and intra-cellular fluid, respectively. The major function of electrolytes is to control fluid exchange within various fluid compartments of the body. When the body sweats a great deal in vigorous exercise, it loses electrolytes in the sweat. This may retard optimal body functioning and lead to fatigue, muscle cramps, or other body impairments.

Sodium is found in most foods (see table 14.5) and does not need to be added to the American diet. In fact, there are risks to large sodium intakes because they serve to raise blood pressure and predispose one to heart disease and strokes. It has been calculated that the body can get along nicely on 200 mg. of sodium a day, although, in reality, humans may consume 4,000 –12,000 mg. per day.

Potassium is found in many foods, but is widely distributed in meat, milk, and fruits. Beer is an additional source of potassium.

Chloride is the last electrolyte to be discussed and it is an anion found in the extra-cellular fluid. It is a necessary component of gastric juice (it forms hydrochloric acid) and is provided almost entirely in the diet by sodium chloride. Other sources of chloride are milk and commercial salt substitutes.

Table 14.5 Sodium Content in Common American Foods

Typical food	Average sodium content (mg.)	Variations			
Apple	2	Applesauce (1 cup)	6	Apple pie (1 slice, froz.)	208
Bread (1 slice, white)	114	Pound cake (1 slice)	171	English muffin	293
Butter (1 tbsp., unsalted)	2	Butter (1 tbsp., salted)	116	Margarine (1 tbsp.)	140
Chicken (1/2 breast)	69	Chicken pie (frozen)	907	Chicken dinner (fast food)	2243
Corn	1	Corn flakes (1 cup)	256	Canned corn (1 cup)	384
Cucumber (7 slices)	2	Cucumber (w/ salad dressing)	234	Dill pickle	928
Grapes (10 seedless)	1	Grape jelly (1 tbsp.)	3	White wine (4 oz. domestic)	19
Lemon	1	Soy sauce (1 tbsp.)	1029	Salt (1 tsp.)	1938
Milk (1 cup)	122	Dry milk (l/2 cup)	322	Cottage cheese (4 oz.)	457
Pork (3 oz.)	59	Bacon (4 slices)	548	Ham (3 oz.)	1114
Potato	5	Potato chips (10)	200	Instant mashed (1 cup)	485
Steak (3 oz.)	55	Jumbo burger (fast food)	990	Meat loaf (frozen dinner)	1304
Tomato	14	Tomato soup (1 cup)	932	Tomato sauce (1 cup)	1498
Tuna (3 oz.)	50	Canned tuna (3 oz., oil-packed)	384	Tuna pot pie (frozen)	715
Water (8 oz., tap)	12	Club soda (8 oz.)	39	Antacid (in water)	564

Source: Brody, Jane. 1981. *Jane Brody's Nutrition Book*. New York: W. W. Norton & Co.

The American Diet

Diseases Caused by American Diet

The American diet has been implicated in a number of diseases and other degenerative processes. Some of these conditions are:

cardiovascular disease
cancer of breast and prostate
atherosclerosis
cerebrovascular disease (stroke)
diabetes

gout
arterial hypertension
obesity
intermittent claudication
dental caries

constipation	cancer of colon and rectum
varicose veins	appendicitis
gallstones	hiatus hernia

and possibly others (Pritikin, 1979; USDA, 1980; NAS, 1980; DHEW, 1979).

Dietary Guidelines

Due to these relationships between diet and degenerative disease, the USDA (1980) established seven "Dietary Guidelines for Americans." These seven guidelines designed to improve the nutrition and health of the American people are:

1. Eat a variety of foods.
2. Maintain ideal weight.
3. Avoid too much fat and cholesterol.
4. Eat foods with starch and fiber.
5. Avoid too much sugar.
6. Avoid too much alcohol.
7. Avoid too much sodium.

These guidelines provide the basis for a sound nutrition program for the general American, as well as for the American athlete.

Percentages of Fat, Protein, and Carbohydrate in the Diet

Current dietary intake patterns in the U.S. show the following percentages of foodstuffs supplying energy in the diet (NAS, 1980).

fat	42% of dietary energy
protein	12% of dietary energy
carbohydrate	46% of dietary energy
	100%

When the percentage of fat calories contributes such a high proportion of total calories in the diet, the diseases and degenerative conditions noted occur more often in the American population. What can be done to change this?

The Recommended American Diet

Following the dietary suggestions noted previously, one can lower the percent fat in the diet, while at the same time raising complex carbohydrates. Such a modification might look as follows:

fat	32–37% of total calories (a reduction of 5–10%)
protein	12–15% of total calories (little or no change)
carbohydrate	56% of total calories (an increase of 5–10%)

This modification of the diet will reduce fat, while increasing carbohydrate intake. The carbohydrate intake should be *complex carbohydrates* (fruits, vegetables, and whole grains). It is difficult to manipulate the protein intake in the diet, other than by artificial means. A more severe modification in the diet is to restrict fat intake to an even greater extent. One could call this new diet the American athlete's diet.

The American Athlete's Diet

fat	20–30% of total calories
protein	12–15% of total calories
carbohydrate	68–55% of total calories

Since the athlete engaging in vigorous total body exercise uses muscle glycogen, glucose, and fat for fuel, it may make sense to increase the total percent of carbohydrate in the diet. In intense physical activity at 85 to 95 percent of maximal output, carbohydrates supply the energy for intense muscular contraction. Therefore, this American Athlete's Diet recommends including 55–70 percent of the total calories from complex carbohydrates (Locksley, 1980; McArdle, Katch, & Katch, 1981).

The Pritikin Diet Plan

One final modification of the diet has been proposed by a group of California researchers (Pritikin, 1979). They have been studying a group of older people who have severe medical problems. These people were admitted to the Longevity Institute and were placed under strict medical supervision. These individuals were placed on the following diet:

fat	10% of the total calories (two-thirds of these fat calories are of the unsaturated variety)
protein	10% of total calories
carbohydrate	80% of total calories (carbohydrate calories of the complex variety—no refined sugars, etc.)

This final dietary modification is *quite severe* and *should only be attempted under strict medical supervision,* such as when a person is admitted to a hospital or an institute. However, it must also be noted that when the above dietary program is combined with an exercise program, patients have markedly improved their total health (Horton, 1982).

In summary, as fats are lowered in the diet, the athlete should increase intake of good carbohydrates (whole grains, vegetables, and fruits). As this dietary modification is followed, the athlete can choose among excellent food sources for his/her increased energy expenditure and also stands to take in more vitamins and minerals in these wholesome unprocessed foods.

Figure 14.2 Relationship Between Energy Intake and Energy Expenditure. If the total caloric intake equals the total energy expenditure, including the basal metabolic rate (BMR), then weight remains stable. If an imbalance is created, weight gain or loss results.

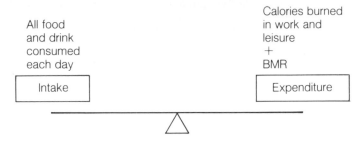

Weight Control and Diet

The healthy body needs energy for various metabolic processes. Food (calories) must be constantly supplied to provide for growth and maintenance of body tissues, as well as to maintain body temperature. A calorie is a unit of heat used to express the energy value of food. The largest single expenditure of calories in the body is to maintain the body's vital functions at resting (basal) conditions. This is termed the *basal metabolic rate* (BMR). The BMR is that necessary resting metabolism which is required for cardiovascular function, respiration, and other ongoing body functions. The BMR is highly dependent on sex, body size, and age. As energy expenditure increases during daily activities, such as working, going to school, or in sport activities, calorie intake must also increase.

The fundamental law of nature regarding body weight states that maintaining desirable body weight is achieved through a balance of energy intake (food) and energy output. Growing youngsters participating in sports may need extra food to provide energy for their daily energy expenditure and to account for their individual growth. The adult must make certain that food intake from all sources (alcohol included, since alcohol furnishes 7 calories/gram) equals energy expended. If there is an imbalance (see figure 14.2), the person will begin to gain or lose weight. Table 14.6 shows the energy expenditures of some examples of human activities. Note that one has to engage in very heavy activities, like running, swimming, or walking uphill to significantly increase caloric expenditure. Running or walking one mile will burn about one hundred calories. The obvious value to the runner is that these one hundred calories are burned in a shorter period of time. Also, some extra calories are burned off in the rest phase after the mile run, since body temperature and overall metabolism may be raised in the runner. This is not likely to occur in the person who takes a leisurely stroll.

Table 14.6 Average Daily Energy Expenditures of Women and Men in Light Occupations

Activity category	Time (hr)	Man, 70 kg		Woman, 58 kg	
		Rate (kcal/min)	Total kcal (kj)	Rate (kcal/min)	Total kcal (kj)
Sleeping, reclining.	8	1.0–1.2	540(2270)	0.9–1.1	440(1850)
Very light Seated and standing activities, painting trades, auto and truck driving, laboratory work, typing, playing musical instruments, sewing, ironing.	12	up to 2.5	1300(5460)	up to 2.0	900(3780)
Light Walking on level at 2.5–3 mph, tailoring, pressing, garage work, electrical trades, carpentry, restaurant trades, cannery work, washing clothes, shopping with light load, golf, sailing, table tennis, volleyball.	3	2.5–4.9	600(2520)	2.0–3.9	450(1890)
Moderate Walking at 3.5–4 mph, plastering, weeding and hoeing, loading and stacking bales, scrubbing floors, shopping with heavy load, cycling, skiing, tennis, dancing.	1	5.0–7.4	300(1260)	4.0–5.9	240(1010)
Heavy Walking with load uphill, tree felling, work with pick and shovel, basketball, swimming, climbing, football, running.	0	7.5–12.0		6.0–10.0	
TOTAL	24		2740(11,500)		2030(8530)

Source: Durnin, J. V. G. A., & R. Passmore, 1967. *Energy, work, and leisure*. London: Heinemann Educational Books.

Maintaining Desirable Weight for Adults and Children

For an adult to maintain desirable weight (see table 14.7), constant attention to detail is necessary. Looking up recommended weights on a height/weight table, one is likely to see ranges of body weight listed. The reason for this is that most people have different body types. An easy way to ascertain your own body type is to try to place the thumb and middle finger of your right hand around your left wrist. If both of these fingers merely touch, you are of average bone size or body type. If your thumb and middle finger do not touch, you are of large frame. If these two fingers overlap slightly, you are of small frame.

Table 14.7 Desirable Weight Ranges for Adults

Height[a]		Men			Women		
in.	cm.	lb.		kg.	lb.		kg.
58	147	———		———	102	(92–119)	46	(42–54)
60	152	———		———	107	(96–125)	49	(44–57)
62	158	123	(112–141)	56	(51–64)	113	(102–131)	51	(46–59)
64	163	130	(118–148)	59	(54–67)	120	(108–138)	55	(49–63)
66	168	136	(124–156)	62	(56–71)	128	(114–146)	58	(52–66)
68	173	145	(132–166)	66	(60–75)	136	(122–154)	62	(55–70)
70	178	154	(140–174)	70	(64–79)	144	(130–163)	65	(59–74)
72	183	162	(148–184)	74	(67–84)	152	(138–173)	69	(63–79)
74	188	171	(156–194)	78	(71–88)	———		———
76	193	181	(164–204)	82	(74–93)	———		———

Source: Bray, G. A. ed. 1975 *Obesity in Perspective* vol. 2. U.S. Department of Health, Education, and Welfare. Publication No. (NIH) 75–708.
[a]Without shoes.
[b]Without clothes. Average weight ranges in parentheses.

Recommended Body Weight for Children

Since individual variability also manifests itself in children's height/weight tables, the data in table 14.8 are merely suggestive guidelines. Please note the ever increasing energy needs from age three until maturation. It is extremely important that the young athlete include quality and quantity in the diet to continue to grow optimally, and to achieve maximum performance in athletic competition. This good diet may be difficult for parents to follow, especially if the child is off to early morning dance or swim practice. However, by providing excellent snack materials such as fruits, vegetables, seeds and nuts, the parents may feel more at ease knowing their youngster is getting a wholesome variety in the diet.

Gaining and Losing Weight

Gaining Weight

The problem of weight gain in athletics is not as great as weight loss, but it still rates some concern for the underweight adolescent trying out for the football, hockey, lacrosse, or basketball team. In these sports, body size may be a definite advantage. The wisest advice any coach or team physician can give to the growing athlete who wants to gain weight is to *eat often* and to eat foods high in calories. Of course, the athlete must continue to

Table 14.8 Mean Heights and Weights and Recommended Energy Intake

Category	Age (years)	Weight (kg)	Weight (lb)	Height (cm)	Height (in.)	Energy needs (with range) (kc 1)		(MJ)
Infants	0–.5	6	13	60	24	kg x 115	(95–145)	kg x .48
	5–1	9	20	71	28	kg x 105	(80–135)	kg x .44
Children	1–3	13	29	90	35	1300	(900–1800)	5.5
	4–6	20	44	112	44	1700	(1300–2300)	7.1
	7–10	28	62	132	52	2400	(1650–3300)	10.1
Males	11–14	45	99	157	62	2700	(2000–3700)	11.3
	15–18	66	145	176	69	2800	(2100–3900)	11.8
	19–22	70	154	177	70	2900	(2500–3300)	12.2
	23–50	70	154	178	70	2700	(2300–3100)	11.3
	51–75	70	154	178	70	2050	(1650–2450)	8.6
Females	11–14	46	101	157	62	2200	(1500–3000)	9.2
	15–18	55	120	163	64	2100	(1200–3000)	8.8
	19–22	55	120	163	64	2100	(1700–2500)	8.8
	23–50	55	120	163	64	2000	(1600–2400)	8.4
	51–75	55	120	163	64	1800	(1400–2200)	7.6
	76+	55	120	163	64	1600	(1200–2000)	6.7
Pregnancy						+300		
Lactation						+500		

Source: National Academy of Sciences, National Research Council. 1980. Recommended Dietary Allowances 9th ed.

Note: The data in this table have been assembled from the observed median heights and weights of children, together with desirable weights for adults, mean height of 70 in. for men, and 64 in. for women, between the ages of 18 and 34 years as surveyed in the U.S. population (HEW/NCHS data).

work out so that the weight gain will be a gain in lean muscle tissue. In many cases, sport training may consume an additional one thousand to three thousand calories per day. Two additional cautions are suggested here: (1) the athlete who has a family history of heart disease and has abnormal levels of plasma lipids should be medically evaluated, and (2) the athlete should not consume more than one thousand to fifteen hundred excess calories per day (Smith, 1976). It is vitally important that the athlete count all calories and recall that an excess of thirty-five hundred calories indicates one extra pound of body weight as fat. The main goal of the young athlete is to gain lean muscle mass, not merely body weight. Programs of heavy resistance training for strength gains are given in another chapter. Table 14.9 gives a sample high calorie diet intended to provide approximately six thousand or more calories for the young athlete intent on gaining weight. Since dried fruits (raisins, dates, etc.), nuts of all types, and seeds are easily carried by the athlete, it is suggested that the young athlete continually have them available. These foods are high in nutritional value, as well as caloric value, and should help any athlete gain weight.

Table 14.9 Sample 6000 Calorie Diet for Gaining Weight

Breakfast	Calories	Snack	Calories
1 orange	40	banana or apple	85
1 cup granola	400	1 cup orange juice	45
2 slices whole wheat toast	289	handful of nuts	600
2 tsp. butter	250	(almonds, peanuts, walnuts, etc.)	
2 tsp. jam	272		
2 scrambled eggs	173		
Lunch		**Snack**	
green salad w/ dressing	250	milkshake	250
ham & cheese on rye sandwich	550	canteloupe	30
		nuts	280
Dinner		**Snack**	
baked potato w/ skin & butter	200	sesame seeds	563
carrots	35	sunflower seeds	560
beans	25	soybeans	400
tuna fish	127	ice cream w/ granola	350
1 cup ice milk w/ strawberries	240	Total calories–snacks	3163
Total calories—meals	**2851**	**Daily total calories**	**6014**

One final warning is given. Under *no* circumstances should the athlete use **anabolic steroids** or similar drug substances in an attempt to gain weight. Anabolic steroids can produce cancer and malfunction of the liver and reproductive organs, cause acne, and even lead to diminished overall growth in the athlete (ACSM, 1977).

Losing Weight

For most athletes, losing weight is more of a problem than gaining weight. However, the major consideration is still the equation that was presented earlier in this chapter—energy intake must equal energy expenditure. If energy intake (in the form of food) exceeds energy expenditure, then weight gain will result. The best way to lose weight is to increase energy expenditure, as well as curtail caloric intake. This has been found to be the most expedient way to lose weight (Hanson, et al., 1967).

The largest single expenditure of calories per day is the basal metabolic rate. This was described earlier as that resting rate of energy metabolism which is required to maintain body functions. A general guideline to use in computing the basal metabolic rate is that each person burns one calorie per kilogram per hour. In a 70 kg. person, the basal metabolic rate is calculated to be 70 x 24, or 1680 calories per day. Another general guideline for computing the basal metabolic rate is to take the body weight in pounds and add a zero to the end. For example, in a 125 lb. person, the basal metabolic rate might be *predicted* to be 1,250 calories.

Table 14.10 Contrasting Body Composition

	Subject A (Male age 40)	Subject B (Male age 40)
Height	73 in.	73 in.
Weight	227 lbs.	227 lbs.
Lean body weight	193.2 lbs.	168.4 lbs.
Fat weight	33.8 lbs.	58.6 lbs.
Percent fat[a]	14.9%	25.8%
Suggested weight[b]	189 lbs.	189 lbs.
Recommended weight loss	38 lbs.	38 lbs.
True weight loss objective	0	27–30 lbs.

NOTE: It is important to determine body composition first, then weight loss objective. Somatotype must also be considered.

[a]15 percent body fat is normal.

[b]Bray, 1975.

The basal metabolic rate, as we have noted earlier, is the largest single energy expenditure per day. The person who is more active, will burn off more calories. An energy expenditure of about two hundred to three hundred calories per day (walking or jogging for two or three miles) would be sufficient to effect a weight loss over a period of time. A weight loss of one pound of fat would be effected, if the individual creates a deficit of thirty-five hundred calories per week. This thirty-five hundred calories can be manipulated in any way. Either the individual can increase the energy expenditure by three hundred to five hundred calories per day, or decrease the caloric intake by three hundred to five hundred calories per day. However, the most expedient weight loss regime is to both expend calories via exercise, and decrease the total caloric intake slightly.

Body Composition As It Relates to Weight Loss

Unless one determines the actual lean mass or fat mass in an individual, it is difficult to predict body fatness. Table 14.10 shows the body composition table of two male subjects, of the same age, height, and weight. However, the lean body weight of Subject A is 193.2 pounds. The lean body weight of Subject B is 168.4 pounds. Therefore, the fat percent is 14.9 and 25.8 respectively. If 15 percent body fat in the 40-year-old male is normal, then Subject A does not need to lose any weight, and the true weight loss objective is zero. Subject B, who has 25.8 percent body fat, needs to make a significant weight reduction in the vicinity of thirty pounds to get to the 15 percent body fat.

Initial changes in body weight may be due to water loss. This can be seen in table 14.11, which shows the approximate water percentages in either fat or lean muscle tissue. In an exercise and diet program for weight control, a person may not initially show any weight change, although lean body mass may be changing. This is because there is a large water component in lean (muscle) tissue. Muscle tissue has about 70 to 72 percent water by weight.

Table 14.11 Approximate Water Percentages in Either Fat or Lean Muscle Tissue

Type of Tissue	Protein Component	Lipid Component	Water Component
Muscle (Skeletal)	20–22%	6–8%	70–72%
Fat	6–8 %	72%	20–22%

Food is a source of energy. As such, it can neither be created nor destroyed. Food as energy must be converted in the body through exercise, or it will be stored as fat. It does not matter when calories are ingested. They may be taken in the evening or at mid-day, but all ingested calories must be consumed within the body or stored as fat. Therefore, *physical activity* of the body is stressed in losing fat weight.

Water is the most abundant body constituent, since it may account for about one-half to three-fourths of the total body weight. Age, sex, and body fat percent are major factors which influence this body water component. For example, a person who has 193 pounds out of 227 that are lean muscle mass will have significantly more water than a person also weighing 227 pounds, but only having 168 pounds of lean tissue. The reasons for this are the various components of fat and muscle tissue. Muscle tissue contains a much greater water component than fat or lipid tissue.

Carbohydrate Loading

The use of dietary manipulation has always been a concern for athletes. It is reported that athletes in early times consumed enormous amounts of red meats or drank blood in the hope of making themselves stronger or improving their athletic performance. Even today, many fads and fallacies exist in the area of proper nutrition for the athlete.

A popular topic of discussion today in dietary manipulation involves the **carbohydrate loading** technique. Exactly what does this regimen entail? What are the pros and cons of dietary carbohydrate manipulation and, specifically, how is it practiced in all concerns of the endurance athlete? These questions will be answered in the following section.

Many early studies involving energy metabolism during physical exercise were done by Scandinavian researchers intent on studying both normal and pathological human metabolism. With the discovery of the muscle biopsy technique for muscle sampling (a needle is introduced into a muscle and a tiny slice of muscle tissue is withdrawn for further laboratory study), scientists can tell us whether fats or carbohydrates are the primary source of energy for muscle work.

Essentially, a person at rest burns slightly more fat than carbohydrate, but when that same person becomes active in physical exercise, the skeletal muscles burn mostly carbohydrates (stored glycogen). Very little fat burns at high intensities of exercise. Refer back to the earlier section on durations of human activity to more fully understand this concept. Since mostly carbohydrate is used both in short, all-out bursts of activity, as well as in physical activity sustained at 75 to 95 percent of maximum for longer periods, it is essential that the athlete have large amounts of carbohydrates stored in the skeletal muscles prior to beginning exercise.

Figure 14.3 CHO Loading Scheme. In this diet manipulation and training strategy, the first three to five days are depletion of CHO days. Workouts are heavy to moderate. The three days before the endurance event are loading days—*high carbohydrates, low calories, tapering-off* of workouts.

Source: Morris, A. F. 1981. Carbohydrate loading procedures. *The Physician and Sportsmedicine*. 9:13.

Diet	↓ CHO ↔ Cal	↓ CHO ↔ Cal	↓ CHO ↔ Cal	↑ CHO ↔ Cal	↑ CHO ↓ Cal	↑ CHO ↓ Cal	Little or no CHO
Training level	Heavy	Hard	Moderate	Moderate	Mild	Little or None	Race or Event

Two Swedish medical researchers (Bergstrom & Hultman, 1972) determined that, if the athlete works at a high percent (near 70 percent or above) of maximum for about seventy to ninety minutes, they deplete nearly all muscle glycogen (a carbohydrate) in the skeletal muscles that were active in the exercise. If the athlete continues moderate workouts, while consuming a diet low in carbohydrates for two or three more days, their muscle carbohydrate stores remain very low. Immediately following this depletion phase, if the athlete consumes a high carbohydrate diet, then the skeletal muscles are able to "bind" more carbohydrate to the fibers and, therefore, the muscle fibers are super-saturated with glycogen. They have been found to hold two or more times the normal amounts of carbohydrate. The athlete who is able to begin an endurance event in this super-saturated phase, theoretically would be able to perform better. Slovic (1975) showed a "swing" of from thirty-six seconds to about eight minutes in a summer marathon race run in Oregon.

The entire carbohydrate loading scheme is shown in figure 14.3. It shows that a depletion phase of 2 to 3 days is necessary before loading begins. It is important to load immediately (within hours) of the last depletion effort. And finally, workouts should be curtailed prior to exhaustive endurance events. There are several important considerations to note in carbohydrate loading.

Carbohydrate loading should only be practiced for endurance events lasting ninety minutes or longer. One does not have to load for a bowling or golf tournament.
It is important to eat *some* carbohydrates during the depletion phase. The brain works mostly on carbohydrates.
Workouts may be difficult during depletion phase, since the body is nearly out of carbohydrates.
Water should be consumed liberally throughout the entire period.
When the athlete switches to high carbohydrates, total *overall calories* should be low, since workouts are generally mild or moderate.

The body's skeletal muscles store more water with glycogen loading, hence, a
feeling of heaviness, stiffness or weight gain may be experienced.

Dietary manipulation may be a psychologically positive thing to occur during the final
week of preparation before a major event.

The first time an athlete tries to carbohydrate load, a modified scheme may be tried
(using only one depletion workout or cutting back less severely in carbohydrate
depletion).

Finally, as with most things in sports, the effects of carbohydrate manipulation seem
to be individual in nature. Some people seem to gain more beneficial effects than
others. Like anything else, try a gradual modification of the routine, then build up
to the total six to seven day program (Morris, 1981).

Proper Hydration

It is often said that only heat and dehydration can kill a trained athlete. This is a true
statement. Unfortunately, it was not too long ago that football and other coaches withheld
fluids from athletes working in the heat, and in some cases, athletes died as a result. Some
authorities note (Costill, 1979) that a loss of only 3 percent of body weight through sweating can adversely affect performance. It is too late during an athletic event to begin drinking when one is thirsty, because the thirst mechanism lags behind the body's need for
water.

What can one do to be certain to be properly hydrated for an athletic contest? It's
simple—drink lots of water. If one exercises a great deal in a hot, humid environment one
needs to drink almost continually. There are three good guidelines to use to tell if an athlete
is properly hydrated. These are that the athlete continually feels the need to urinate; that
when the athletes urinate, they pass large volumes of urine; and finally, the urine is mostly
clear. To get to this state, the athlete must drink continually.

Proper Athletic Drinks

The best athletic drink during a contest is probably cold water. Studies done at Ball State
University (Costill, 1979) seem to indicate that cold water (about 39°F) seems to leave the
stomach and get into the system more rapidly than warmer water or drinks with a high
concentration of sugar. Most commercially prepared drinks (Gatorade, ERG, Body Punch,
etc.) are all too high in sugar content, which inhibits stomach emptying. These should
generally be avoided during a game or contest. As a post-event fluid replacement, these
drinks are adequate.

The Pre-Game Meal

A lot of tradition surrounds the pre-game meal. Many coaches like to assemble the team
together and eat privately as a unit before a game. Some coaches still have a traditional
meat, eggs, and potatoes meal before the contest. However, except for the potatoes, this
meal is simply not complementary to a good athletic performance. Since carbohydrates
are the prime fuel for muscular activity, the pre-game meal should be rich in easily-digested carbohydrates.

The athlete should eat a small meal at least three hours prior to the start of the contest. Individual variability is a prime consideration. Some athletes have favorite, easily-digested, good carbohydrates (vegetables, fruits, and whole grains) and these should be eaten as their pre-game meal. Fruit or vegetable juices will provide more of the vitamins and minerals that all athletes need. Milk, if tolerated by the individual athlete, should be OK. Since fats and protein are generally found together in foods, and they take longer to digest, they are not recommended as part of a sound pre-game meal. The athlete should not experiment with new foods prior to any contest.

Liquid Meals

Often, when the athlete is forced to travel some distances on a bus to play a game, the pre-game meal may be difficult or impossible. In these cases, several companies prepare liquid meals that are quite tasty and nutritious for the athlete. Again, individual taste should dictate which particular drink is consumed. A liquid meal containing mostly carbohydrate calories should be best, especially if it has some minerals and vitamins added. Fruits, such as bananas, raisins, oranges, apples, etc., can be taken aboard a bus and consumed as the athlete travels to the athletic contest. Again, do not experiment prior to a game or contest. Try different foods and combinations prior to practices or workouts, then stick with something that works for you. If in doubt about a particular food, *don't* eat it; if in doubt about eating, don't eat until after the game. You can enjoy the food then. Any post-game food is OK, as long as you like it. ■

Summary

This chapter discusses the major areas of diet and nutrition and how they affect and relate to athletic performance. A listing of the six nutrients is given. Those nutrients include fats, carbohydrates, protein, minerals, vitamins, and water.

The next section of this chapter concerns the American diet. The American diet, consumed by the typical person in North America, is high in fat, high in refined sugar and salt, and low in fiber. This may lead to many problems in the cardiovascular system, as well as other areas. Modifications to this diet are suggested. Finally, a section on the athlete's diet is given. Essentially, the athlete's diet should be high in complex carbohydrates, with about 12 to 15 percent of the calories in the diet coming from protein, and approximately twice the percentage of calories coming from fat.

Other areas covered in this chapter are the pre-game meal, weight control, and carbohydrate loading. The pre-game meal should be eaten at least three to four hours prior to the event. Individual preferences and individual differences, in terms of the types and amounts of foodstuffs, have to be carefully monitored through trial and error experience, as the athlete attempts to determine the best pre-game meal. Carbohydrate loading involves a seven day regimen, with approximately three days of depletion; that is, a low carbohydrate diet with intense to moderate activity, followed by a three day carbohydrate loading regime in which the physical activity begins to taper off to a day or two of rest before the event. The calories during this period are very high in carbohydrates, but the total caloric content of the diet is average or low, since the workout schedule is reduced during the three days of carbohydrate loading.

As regards weight control, the individual must consider total caloric intake versus total caloric expenditure. If there is an imbalance in this equation, there will be either weight gain or weight loss. The most efficient and effective way to lose weight in a healthful fashion is to gradually decrease the intake of calories, while at the same time, gradually increasing the expenditure of calories, through an intelligent, well-planned endurance conditioning program.

References

American College of Sports Medicine. 1977. The use and abuse of anabolic-androgenic steroids in sports (Position Statement). *Medicine and Science in Sports*. 9.

Bassler, T. J., & R. E. Burger. 1979. *The whole life diet*. New York: M. Evans & Co.

Bergstrom, J., & E. Hultman. 1972. Nutrition for maximal sports performance. *The Journal of the American Medical Association*. 221:999.

Bogert, L. J., G. M. Briggs, & D. H. Calloway. 1973. *Nutrition and physical fitness*. 9th ed. Philadelphia: W. B. Saunders Co.

Bray, G. A. ed. 1975. *Obesity in perspective*, vol. 2. DHEW Publication No. (NIH) 75–708. Washington, D.C.: U.S. DHEW.

Brody, J. 1981. *Jane Brody's nutrition book*. New York: W. W. Norton Co.

Costill, D. L. 1979. A scientific approach to distance running. *Track and Field News*. Palo Alto, CA.

Durnin, J. V. G. A., & R. Passmore. 1967. *Energy, work and leisure*. London: Heinemann Education Books.

Hanson, D. L., et al. 1967. Effects of fat intake and exercise on serum cholesterol and body composition of rats. *The American Journal of Physiology*. 213:347.

Horton, M. J. 1982. Taking the Pritikin health prescription. *Runner's World*. 17:31.

Locksley, R. 1980. Fuel utilization in marathons: implications for performance. *The Western Journal of Medicine*. 133:493.

Marine Corps Institute. 1977. *Basic nutrition*. Washington, D.C.: Marine Barracks.

McArdle, W. D., F. I. Katch, & V. L. Katch. 1981. *Exercise physiology: energy, nutrition and human performance*. Philadelphia: Lea & Febiger.

Morris, A. F. 1981. Carbohydrate loading procedures. *The Physician and Sportsmedicine*. 9:13.

National Academy of Sciences. National Research Council. 1980. *Recommended dietary allowances*. 9th ed.

Nickerson, H. J., & A. D. Tripp. 1983. Iron deficiency in adolescent cross-country runners. *The Physician and Sportsmedicine*. 11:60.

Pritikin, N. 1979. *The Pritikin program for diet and exercise*. New York: Grosset & Dunlap, Inc.

Slovic, P. 1975. What helps the long distance runner run? *Nutrition Today*. 10:18.

Smith, N. J. 1976. *Food for sport*. Palo Alto, CA: Bull Publishing Co.

United States Department of Agriculture, and United States Department of Health and Human Services. 1980. *Dietary guidelines for Americans*. Washington, D.C.

United States Department of Health, Education and Welfare. 1979. *Healthy people*. The Surgeon General's Report on Health Promotion and Disease Prevention. Washington, D.C.

Drugs and Athletic Performance

Outline

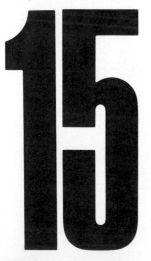

Introduction

This chapter is on the relationship of drugs to athletic performance. Drugs are defined and the popularity and habit-forming nature of many drug substances will be discussed. Certain aspects of drug terminology, such as addiction, habit-forming, habituation, and drug dependence are defined. Drug interactions and the placebo effects of drugs are covered. The individual nature of drug tolerance will be described in another section.

There are always trade-offs in taking drugs. One hopes to balance the desired beneficial effect from the medicine within the particular drug against the potential side effects, which *all* drugs possess. Also, various classifications of drugs, such as stimulants and anabolic steroids, are banned by the International Olympic Committee.

The drug DMSO is discussed in a third section in this chapter. Various side effects and precautions are listed. Finally, there is a section on blood doping, and on the effects of alcohol on athletic performance. This section concludes with the negative effects of smoking and marijuana on athletic performance.

Drugs Defined

A drug is a *medicinal substance used in the treatment of a disease* (Thomas, 1963). Since this is the generally accepted clinical definition of a drug, and since most athletes are not sick or suffering from a disease or illness, there should be little use of drugs in athletes. Unfortunately, this is not the case. It is estimated that many, if not all athletes, take drugs during some phase of their athletic career. If one considers alcohol a drug (as it should be), almost all athletes have become involved in drug consumption at one time or another. Even the consumption of vast quantities of vitamins or minerals may be considered a form of drug usage, leading to negative aspects of physiological functioning.

Popularity of Drugs

Why are drugs so popular in our culture today? Modern Western society consists of hard, fast-paced living. Because of this, there may be many reasons for drug consumption. However, three main reasons for the use of drugs are listed below:

1. Drugs are popular in Western society because of our emphasis on *narcissism*. That is, we tend to live in a "now" or "me" generation. The American public is constantly being told to "go for it," enjoy all the "pleasure/gusto" that one can get at the present time and not to worry about the future. The public is constantly informed by the media that drugs can manipulate our moods. Examples of this are the advertisements for various forms of alcohol or other mood-altering drugs.
2. A second reason why drugs are popular stems from the fact that popular opinion tells us to eat, drink, or play to excess and then just pop a pill ("plop-plop—fizz-fizz") to whisk away your discomfort. There seems to be a widespread belief among the general public that modern science or clinical medicine has produced a pill to cure almost any illness of human excess. That simply taking a pill will remedy the discomfort caused by the excesses that we have subjected our bodies to. *This, unfortunately, is not true.*
3. Finally, the third major reason for drug abuse is that so much media attention and literature seems to favor the quick, easy drug solution. One merely has to read a sample of a recent issue of a prominent sports medicine journal, like *The Physician and Sportsmedicine,* to note that nearly one-half of all the pages in a single issue relate to drug advertisements. The same is true of popular periodicals like *Sports Illustrated, Time,* or *People.* The media attention directed to promoting drug products, alcohol, tobacco, etc., in our society is tremendous. And, of course, this advertising eventually reaches many people, especially the young, impressionable ones.

Drug Terminology

Before we get into an extended discussion of drugs and the athlete, there are several terms which will be operationally defined so that this presentation on drugs can be meaningful.

The first three terms, *addiction, habit-forming* or *habituation,* and *drug dependence,* are difficult to define. Even medical experts in this field differ as to precise definitions. Below are operational definitions for these terms.

> **Habit-Forming** A habit (**habituation**) is a condition resulting from the repeated consumption of a drug. Its characteristics include:
>
> 1. a desire to continue taking the drug for the sense of perceived well-being it provides.
> 2. little or no tendency to increase dosage.
> 3. some degree of psychic dependence on the drug, but absence of physical dependence.
> 4. detrimental effects are possible. (Example: tobacco, amphetamines.)
>
> **Dependence and Addiction** These two terms are often used interchangeably and will carry the same definition for our purposes. **Addiction** is a state of psychic or physical dependence, or both, on a drug, arising in a person after periodic or continuous consumption of that drug. Drug addiction characteristics include:
>
> 1. an overpowering desire or need to continue taking the drug.
> 2. a tendency to increase dosage.
> 3. a psychological and often physical dependence on the drug.
> 4. probable detrimental effects on the individual and society. (Example: narcotics, barbiturates, and alcohol.)
>
> **Generic Drugs** Generic drugs denote a type or category of drugs. Examples are aspirin, tranquilizers, or steroids. The generic name is the public, scientific, and established name for the drug.
>
> **Brand Drugs** Brand drugs are trade-name drugs. The brand drug name is the labeler's package of a brand of a particular drug product, like *Bayer*® aspirin, *Valium*® as a tranquilizer, or *Dianabol*® as a steroid.
>
> **Drug Interactions** A drug is given to *a specific individual* in *a specific dosage* for *a specific condition*. If an athlete *mixes* drugs (i.e. alcohol and aspirin) serious, harmful side effects (called reactions) can occur. Even mixing certain vitamins, like vitamin C with aspirin, can cause severe stomach irritation and upset. With certain drug *interactions* death may be the end result.
>
> **Placebo** An *inactive substance* given to satisfy a patient's request for some medicine. Generally, this placebo has no physiological effect on the body. The person may believe that the placebo ("pill") has a positive effect. (Example: sugar or bread pill.)

Prescription Drugs These drugs are chemically active medicinal substances *ordered* by a physician for specific purposes in treating a specific disease or condition of an individual. The patient or athlete must get these directly from the physician or a registered pharmacist. These are legally controlled drugs.

Over-the-Counter Drugs (OTC) These drugs are sold over-the-counter *without a doctor's prescription*. Typically, these **OTC drugs** are of the type that can be used with relative safety without a doctor's supervision, if the labels are strictly followed. It is important to note that most OTC drugs attempt to alleviate the symptoms (subjective feelings of pain or discomfort) and not actually "cure" the underlying cause of the disease. Some examples of OTC drug categories are: aspirin, analgesics, cough preparations, antacids, laxatives, hypnotics, and some antihistamines (Hafen & Peterson, 1978).

Drug Administration The process of introducing a drug into the body may be varied. Examples of administration of drugs are: swallowed, inhaled, or injected. The type of covering on a drug might be important. If the drug is given in capsule form, it may be impossible to tell via taste what type of drug a person is ingesting. Many pills have a distinctive taste so that the person knows that they are ingesting a specific substance (for example, vitamin C generally has an acidic taste, since it is ascorbic acid).

Before a detailed description of the types of drugs that athletes consume is discussed, two important considerations regarding drug usage must be presented. The first crucial consideration in drug prescription is *individual* tolerance, while the second is the *trade-off* (risk) nature of using drugs as a therapeutic modality.

Individual Tolerances

Individual tolerances are described as the particular response to a certain dose of a specific drug as a person continues to take that drug. Each and every person differs chemically. They also differ significantly in age, sex, and body build. Since medicines do not produce the same effects in all people, one should never take drugs prescribed for a friend, even though symptoms may appear similar. It must be understood that each athlete may respond differently to the same type of drug. That is why the physician questions the patient carefully and monitors adverse reactions which may develop from drug usage. This is called the *individuality principle* regarding drug tolerance.

In addition, it is important to note that a person's response may increase or decrease with repeated dosages of the drug. Athletes who are physically active may affect the workings of a specific drug. Moreover, all individuals differ in their reactions to a combination of several drugs. The physician should know *all medications* that the athlete is taking. It is only in this way that possible complications may be avoided if the athlete is taking two or more medications at the same time.

Trade-Off in Drug Taking

Finally, one must consider the trade-offs in taking drugs. Fifty to seventy-five years ago, physicians used surgery or simply "tincture of time," with the body healing itself, to attempt to cure diseases. Now, polio and other horrible diseases may be cured with the proper administration of drugs. Although these advancements are significant, there is still some risk involved in most drug taking. These risks must be balanced against the advantages in taking the particular drug. The positive versus negative outcomes of the particular drug must be carefully weighed in deciding whether or not to take it. The risk of overdose is present, if directions are not followed. Adverse reactions may also occur. Finally, adverse side effects of drugs may affect the individual in the long run. Since most of the prescriptions written today are for drugs that were not even on the market twenty-five years ago, such long term effects could prove harmful in the future. *All drug taking involves risks.* The doctor and the athlete must weigh all possible advantages with the possible disadvantages of the drug. It is only when the benefits *far outweigh* the risks involved that the athlete should resort to drug therapy. This is a most important area, legally and morally, for both the athlete and the doctor (Ryan, 1983).

The next section discusses **doping**. Some broad categories of drugs common in athletic circles are discussed and restrictions on these drugs by the various sport governing bodies limiting these drugs are also covered.

Doping

The illegal use of drugs in sports, often referred to as **doping**, has been strictly defined by the International Olympic Committee (IOC) as "the administration of or the use by a competing athlete, of any substance foreign to the body, or of any physiologic substance taken in abnormal quantity, or taken by an abnormal route of entry into the body, with the sole intention of increasing, in an artificial and unfair manner, his/her performance in competition."

A note about competition is important here. Sport should be a controlled trial—person versus person, or team versus team—within a constant rigid framework of rules. If a competitor tries to cheat by using a performance-enhancing substance (a drug), the underlying structure of the sporting activity is destroyed. Despite this contention, humans, throughout history, have expressed a desire to take medicines or drugs in order to attempt to improve their performance. In the sixteenth century, explorer Juan Ponce de Leon reportedly found the legendary "Fountain of Youth." This reported spring of running waters was said to be of such extraordinary nature that the water drunk from it made old men young again. Unfortunately, it did not aid Mr. Ponce de Leon, since history records that he died shortly after discovering the fountain, from a festering arrow wound from an unfriendly Indian.

Early Doping History

Dr. Hanley (1979) tells the tale of Scandinavian warriors using an extract of roots that may have produced hallucinations. These fighting men were said to go "berserk" when they ingested this special potion. Berserk is derived from "berserkr," which was Old Norse for "bear's skin." Throughout recorded history there has been mention of athletes using special foods or drink in the hopes of improving athletic feats.

The first internationally reported case of doping was noted in 1865 among certain canal swimmers in Europe. The practice of ingesting drugs soon became more widespread. In 1879 participants in a six day bike race were found to have used alcohol, caffeine, ether-soaked sugar cubes, cocaine, opium, strychnine pills, and nitroglycerine (Hanley, 1979). This is a staggering assortment of artificial aids designed to give an athlete an edge over the competitors. In 1886 the first recorded drug fatality, an English cyclist, was found after reportedly overdosing on a stimulant administered by the coach. Since these early incidents, there have been over one dozen documented *deaths* in athletic activities because of the unwise use of drugs.

Today there are literally hundreds of ingredients (vitamins, red blood cells, iron, steroids, hormones, etc.) that athletes ingest in the hope of improving their performance. Also, many of the above listed substances are mixed or tried in varying proportions, adding to the hazard that may be created within the human body. Dr. Daniel F. Hanley, U.S. Olympic team physician, notes that no substance, or mixture of substances, has been shown to consistently improve performance in a normal, well-conditioned, healthy athlete. Increased performances only accrue from superior, intelligent, hard work and training.

Classes of Drugs Banned by IOC

There are several categories of drugs which are banned by the International Olympic Committee (IOC). This list is continually changing as new drugs are added to the scene and as newer methods of drug detection are established. The four major drug classes follow. To underscore the point that new agents are currently being added to the list, the final entry under each category is labeled "and related compounds."

Psychomotor Stimulant Drugs

This common category of drugs includes the amphetamines. This class may be better known as stimulants. It is believed to be the largest class of drugs used by athletes. These drugs stimulate the central nervous system. Pulse rate and blood pressure are increased. The *sensation* of fatigue may be depressed and appetite decreased. Hence, many "diet pills" are amphetamine types. Other side effects of these stimulant drugs include headache, stomach upset, excitation, hyperactivity, constipation, euphoria, libido changes, insomnia, and others. The person taking these drugs almost always has some impairment of rational judgment. Typically, they think they are performing better than they are. In some people, symptoms of aggressiveness, hostility, and irritability result. With continued use, psychomotor stimulants may produce delusions, confusion, hostility reactions, hallucinations, and eventually psychosis.

Many experts describe amphetamines as habit-forming and potentially addictive. Certainly the potential for psychological addiction is present. The person who starts on these drugs may seek an ever increasing dose to get the desired effect. An overdose of these drugs would be fatal. Dr. Gabe Mirkin (1978) has decried the use of amphetamines because they impair judgment and, to a degree, mask pain. Hence, the athlete may be more susceptible to injury because the natural pain feedback system may be malfunctioning.

Many common, illicit "street drugs" are amphetamines. The list of doping substances of the psychomotor stimulant type are:

1. Amphetamines (Benzedrine)
2. Benyphetamine
3. Cocaine
4. Diethylpropion
5. Dimethylamphetamine
6. Ethylamphetamine
7. Fencamfamine
8. Methylamphetamine
9. Methyphenidate
10. Norpsuedoephedrine
11. Phendimetrazine
12. Phenmetrazine
13. Prolintane
14. Related compounds

Sympathomimetic Amines

A second category of banned doping substances is *sympathomimetic amines*. The drugs in this category are typically nasal decongestants and those used in the treatment of asthma. These drugs affect sympathetic nervous action and, therefore, produce increases in pulse rate, blood pressure, and cardiac functioning. They mimic the effect of adrenaline (epinephrine), thereby producing anxiety and uneasiness. Some specific physiological responses are constricted peripheral blood vessels and relaxed bronchial muscles, hence, they may aid in breathing.

An unfortunate use of this type of drug occurred in the 1972 Olympic games in Munich. An American swimmer, who was an asthmatic, was taking a prescription drug which contained small amounts of ephedrine. The swimmer won a gold medal in the 400m freestyle. He had to forfeit his medal, however, when a urine sample revealed traces of this banned substance in his system. Perhaps if his team physician had reported his asthma condition and the medication that he was taking, this unfortunate situation could have been avoided.

Some common sympathomimetic amines which are banned include:

1. Ephedrine
2. Methylephedrine
3. Methoxyphenamine
4. Related compounds

Miscellaneous Central Nervous System Stimulants

This category of drugs is similar to the stimulants noted earlier in Class I. They act specifically on the central nervous system (the brain and spinal cord). Since excitability of the spinal cord is affected by these drugs, certain athletic skills may be affected, resulting in unpredictable movements and uncoordinated actions. Taken to the excess, these drugs may lead to severe muscle spasms and convulsion, which could lead to death. As in the other categories that we have examined, an erroneous dose or overdose could be critical. The person experimenting with these classes of drugs is virtually sitting on a powder keg just waiting for an explosion.

Major central nervous system stimulant drugs currently banned by the IOC include:

1. Amiphenazole
2. Bemegride
3. Leptazol
4. Nikethamide
5. Strychnine
6. Related compounds

Narcotic Analgesics

This class of narcotic analgesics is usually taken to make the body insensitive to pain. It is rumored that a former professional quarterback took some types of anti-inflammatory and/or narcotic analgesics to reduce pain from his battle-scarred knees. The popular media would have us believe that this practice is widespread in professional contact sports where athletes are supposed to be "paid to play with pain." Also included under narcotic analgesics are compounds containing *codeine*. In fact, some popular cold and cough products (Vicks®, St. Joseph's®, Dristan®, Pertussin®, Coldene®, Coryban D®, and others) are known to contain some narcotic analgesics.

The "hard" narcotics are heroin, morphine, opium, and methadone. These prescription drugs are useful when used under strict physician's control in medical emergencies, surgery, or other cases, however, their indiscriminate use in athletes or recreational activities can never be condoned. These drugs are *addictive*.

The most common narcotic analgesics include:

1. Heroin
2. Morphine
3. Methadone
4. Dextromoramide
5. Dipipanone
6. Pethidine
7. Related compounds

Before moving on to the last category—anabolic steroids—some further comments must be made concerning anti-inflammatory agents, such as salicylates, cortisone, phenylbutazone, indomethacin, and the analgesics of ethyl chloride spray, procaine, and lidocaine, which are often used in sports to reduce inflammation and/or pain. It must be emphasized here that pain is a natural, normal bodily reaction that serves useful functions. If athletes did not perceive pain, serious body injury could result. Pain should be considered a useful cue that something is wrong and that cessation of the activity is needed, until the reason for the pain is determined. Pain that produces a muscle spasm, limp, or other physiological manifestation might protect the body from further injury. Unlike an animal, which can get along on three legs, humans are rendered immobile if an injury occurs to the lower extremities. The animal may also be smart enough to realize that pain should signal a cessation of activity. Man, on the other hand, will sometimes try to "work through" leg or foot pain, risking further injury, as in stress fractures. An animal, left to its own in the wild, will never get a stress fracture. (This is unlike the racehorse or the racing dog that will get a stress fracture—but only if the trainer pushes the animal too much to work with pain).

There may be a legitimate situation where an anti-inflammatory agent may be prescribed by a physician to control inflammation and thus aid rehabilitation. Anti-inflammatory medications, when properly prescribed, do have a place in sports medicine.

Anabolic Steroids

The final category of banned drugs includes the anabolic steroids. This category is a subject of much concern in sports today. These synthetically produced drugs were designed to promote body growth, while attempting to minimize harmful side effects. Recall that, for every drug ingested, there may be beneficial or positive effects, but there also may be harmful or negative side effects. The anabolic steroids are made from testosterone derivates. Testosterone is a normally occurring hormone found in both males and females. Around the time of puberty in males, the body is quite active in naturally producing testosterone, and that is when common androgenic (masculinizing) characteristics appear. Common signs are increases in body hair on face, legs, and abdomen, a deepening of the voice, and an increase in muscle definition in the male. Muscle definition is much more common in the male if strength training activities are followed. Many more subtle changes also occur.

Since most athletes believe that an increase in strength and power would aid them in their performance, many unwise athletes resort to taking anabolic steroids. This seems to be the case in sports which emphasize size or strength. Football players, and field event performers in track (shot, discus, hammer, javelin), as well as participants in other contact sports, may resort to taking steroids. In fact, many athletes think that to get stronger they must ingest steroids.

What is known about anabolic steroids? Scientific and medical evidence shows that anabolic steroids definitely have masculinizing properties and that steroids decrease normal body production of testosterone, cause fluid retention, cause personality changes, increase incidence of gastric ulcers, and could lead to kidney and liver tumors (cancers). These are only a few of the harmful steroid side effects.

Other documented harmful side effects are:

1. Increase in acne
2. Growth retardation in young athletes
3. Atrophy of testicles
4. Possible intestinal bleeding
5. Decreased sperm count
6. Bone thinning
7. Muscle wasting
8. Increase in facial hair
9. Liver dysfunction

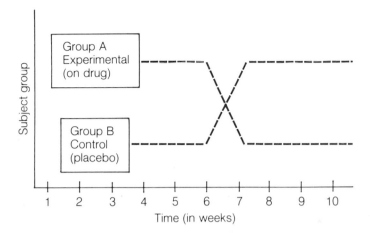

Figure 15.1 Example of a cross-over drug-type experiment. Note that Group A started on the drug and progressed for four to six weeks; went off the drug for two weeks; then took the placebo for four to six more weeks. Group B started out on the placebo, then crossed-over and became the experimental group.

There are some limited, genuine, medical emergencies in which the administration of steroids under the guidance of a competent physician may be indicated. These situations might include serious injury or burns where the natural antibody production is temporarily defective. In other serious or life-threatening conditions, such as major endocrine disturbances, starvation, severe anemia, breast cancer, or pituitary dwarfism, certain steroid treatments may be necessary. Recall, however, that all chemotherapy (drug therapy) is often a delicate balancing act. The medical doctor attempts to control a serious condition while considering potential harmful side effects, both short term and long term. Many grave side effects of steroids might involve long term complications.

Many studies have been reported on the effectiveness of anabolic steroids and performance. Some of these studies did not have proper controls, nor was care taken to use blind or double-blind procedures. In a blind procedure, the subjects do not know whether they are taking a real drug or a placebo. A double-blind study keeps both the subjects and the investigator "blind" as to the treatment until the experiment is over. Another effective technique in drug experimentation is the use of the cross-over technique, in which one group of subjects starts out by taking the drug, then goes off the drug, while the control begins taking the drug and vice versa. See figure 15.1 for further explanation. It is important that the experimental group be on the drug long enough for the drug to be effective. Then, the experimental group must go through a control period with no drug to see what effects are portrayed.

In 1976 the American College of Sports Medicine evaluated all the scientific literature and made a position statement on steroids that is included as Appendix 4. Essentially, these top medical minds in the sports medicine field reported that there was no reliable evidence that anabolic steroids increased performance, and that because of the potential side effects, athletes should refrain from ever taking these substances. Finally, steroids are illegal and are not tolerated in international or national competitions.

A listing of documented harmful side effects of steroids appeared earlier in this section.

Some names for anabolic steroids are listed below:

1. Methandienone
2. Stanozolol
3. Oxymetholone
4. Nandrolone Decanoate
5. Nandrolone Phenpropionate
6. Related compounds

Some common trade names for popular steroids include Anavar®, Durabolin®, Dianabol®, Maxibolin®, and Winstrol®.

DMSO

In the early 1980s some athletes and athletic doctors reported on the beneficial effects of dimethyl sulfoxide (DMSO). Unfortunately, as with the use of many drugs, the positive effects are more favorably advanced than negative side effects (Percy & Carson, 1981). What is presently known regarding DMSO? How does it work? When is its use suggested? And what are the negative side effects? These questions and other comments are presented in the following section.

What is DMSO?

DMSO, a by-product of paper manufacturing, was discovered in the last century. It is used as a degreaser, paint solvent, antifreeze product, and as a registered drug to relieve pain and "promote healing" *in animals*.

How Does DMSO Work?

This is where the problem lies. Apparently DMSO selectively blocks nerve pain fibers and prevents swelling. It is not totally clear what else it does, other than that it very quickly enters the blood stream and can act as a carrier, taking with it the impurities that it contains, or the impurities on the skin. DMSO is ordinarily cut (diluted) with sterile water to reduce its tendency to burn the skin. DMSO seems to work best on nagging injuries of tendinitis, muscle strains, slight sprains, contusion injuries, and bursitis problems. Proponents suggest that it helps to control swelling, relieve pain, and prevent buildup of waste products in an injury site. In relieving pain it can block the pain impulses transmitted in the unmyelinated C nerve fibers without numbing the area, as would be the case with the use of xylocaine, for example. There is some evidence that DMSO can prevent swelling, if administered quickly.

When is DMSO Used?

Athletes use it, on injured areas, after workouts or races in combination with the usual RICES (rest, ice, compression, elevation, stabilization/support) treatment. Some use it prior to exercise. This presents the usual problem of a pain reliever, which is that the athlete cannot feel the damage being done to an injured part of the body. Pain is an important warning to be felt and responded to in the correct manner. For example, if your ankle hurts when you run, there is a good chance you should not be running until your ankle stops hurting—the pain is there for a reason. The pain blocking effect of DMSO allows some athletes to compete while injured. This decision to compete while injured is one to be evaluated very carefully by the athlete, the coach, and the medical consultant.

Side Effects

DMSO has had the following side effects in users: burning of the skin at the site of application, bad breath, body odors, garlic or onion taste in the mouth, burning sensation in the mouth, burning on urination, light-headedness, blurred vision, and some other variations of these. There is a report that eye damage was found in an experiment with animals. Also, there is little known of the adverse long term side effects.

Precautions for Those Who Use It

If DMSO is used by prescription in one of the ten states where the state law allows for its medical use, then the following information should be known. The site of application should be washed with soap and water thoroughly and dried. Properly diluted DMSO, of medical purity, is then rubbed into the area and allowed ten to fifteen minutes in the open air before wrapping with clear plastic or white gauze wrap and applying clothing over that. After one hour, the wrap should be removed. Both the skin area and the wrap should be sterile and free of dyes (which in some cases are carcinogenic and can be carried into the skin with DMSO). The DMSO should be prescribed by a competent medical source and directions should be followed closely.

Recommendations

Since there have been no human studies to determine the long term effects of use, and since several of the side effects are quite significant, one cannot recommend the use of DMSO unless administered by competent medical authorities in an area of use approved by the FDA. If the body is in pain, there is a reason, and professional care should be sought, if *conservative* self-treatment does not work. Certainly, based on the evidence as we know it, conservation in the use of this substance is in order, and the indiscriminate issuance of it to young athletes by coaches is irresponsible. Until more evidence is in, it would be recommended that each potential user carefully weigh the *benefits* versus *risks,* before deciding whether or not to join the ever-growing group of users, which includes some big-name athletes.

DMSO Evaluation

DMSO has been the topic of concern of several international conferences in the past two decades. The conclusions, after much presentation of material, have been that DMSO is indeed a remarkable substance. Inexpensive, fast-acting, and applicable to the injured extremity in a noninvasive manner, DMSO has great appeal for these reasons alone as a possible agent of pain relief and swelling reduction. In reviewing the remarks within the conclusion from these conferences on DMSO, it is apparent that enough information exists to warrant a well-controlled study of this drug to find its proper place in therapeutic medicine. One such study (Percy & Carson, 1981) showed no beneficial effects of DMSO over conventional treatment for tennis elbow. Until more studies are reported, it is still a drug of controversy, and an appropriately conservative stand must be taken on its use. There is no question, however, that the indiscriminate use of DMSO or any drug by athletes of any age or condition, is unwise and can lead to problems far greater than the cause or treatment.

Blood Doping

A recent topic of concern to the sports medicine practitioner is the controversial subject of **blood doping**. Simply stated, blood doping may be defined as the process of withdrawing an athlete's blood, holding it out for six to twelve weeks in which the body generates more blood, then reintroducing the withheld blood back into the athlete's body. It is a most controversial procedure, which is ethically wrong, and at present, illegal. Sports should be a place for objective competition and evaluation in a rigidly controlled atmosphere. With blood doping, as with the use of other drugs, a match or contest is likely to result in an unfair advantage to one contestant, thus rendering the underlying theme of sport inappropriate.

Factors Involved With Blood Doping

There are many interlaced and complex factors which make blood doping a risky procedure. Some of these factors are:

1. When should the athlete's blood be withdrawn?
2. How much blood should be withdrawn?
3. What should be the time interval between blood withdrawal and reinfusion?
4. How intensely should the athlete work out after the blood is withdrawn?
5. Precisely what substance should be reinjected? Whole blood, or merely frozen red blood cells (RBC)?
6. How close to the time of actual competition should the athlete's blood be reinjected?
7. How much blood should be reinjected?
8. Finally, absolutely sterile procedures must be maintained in blood withdrawal and reinfusion, since the athlete could become quite sick, if infected. Also, storage procedures for the blood, or RBC, must be carefully monitored.

Remember that this entire procedure is still *illegal!*

Dr. Melvin H. Williams, Director of the Human Performance Laboratory at Old Dominion University in Virginia, and a leading researcher in blood doping, noted that early studies (prior to 1975) had reported no consistent physiological effect on human endurance performance with blood doping. Williams, in a later review (1981), now reports that there may be a possibility that when proper amounts of blood are withdrawn and then infused prior to performance, endurance activities, such as running distances of 5km, 10km, or the marathon, may be improved.

Rationale for Blood Doping

The theoretical rationale behind blood doping is as follows. The packed RBCs, which are prepared and infused into the athlete, should raise hemoglobin concentration in the blood. (Hemoglobin is the compound that carries oxygen in the blood). Hence, the blood should be capable of carrying more oxygen for delivery to the working skeletal muscle tissues. To find out if this blood doping procedure works, scientists must make certain that the factors listed in the initial discussion are accounted for, and that other adequate laboratory and experimental controls are strictly followed. If possible, the athlete and the experimenter should be blind to the procedure being done. There should be no training effect. The work task being evaluated should be appropriate, and other considerations of safety and adequate controls must be observed.

Williams (1981), in his latest report, notes that maximum oxygen consumption increased and running time to exhaustion was longer in subjects who had received blood infusion. In another study, treadmill running time for five miles decreased an average of forty-five seconds. Do these laboratory findings necessarily predict success on the track in the real world? It is a rather large jump to interpolate laboratory research findings to the practical athletic situation.

Finally, remember that blood doping is still dangerous (as are all drugs) and it is *still illegal!*

Alcohol

Alcohol is not specifically listed among the named drugs which are banned by the IOC, nevertheless, problem drinking is of major concern in our society which, of course, affects the athlete. We have indicated previously that Western society appears to be a society of drug takers. When the cost, in terms of disability, death, violence, and shattered lives is taken, alcohol is the most common, readily available drug. The use and abuse of alcohol is not merely a physiological problem. Complicated by social pressures on athletes, their parents, coaches, and school administrators, the question of drinking affects nearly every adult in our society. What is known about alcohol and the athlete? Exactly how does alcohol affect human performance? And is there any place for alcohol in athletics?

Early History of Alcohol

In the oldest of civilizations, among the most primitive peoples, alcoholic beverages have been made by fermentation. A mass of fruit or berries, left exposed to airborne yeast spores in a warm environment, could be fermented into crude wine. The early consumers of this drink soon realized the feelings of well-being, sedation, intoxication, and even unconsciousness which it produced.

In the fifteenth century in Europe, the refinement of the distillation process produced a new and even stronger drink—the spirit of wine. With more development, the spirits of any fermented fluid from other sources, such as grains and tubers, could increase the alcoholic content from 6 to 14 percent, to upwards of 50 to 75 percent. These basics of alcohol have remained essentially the same throughout countless generations. Today, bottles of wine and liquor are brightly packaged and advertised for mass consumption. The media push to advertise and sell these beverages is phenomenal. Since alcohol consumption in many families is part of religious or cultural functions, many people are introduced to alcohol while very young. With alcohol's easy availability, and pressures of society to conform and be part of the group, many young people become involved with alcohol at early ages. What are some of the effects of alcohol on the human body? How can alcohol affect sports performance?

Determinants of Drinking Behavior

Several factors interact to determine specific effects of alcohol on a person. Among the factors which affect how quickly alcohol is absorbed into the bloodstream are the following:

1. What type of beverage is drunk. All alcoholic beverages have one significant ingredient: *alcohol*. Beers and wines typically have an alcoholic content of about 6 to 15 percent. Liqueurs and other hard, distilled spirits may have an alcohol content of 50 to 85 percent.
2. The speed of drinking is significant. The more rapidly an alcoholic beverage is consumed, the higher the blood-alcohol levels will be.
3. A person's body size and weight is important to resultant alcohol effects. A professional wrestler weighing 374 pounds can consume more alcohol than a young 84 pound gymnast.
4. The presence of food in the stomach affects alcohol absorption. If alcohol is consumed at mealtime with a large food intake, most likely the person will also take longer to imbibe the alcohol, and the effects of the alcohol may be reduced by nearly 50 percent. Conversely, the person who consumes lots of beer quite rapidly after a hard 10 or 20km race in a hot/humid environment, early in the day, after having no breakfast, is likely to be inebriated quite rapidly.
5. Finally, a person's individual body chemistry and drinking history may affect alcohol absorption. A person may actually develop a tolerance and be able to consume more alcohol before effects begin to take place.

There are other factors which influence specific alcohol effects on the body. These might include whether the alcoholic beverage is mixed with another liquid, such as water, which may dilute the alcohol and slow absorption. However, certain carbonated mixers may actually speed alcohol absorption.

Specific Alcohol Effects on the Body

Alcohol is believed to be a stimulant at low dosages. However, as the dose increases, alcohol acts as a brain depressant. Alcohol is unique in that it is absorbed quickly into the bloodstream directly from the stomach or small intestine. It is then rapidly carried to the brain. It is this adverse action on the brain that enables alcohol in larger dosages to produce adverse effects on motor control and cause unconsciousness.

Let's examine some specific physiological effects which might occur to a 150 pound man taking several drinks.

At an initial consumption level of two drinks in quick succession, the blood-alcohol level may rise to between 0.03 and 0.05 percent—that is, 1 part of alcohol to 2000 parts of blood. Some scientists have reported that a blood-alcohol level (BAL) of this amount—0.03 to 0.05 percent—could begin to distort complex skills controlled by the nervous system. This may occur with only *two quick drinks!* This person might begin to feel carefree, released from ordinary tensions and inhibitions, and begin to "loosen up." This is the reported "pleasant state" that many people seek to achieve when drinking in moderation.

As more alcohol enters the bloodstream with more drinking, a definite "short-circuiting" effect on the brain occurs. Here, the BAL may be 0.05 to 0.10 percent and simple reaction time seems to be adversely affected. Other studies have shown that balance, visual tracking with hand movements, and other psychomotor tasks are adversely affected.

With continued drinking, blood-alcohol continues to be elevated 0.10 to 0.20 percent —now 1 part alcohol to 500 parts of blood and the entire brain motor area is affected. The person may stagger. Emotional behavior is severely affected. The person may become loud, easily angered, uncontrollable. The person may lie down, even pass out—the person is "drunk."

If the BAL goes still higher to 0.20, 0.30, or 0.50 percent, this is an extremely dangerous time. These very high BALs could block the lower brain centers and breathing and heart rate could be affected. The person may lapse into a coma. Death is a distinct possibility.

It is crucial to realize that alcohol is a *DRUG,* with possible actions like any prescription drug, when taken in overdose. It is hard to realize that this familiar aspect of our social life could be so dangerous, but it is.

Another adverse side effect of alcohol consumption should be noted. Taking several drinks of alcohol before sleep may decrease REM (rapid eye movement) sleep. This REM is dream sleep, and is the restful type of sleep that the individual needs most (Morris, 1982). REM sleep deprivation may lead to impaired concentration and memory, anxiety, tiredness, and general irritability.

The final caution that needs to be emphasized is the dreadful effects of mixing alcohol with other drugs. These other drugs, such as tranquilizers, amphetamines, pain relievers, cold medicines, and others too numerous to note, when mixed with alcohol, may have explosive effects. Almost weekly, the newspapers report death overdoses due to mixing alcohol with other drugs. This unfortunate occurrence is not always limited to Hollywood personalities, but to many unknowing, unfortunate individuals.

Conclusions on Alcohol and Sports

By way of summary, it may be said that alcohol has no beneficial effect on sports performance (Williams, 1983). Some early reports on the steadying effects of alcohol on pistol shooters (Ryan, 1979) appear to be perfunctory. Other athletes who attempt to relax by drinking alcohol may be risking potential long term effects, because alcohol is certainly addictive when consumed in large quantities over a period of time.

Smoking

For years, scientists have expressed the adverse effects of tobacco. Today, it is known that cigarette smoking is one of the three primary risk factors of coronary heart disease (CHD). In addition, the connection between cigarette smoking and lung cancer seems to grow as the evidence is evaluated. Klafs & Arnheim (1981) list the many adverse relationships between smoking and physical performance:

1. Inhalation of cigarette smoke may cause a decrease of airway conductance of nearly 50%. This has been observed in smokers, as well as in nonsmokers who are exposed to cigarette smoke-filled rooms. (This is the passive smoking effect).
2. The oxygen-carrying capacity of the blood is reduced in the smoker.
3. Smoking unnecessarily accelerates heart rate by causing overstimulation of heart muscle cells.
4. Total lung capacity is most likely reduced in chronic heavy smokers.
5. Pulmonary diffusing capacity (the ability of the O_2 to get through the lungs into the bloodstream) is greatly diminished.
6. Smoking cigarettes significantly increases one's risk of CHD and lung cancer.
7. Smokers show more coronary atherosclerosis (buildup of fatty plaque in coronary arteries) than nonsmokers.
8. Blood pressure is stimulated unnecessarily in cigarette smokers.
9. Cigarette smoke may damage cilia, the microscopic hairs that line the airways of the lungs, thus predisposing the individual to increased inhalation of dust particles and bacteria.
10. In certain people, it may cause another whole constellation of symptoms, such as eye irritation, sneezing, coughing, sore throat, headaches, nausea, and hoarseness, among others.
11. Smokers are more prone to attacks of bronchitis, pneumonia, and tonsillitis.

All these adverse effects of cigarette smoke are listed to show the potential harmful effects of smoking. Only the major, documented, adverse conclusions have been listed. When smoking dramatically increased in this country in the 1920s and 1930s, people felt that it was a relatively innocuous habit. Now, a half century later, we are discovering the effects of this deadly habit. Marijuana is presently being touted as innocuous and harmless. Will it take another dozen years to carefully document the adverse side effects of this drug?

Marijuana

During the past fifteen to twenty years, marijuana use has increased in the United States. In addition, more youngsters in their teens and even in the pre-teen years, have been experimenting with this drug. An additional consideration is that most authorities believe that the marijuana being consumed is of the more potent variety, or has more impurities, which could harm the user. This would lead any intelligent person to conclude that smoking marijuana is both foolish and physically dangerous.

Marijuana is obtained from a hemp-like plant, cannabis sativa, which grows freely as a weed in almost any climate. The active ingredient, delta-1-Tetrahydrocannabinol, or THC, was first isolated in the early 1960s. It appears that the THC produces all the reported mind-altering effects of eating or smoking marijuana.

This cannabis plant has been used in India and China for thousands of years, and it is believed that marijuana was probably brought from Egypt by Napoleon's troops. Marijuana was named in Mexico, and began to be smuggled into the United States in significant quantities around the turn of the last century. As its use grew, all states passed laws making use, possession, and sale of this drug a criminal offense. Today, it is still illegal, but many states have imposed stiffer penalties on dealers, and not users or possessors.

In the scientific and medical community, marijuana has been tried experimentally in treatment of glaucoma, an eye condition, and in combating the nausea that often accompanies cancer drug therapy. In both of these instances, the benefits have been contrasted with the risks, and this form of drug therapy is advocated.

Users of marijuana generally report enhanced feelings of well-being, some mind-altering states (a high), a loosening of inhibitions, and a change in perception and sensation, possibly without true hallucinations. Variations in these subjective feelings and reports occur widely among users. The drug's subjective effects reportedly may occur quickly, and last for two or three hours. While the above changes are those reported for the mind-altering effects of *subjective* feelings, there are definite *objective* changes which can occur. These physical bodily changes have been documented in carefully controlled scientific studies, and they include: slowed reaction time, distorted perception of passing time, decrease in attention span, decrease in arithmetic ability, decrease in short-term memory, and general clumsiness (although the user may reportedly feel quite graceful). Also, driving and/or piloting skills have been shown to be decreased under the influence of marijuana. This decrease in manual physical performance may last for hours, even after the "high" sensation has passed. Therefore, one could expect athletic skills to be lessened.

Specific Effects of Marijuana on Users

Effects of the harmful nature are generally categorized into two components—those of short duration and those with longer term consequences. Unfortunately, we do not have any fifteen or twenty year, long-term studies on this drug. However, if they prove similar to cigarettes, the potential harmful effects could be significant.

What are some specific findings with regard to marijuana use and human functioning? These negative effects will be grouped according to the organ or system adversely affected.

Effects on the Lungs

Most scientists note that there is no direct connection or association between marijuana and lung cancer, as of the present time. However, it took decades to confirm the negative aspects of cigarette smoking. It is known that there are more cancer-causing agents in marijuana than in tobacco. Also, it is pointed out that most marijuana users tend to *inhale more deeply* and *to hold* the smoke longer than regular tobacco users. It is known that a person who uses both tobacco and marijuana is more at risk for lung cancer. Lung function is definitely impaired in chronic marijuana users, as it is in tobacco users.

Reproductive Effects

Both animal and human studies suggest that continued use of marijuana may adversely impair aspects of reproduction function. In women, menstruation may be disrupted and fertility reduced. In males, testosterone is reduced and male sperm can be reduced, thereby impairing reproductive function.

Far more serious effects of marijuana may happen in pregnancy. Women who are pregnant and use marijuana may miscarry or have a child with birth defects.

Effects on the Brain

There has been much controversy over marijuana use and brain damage. Early reports noted that there was some "atrophy" or shrinking of the brain among chronic marijuana users. These studies have not been confirmed. However, researchers have noted abnormalities of brain wave function in monkeys and in man after marijuana use. Many scientists who have studied behavior and marijuana note a condition which they label "brown out"— a condition in which the marijuana user becomes increasingly unaware of or disinterested in their surroundings. Also, flashbacks and panic reactions have been noted in isolated cases.

Effects on the Heart

Adverse effects on the heart include a speeding of the heart rate similar to that caused by cigarette smoke. Also, an increase in blood pressure may be detected. Both these responses could be detrimental over the long term.

Immune Response Effects

Some studies have shown lower resistance to infection among chronic marijuana users. Since a correctly functioning immune system is crucial in the athlete, anything which might interfere with it could be counterproductive to the athlete. Also, it has been reported that one of the major systems to deteriorate with aging is the immune response. So here again, any foreign substance (marijuana) which adversely affects the immune response could be harmful to the person.

Evaluation of Marijuana Effects

From an objective evaluation of the specific effects of marijuana on habitual users, it may be seen that certain potential serious side effects have been documented in the literature. Because of this information, the use of marijuana in a sport situation is definitely contraindicated. If the athlete seeks to achieve optimal performance, then he or she should train more intelligently and not resort to outside artificial aids. ■

Summary

In this chapter, the role of drugs in sports medicine is covered. Specific drug terms are defined and described in the initial section. Essentially, drugs are defined as a medical substance used in the treatment of disease. A habit-forming drug is a drug to which the person quickly becomes either physically or psychologically addicted. Addiction relates to an overpowering need or desire to continue taking the drug, and a further inclination to increase the drug dosage, until finally, a physical and/or psychological dependence on the drug is formed. Generic drugs are defined as a specific type or category of drugs. An example is aspirin. Brand name drugs are trade name drugs. An example is Bayer® aspirin. Drug interactions are listed, as well as individual tolerances, and the trade-offs of the beneficial effects versus the negative effects of drug taking are listed.

Doping is defined as the illegal use of drugs. The International Olympic Committee has banned four main categories of drugs. These four main areas are: (1) psychomotor stimulant drugs, (2) sympathomimetic amines, (3) miscellaneous central nervous system stimulants, and (4) narcotic analgesics. Anabolic steroids are another category of drugs which are banned by the IOC. Some of the documented negative effects of anabolic steroids are listed, and it is pointed out that there is no conclusive evidence that anabolic steroids help athletic performance by increasing either strength, or muscle mass. Adverse side effects of anabolic steroids affect both male and female athletes. DMSO (dimethyl sulfoxide), a very new and controversial drug, is discussed. DMSO is generally used in the healing of soft tissue (muscle, tendon, or ligament) injuries. In one well-controlled study which was cited, there was no beneficial effect of DMSO over the conventional therapy for the treatment of a common injury (tennis elbow).

The next issue concerns blood doping. It is pointed out that blood doping involves withdrawing blood, and later reinfusing it in the athlete. It is an illegal procedure. Earlier studies indicated that blood doping had no effect on performance. However, later studies, when more blood was withdrawn and subsequently reinfused in the athletes, showed slight improvements in performance on laboratory tests. Whether improvements will hold in the athletic arena still have to be determined. It must be remembered that blood doping is an illegal procedure.

Comments regarding alcohol usage and smoking marijuana are listed, as they relate to athletic performance. It is noted that, in no way can alcohol, tobacco, or marijuana aid the athlete, and consequently, these substances should be discouraged for use by all athletes.

References

Hafen, B. Q., & B. Peterson. 1978. *Medicines and drugs.* 2d ed. Philadelphia: Lea & Febiger.

Hanley, D. F. 1979. Drug use and abuse. In Strauss, R. H. ed. *Sports medicine and physiology.* Philadelphia: W. B. Saunders Co.

Klafs, C. E., & D. D. Arnheim. 1981. *Modern principles of athletic training.* 5th ed. St. Louis: C. V. Mosby.

Mirkin, G., & M. Hoffman. 1978. *Sports medicine.* Boston: Little Brown & Co.

Morris, A. F. 1982. Sleep disturbances in athletes. *The Physician and Sportsmedicine.* 10:75.

Percy, E. C., & J. D. Carson. 1981. The use of DMSO in tennis elbow and rotator cuff tendinitis: a double blind study. *Medicine and Science in Sports and Exercise.* 14:215.

Ryan, A. J. 1979. Alcohol and athletes: a roundtable. *The Physician and Sportsmedicine.* 7:38.

Ryan, A. J. 1983. Drug testing for athletes—pro and con. *The Physician and Sports Medicine.* 11:131.

Thomas, C. L. ed. 1963. *Taber's cyclopedic medical dictionary.* 9th ed. Philadelphia: F. A. Davis & Co.

Williams, M. H., et al. 1973. The effect of blood reinjection upon endurance capacity and heart rate. *Medicine and Science in Sports.* 5:181.

Williams, M. H. 1981. Blood doping: an update. *The Physician and Sportsmedicine.* 9:59.

Williams, M. H. 1983. Alcohol-sport position statement. *The Physician and Sportsmedicine.* 11:25.

Environmental Factors in Athletic Training and Sports Medicine

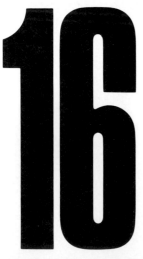

Outline

Introduction

This chapter considers environmental factors as they impact on the athlete. The various factors of weather, temperature, humidity, and wind velocity are detailed as they adversely affect the athlete.

As the athlete performs in longer endurance activities in hot, humid climates, sweating and the accompanying loss of fluid become significant factors in performance. Proper fluids to ingest to maintain adequate hydration are given in this chapter. Essentially, cold water is the best thing the athlete can drink during activity. Various commercial athletic drinks are evaluated, and it is noted that most of these are too high in concentration to aid the athlete during the event. Guidelines for proper hydration are given.

Another section of this environmental chapter deals with heat problems. Heat cramps, heat fatigue, heat exhaustion, and finally, heatstroke, are defined; prominent symptoms given; and prevention and treatment for these heat problems discussed.

Another section concerns the cold environment. Physiological reactions to cold and proper precautions that the athlete may take when participating in the cold are given.

Finally, there is a small section on performing at high altitudes; the acclimatization to altitude; and the effects of air pollution on athletic performance.

Weather and the Athlete

The athlete cannot perform in a vacuum. Although many conditions of the *training* environment may be controlled by the athlete, this is not always true in *competition*. For example, in training the athlete may decide to train indoors to avoid inclement weather. However, during formal competition, if an event is scheduled outdoors, then that event generally goes on regardless of the type of weather conditions.

There are eight major elements of weather and environmental factors that concern the athlete when performing outdoors (USMC, 1979). These eight elements are noted here, followed by a short comment on each. The eight elements of weather are *temperature, humidity, wind velocity, barometric pressure* (air density), *air pollution* (fog, haze, and smoke), *precipitation, clouds,* and *light data.* These elements are not listed in any particular order; however, *temperature* and *humidity* are two prime factors of environmental conditions that all athletes must face in sports.

Temperature

Temperature affects athletic performance a great deal. The runner knows that a fast pace cannot be maintained in extremely hot weather. An example of this would be the running times in the Honolulu marathon. This race is generally run in extremely hot and humid conditions, even though it takes place during December. The extremely high temperatures, combined with high humidity in Hawaii, certainly affects runners' performance, and of course, slows them down.

Temperature may be an indirect factor as it relates to other conditions. For example, for the cross-country skier, the particular surface of snow is greatly affected by the temperature.

Humidity

Humidity may be defined as the amount of water vapor in the air. Saturated air or air with a very high percentage of humidity, is going to impede evaporation of the athlete's sweat into the environment. In environments where the humidity is quite high, it is very difficult for the athlete to perform well. The previous example, relating to marathon running in Hawaii, is also an appropriate example here. The fact that Hawaii is surrounded by water generally indicates that the humidity is quite high. Although the Hawaiian marathon race is started very early in the morning in an attempt to avoid some of the extremes of temperature, the humidity is still often very high, occasionally 80 or 90 percent. This, obviously, affects long distance performance of an endurance nature because the evaporation of sweat is reduced during periods of high humidity. The two graphs in figure 16.1 show how high humidity interacts with high air temperature to produce conditions in the environment that are unsafe or dangerous to athletes. Note that in a stop-and-go activity like football the interaction of humidity and air temperature may be somewhat lower than in a continuous, all-out exertion, such as a ten mile road race.

Figure 16.1 Cumulative Effect of Heat and High Humidity on Athletic Activity.

Source: Morris, A. F. 1981. The effects of heat and cold on athletes. *Potomac Valley Newsletter.* Washington, D.C.

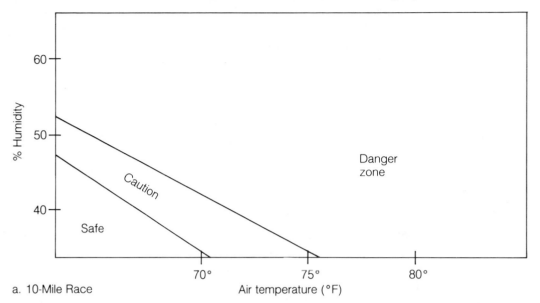

a. 10-Mile Race

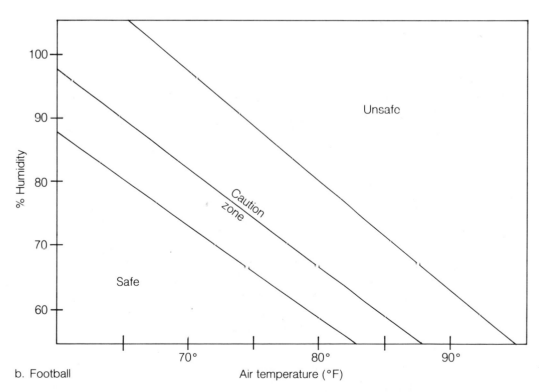

b. Football

Wind Velocity

Wind velocity affects athletes. Long distance cyclists are greatly affected by adverse wind conditions. Long distance runners, cross-country skiers, rowers, and even kayakers, are obviously adversely affected by extremes of wind velocity. Or, alternatively, in some of the longer distance events, wind may aid participants. Wind sometimes aids by evaporating sweat, which has a cooling effect; or wind may aid directly in long distance running events by coming from behind the runners and giving them a slight push. Since this is the case, many of the records established on point-to-point marathon courses are not officially accepted as world records because of the fact that the wind velocity may have aided the runner.

Barometric Pressure

Barometric pressure and air density can affect athletic performance. An example of this is seen in the outstanding long jump performance of Bob Beaman in the 1968 Olympics. Those games were held in Mexico City at an elevation of approximately twenty-two hundred meters. This altitude reduces the air density and, consequently, may enable an athlete to jump longer. Obviously, air density may affect performance in some of the running events, in that the percentage of oxygen in the air is reduced at this higher elevation. Performances in events over ten kilometers, especially the marathon, are often reduced at lesser air densities.

Air Pollution—Fog, Haze, Smoke

Factors of *fog, haze, smoke,* and *extremes* of *air pollution* will adversely affect performers. Very often, these conditions of air pollution are found in conjunction with extremes in temperature and humidity. There are various factors involved in air pollution, and this text will not go into a detailed discussion of them. In addition to air pollution, when pollen counts or readings of sulphur dioxide or other pollutants are extremely high in the atmosphere, the quality of athletic performances will be reduced (McCafferty, 1981). Fog, haze, and smoke also may affect performances in events which require the athlete to be able to see long distances.

Precipitation

Precipitation refers to rain, snow, sleet, or hail, which may fall on the athletes as they compete in their events. Extreme amounts of snowfall, rain, sleet, or hail impede athletic performance. Snow conditions are extremely crucial in long distance cross-country skiing events. Heavy rain may affect the long distance runner. Hail and sleet affect different types of athletes in different sports to varying degrees.

Clouds

Clouds, as an element of weather, are important because they affect the amount of sunlight falling directly on the athlete. In extreme sun, athletes may have to make adjustments by wearing sunglasses, sunscreens, caps, or provide some other type of shade. The clouds indirectly affect the surfaces on which athletes perform.

Light Data

The hours of daylight, or length of daylight on a particular day may affect the athlete. It may affect the athlete indirectly as it influences the light and dark cycles, affecting biorhythms to a degree. More importantly, in long distance sports where visibility is crucial, the light data may be important to the athlete.

Exercise in Heat

The hypothalamus, located deep within the temple region of the brain, is the thermoregulatory mechanism, or the heat control center, for the athlete. This center governs dissipation of body heat. By sensing heat from various thermoreceptors in the skin, as well as core organs, the body begins to make changes to rid itself of this rising internal heat. Skeletal muscles, which suddenly become active in vigorous activity, may increase heat production by as much as fifteen to eighteen times over basal or resting levels. The heat they produce must be dissipated. Figure 16.2 shows the effects of heat and high body temperature on human functioning. Most body heat is given off through the skin. Evaporation of sweat from the skin produces a cooling effect. In addition, heat may be dissipated through the lungs, or even via conduction, radiation, or convection to the environment. Conduction is defined here as the transmission of heat from particle to particle. In this case, heat from the athlete's body may be lost to the environment if body temperature is higher than the environmental temperature. Radiation is defined as a process of sending out rays of heat from the body as it is produced in the body through exercise. Convection is defined as transmitting heat by mass movement of heated particles. By far, *the most important cooling mechanism that the human body possesses is evaporation of sweat.*

The Content of Sweat

Sweat is about 90 percent water. It is faintly alkaline and contains some sodium chloride (salt), sugar, organic nitrogen, and waste products. If excessive amounts of any of the above components show up in the sweat, there is an indication that something abnormal is taking place within the athlete's body.

Factors in Sweat Loss

There are several factors involved in sweat loss. Most sweating occurs from the head, neck, and trunk. Therefore, it is important to keep these body areas cool by wearing no covering or extremely light clothing. The skin must be bare to dispose of sweat in an attempt to cool the body during performance in the hot weather.

Figure 16.2 Effect of Heat and High Body
Temperatures on Humans.
  Source: DuBois, E. F. 1948. *Fever and regulation
  of body temperature.* Springfield, IL: Charles C.
  Thomas. Reprinted with permission.

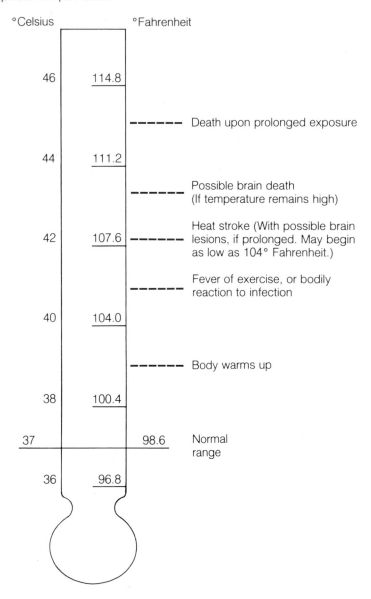

Another major factor in sweat loss is *humidity*. When humidity is high (60 to 100 percent), the ability of sweat to evaporate from the body is diminished, therefore, the ability of sweat to cool the body by evaporation is greatly lessened. Sweat simply rolls off the body if the humidity is high. If the athlete is not taking additional water or other fluids during performance to replace the water loss, there will be a decrement in performance. Some beneficial fluids to ingest are listed in the next section.

Fluids to Ingest to Maintain Proper Hydration

In an earlier section it was suggested that, under extreme conditions of high heat and humidity, the athlete may be in *grave* danger. It was also noted that the best way that athletes can insure that they won't fall victim to the heat is to ensure that they are properly hydrated before the event and that they drink continually during the athletic event. It is known that the best fluid to ingest during an athletic contest appears to be cold water (Costill, 1979). What is the usefulness of some of the commercial athletic drinks that have found their way into the marketplace? The next section answers this important question.

Commercial Athletic Drinks

To begin to analyze the question of which athletic drink is best for the athlete, one needs to know a little concerning the composition of sweat. Sweat is more than just plain water. It is composed of sodium, potassium, calcium, phosphate, magnesium, and slight traces of other components. The above minerals are often referred to as *electrolytes*, because, when they are found in fluids, they can conduct an electrical current. So, electrolytes are substances which may be dissolved in water and can make water conduct an electrical current. This conduction property is important in the human body because nerve impulses must be conducted along nerve fibers and to skeletal muscles in order to cause human voluntary movement. Whenever there is a breakdown in conduction of impulses in the body, we get abnormal functions in the form of irregular heartbeats, or misinformation to skeletal muscles, perhaps causing a cramp.

Since it was found that electrolytes are lost in sweat, some scientists began experimenting to try to determine exactly what important electrolytes were lost in sweat and in what amounts. Dr. Robert Cade conducted studies of football players and marathon runners at the University of Florida, which revealed that the ideal electrolyte replacement drink should have some potassium, sodium, and, obviously, water. Also, it was determined that the replacement fluid might be artificially sweetened, or at least contain some sugar (glucose or sucrose) replacement for the body sugars burned during exercise. Dr. Cade's original drink, called "Gatorade" (after the University of Florida's Gators) included sodium, potassium, and some artificial sweeteners to improve taste. The artificial sweeteners were added to the drink because electrolytes and water were found not to be very palatable to a hot, dry, thirsty athlete.

Soon, other developers got into the fluid replacement game. Electrolyte replacement with glucose (ERG), first produced in the late 60s, is similar to Gatorade, except it has more potassium (42 mg% to 24% for Gatorade) and less sodium (32 mg% to 130% for Gatorade). Again, some flavoring is added to make the drink taste better. The object is to get the athlete to drink something. If the fluid replacement drink is tasteless and, therefore, not consumed, the athlete is more susceptible to dehydration and subsequent overheating. Currently, there are dozens of athletic drinks available to the athlete for consumption during competition in hot weather. Some general suggestions for proper hydration are listed below.

Guidelines for Proper Hydration

1. First of all, the athlete should begin the activity in a well-hydrated state, which is indicated by *frequent urination of large volumes of relatively clear urine.*
2. During continued exercise in hot, humid conditions, the athlete should begin to drink before the actual thirst mechanism is triggered. If the athlete delays, it will be too late, and the core body temperature will rise (see fig. 16.3). A loss of 2–3 percent body weight, via sweating, may impair performance. A 4–5 percent loss of body weight due to sweating, coupled with continued high levels of exertion, is dangerous and definitely affects performance.
3. It has been *shown* that a cool (39° F) drink of water may be the best replacement fluid. This cool and unconcentrated solution will get from the stomach into the system to promote cooling better than a warmer, concentrated drink which contains much sugar or a heavily concentrated juice.

Figure 16.3 Effect of Fluid Intake on Rectal Temperatures During Prolonged Running.
Source: Coote, J. H. 1975. Physiological significance of somatic afferent pathways from skeletal muscle and joints with reflex effects on the heart and circulation. *Brain Res.* 87:139.

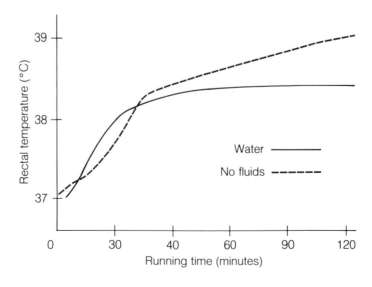

4. Frequent drinks of lesser amounts appear to be tolerated better than large amounts taken less frequently. A good guide seems to be to consume four to eight ounces to each five to fifteen minutes of activity.

5. Continued fluid replacement must be made immediately after the competition, and this replacement fluid may contain some electrolytes and sweetened solution. It is important to get any fluid replacement in the post-event recovery phase. At this point, the athletes usually take whatever drink is most acceptable to them. This seems to be a highly individual characteristic.

Heat Problems—Dehydrated and/or Overheated

There are several problems which can occur to the athlete due to unaccustomed exertion and unpreparedness when working out in a hot, humid environment. Four recognizable disorders that occur under these conditions are *heat cramps, heat fatigue, heat exhaustion,* and *heatstroke.* Several of these problems are major medical emergencies, especially *heat exhaustion* and *heatstroke.* When these conditions exist, the athlete must be seen immediately by trained medical emergency personnel and, if necessary, transported to a hospital or similar facility (Hanson, 1979; 1982).

Heat Cramps

Heat cramps are painful involuntary spasms of skeletal muscle. Most often, these cramps occur in the muscles of the lower limb. For years, the literature has suggested that this problem in athletes was due mainly to salt loss (Murphy, 1963). However, a recent suggestion is that heat cramps are more likely caused by a fluid volume problem. It has been suggested that heat cramps may be prevented by providing large amounts of water to the athlete throughout the entire exercise period (Nicholson, 1981). The treatment for heat cramps is for the athlete to refrain from the activity and to rehydrate properly.

Heat Fatigue

This particular problem affects many athletes after they have exercised in a hot, humid environment. Murphy (1979) characterizes this syndrome as simply a feeling of weakness and tiredness. This condition usually will improve promptly with rest and replenishment of lost body fluids.

The next two conditions, heat exhaustion and heatstroke, are very serious medical problems. As was noted above, these are genuine medical emergencies which must receive proper, immediate medical attention.

Heat Exhaustion

Heat exhaustion is defined as a physical condition characterized by extreme weakness, stupor, headache, and nausea, following unaccustomed exertion in a hot, humid environment. Dizziness, as well as headache and profuse sweating, are usually present in the heat exhaustion victim. These symptoms occur mainly because of a decrease in blood volume. With severe sweating, the body fluid level drops, causing a decrease in total blood volume. Murphy (1979) notes that the key features which differentiate heat exhaustion from heatstroke are (1) sweating, and (2) normal body temperature. Other symptoms which may occur are that the skin of the athlete appears cold, wet, and often ashen in color; pulse is mostly rapid; blood pressure is extremely low; and finally, a general feeling of fatigue, faintness, nausea, headache, cramps, and blurring vision. An important consideration at this point is that, if the heat exhaustion condition is allowed to continue, the distinct possibility of a heatstroke and worse complications is present (Appenzeller & Atkinson, 1981).

The Treatment for Heat Exhaustion

The treatment for heat exhaustion is that the athlete should be *immediately withdrawn from further activity for the remainder of the day.* The athlete should be made as comfortable as possible, and fluids should be given by mouth when the athlete is able to swallow. If unconsciousness or semi-consciousness is present, the administration of fluids via the mouth is not advisable. If the athlete is vomiting and unable to consume fluids, hospitalization with intravenous administration of fluids is most likely necessary. Murphy (1979) further suggests that the athlete's fluid intake, especially water, should be reviewed before more strenuous exercise in the heat is undertaken in succeeding days.

Heatstroke

Heatstroke is an acute medical emergency. It is characterized by a dangerously high core body temperature, due to a failure of the temperature regulatory mechanism. A heatstroke victim has severe central nervous system disturbance. Heatstroke may occur suddenly, without being preceded by any of the other clinical symptoms which were listed for heat exhaustion, heat cramps, or heat fatigue. In the condition of heatstroke, the athlete may become unconscious. Some of the more common symptoms of heatstroke are listed below (Noble & Bachman, 1979).

Heatstroke Symptoms

The skin of the heatstroke victim tends to be hot, red, and dry. Perspiration may be present. The core temperature is extremely high—it may be in the range of 103° to 109°F (above 40°C). Blood pressure tends to be low. The pulse may be strong and rapid, but also the heart may be diminishing in its beat. The eyes and pupils may be dilated or contracted. Breathing may be deep or rapid. There is a general feeling of confusion, headache, and extreme hotness. The brain, as well as other vital organs, may begin to shut down because of the rapid depletion of body fluid, as well as the high heat which is present. The victim may exhibit combative delirium, vomit, and lapse into convulsions and coma.

Table 16.1 Common Symptoms of Physical Exertion in Hot, Humid Environments

	Heat exhaustion	Heatstroke
Dominant symptoms	Fatigue; nausea; headache	Disorientation; headache
Mental status	Usually conscious (but supine); disoriented	Marked alteration of mental status or unconscious; blurred vision; disorientation
Rectal temperature	$\approx 40°C$; $\approx 102°F$	$\approx 41°C$; $\approx 103°F$
Skin/sweat	Vasoconstricted (mostly); active sweating in most cases	Vasodilated (mostly); active sweating may be present, but sweating may stop
Blood pressure	Narrow pulse pressure; orthostatic drop severe	Wide pulse pressure; diastolic low
Pulse	100 to 140 BPM; pulse mostly rapid; narrow, slight pulse	120 to 160 BPM—sometimes strong, sometimes weak and bounding

Sources: Hanson, P. G. 1982. Coping with the elements: cold, heat, wind, rain. Paper presented at the American Medical Joggers Assoc. Symposium. Chicago. Luce, J. M. 1979. Respiratory adaption and maladaption to altitude. The physician and sports medicine. 7:54.

Heatstroke Treatment

Treatment for the heatstroke victim involves *immediate, rapid cooling* and *transfer to a hospital* where cooling continues. Often, the body is covered with ice or immersed in cold water to effect immediate cooling. Other medical doctors suggest using ice to massage the head, neck, and extremities to effect rapid cooling. Until the athlete is able to be transported to the medical facility, a trainer, or any other supervisory athletic personnel, must attempt to lower body temperature *immediately* by removing clothing, drenching the athlete with cool water, using ice packs, and massaging the head, neck, trunk, and extremities. The object, of course, is to lower the body temperature *as quickly as possible*. This must be done immediately because death or serious damage could occur, literally within a matter of minutes. As the rectal temperature (core temperature) rises to 105° or 106°F, for even a few minutes, there is the possibility of irreversible damage to the liver, brain, or kidneys. In heatstroke, very high temperatures can be reached very rapidly. Table 16.1 indicates some of the common clinical findings connected with exertion in the heat. Both heat exhaustion and heatstroke are reported.

Practical Tips for Performing in the Heat

1. Be well hydrated to start.
2. Wear minimal clothing.
3. Drink continuously.
4. Drink cold fluids.
5. Cease activity, if possible.
6. Be alert to danger signs.

Cold Environment

There are many sports that require the athlete to compete in a cold environment. Cross-country and downhill skiing, mountain climbing, sailing, ice hockey or skating, hiking or backpacking, kayaking, hunting and fishing, cave exploring, and others. In many northern sections of North America and Europe, sportsmen are exposed to low temperatures during the late fall and winter seasons. American football is sometimes played on snow covered fields in a windchill factor of −30° to −50°F. Runners in the northern United States in the winter are exposed to bitterly cold conditions. How does the body react to these extreme cold temperatures? What can be done to enable the athlete who chooses to perform in the cold to do so safely?

The next section looks at some of the physiological responses to the cold. Also, the topics of hypothermia and frostbite are considered and some practical tips for fighting the cold are offered.

Animals living in cold climates often have specific adaptations to protect them from severe cold. Most cold weather creatures have developed thick layers of fat to insulate them against the cold. The polar bear has a unique membrane that passes over its eyeball to wipe away slush. The fur on many animals doubles in length during the cold season. These are some of the adaptations which may be necessary for certain animals to survive in the cold winter seasons. The human organism can make some physiological responses to a cold environment. For example, long distance (e.g. English Channel) swimmers tend to have more body fat than pool swimmers.

Physiological Reactions to Cold

There are several things which happen when the body begins to get chilled. These reactions are noted in figure 16.4 and table 16.2. The main physiological reactions to the cold generally occur in the following sequence. When first chilled, the body begins to close down circulation to the skin. If cold is continued, circulation to the extremities—the hands

Table 16.2 Effects of Hypothermia

Water temperature (degrees Fahrenheit)	Onset of exhaustion, leading to possible blackout	Estimated time of survival with continued exposure[a]
32.5	Under 15 min.	Under 15 to 45 min.
32.5 to 40	15 to 30 min.	30 to 90 min.
40 to 50	30 to 60 min.	1 to 3 hrs.
50 to 60	1 to 3 hrs.	1 to 6 hrs.
60 to 70	2 to 7 hrs.	2 to 40 hrs.
70 to 80	3 to 12 hrs.	3 hrs. to indefinite
Over 80	Indefinite	Indefinite

Source: United States Marine Corps. 1979. Cold weather operations handbook. Quantico, VA: USMC Development and Education Command.

[a]These times vary according to age, sex, and fitness level of the individual.

Figure 16.4 Effect of Cold Temperatures on Humans.

Source: DuBois, E. F. 1948. *Fever and regulation of body temperature*. Springfield, IL: Charles C. Thomas. Reprinted with permission.

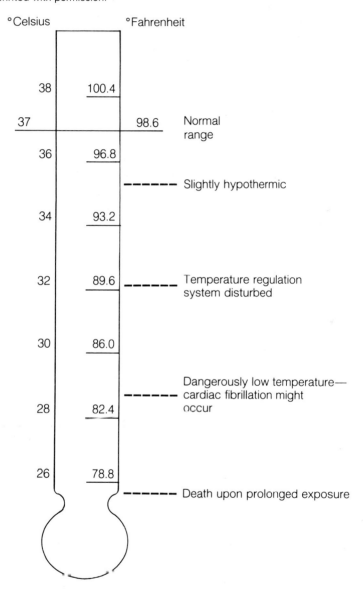

257

and feet—is also reduced. The tips of the ears and nose may also suffer lessened circulation. This bodily reaction tends to conserve core (torso) temperature. Thus, the critical organs (heart, lungs, etc.), are attempting to conserve heat at the expense of the extremities.

If the cold continues, the body begins to shiver. This automatic reaction is another attempt by the body to conserve heat. Upon continued exposure to the cold, the core temperature continues to drop and mental and physical deterioration occur. Mental symptoms of **hypothermia** include anxiety, irritability, apathy, loss of purpose, and dizziness. Prominent physical symptoms, in addition to shivering, are motor difficulties, clumsiness, muscle weakness, and cramps. The body's temperature regulating system begins to malfunction and total body collapse may be imminent. Unless rapid rewarming is accomplished, death may ensue. All this could happen in three hours or less. If a person were suddenly dumped into freezing waters, death could occur within minutes—certainly within one hour. Table 16.2 shows the effects of extreme cold, which may occur when a person is immersed into cold water. One can see that recovery and warming must be quick, if negative effects are to be avoided.

Layering Against Cold

Many people, forced to live and work in Arctic climates, make adaptations in order to be successful in that environment. Military personnel stationed in frigid climates are told to wear *seven* layers of specially-made clothing on their upper bodies. The recommended layering for the lower body is six layers of clothing. This emphasizes the single most important fact of cold weather dressing—*layering* of clothing.

When layering, it is best to choose several layers of different types of material, rather than to simply have a single, large, bulky layer. Cold weather scientists suggest that athletes choose materials of loosely woven fabrics, like wool, since they tend to trap air better. This trapped air, in turn, acts as insulation.

Another unique feature of wool clothing is that it tends to dry from the inside out, thus it is not likely to draw heat from your skin as most wet garments do. Try this experiment to see wool's effectiveness. Wrap a strip of wool fabric tightly around a ruler and then dip it into a glass of water. Note that only the submerged part will hold water. Now try the same experiment with cotton. Observe that the cotton absorbs water and the water actually appears to run up the measuring stick as the cotton material absorbs moisture. Therefore, cotton materials are poor insulating materials, especially when wet. Many synthetics, especially acrylic, can be effective as insulating layers of clothing, but everyone must know their tolerances to this type of man-made material.

A final consideration in layering the body with clothes is to protect the body from the harmful effects of *wind.* As figure 16.5 diagrams, a strong wind may make a chilly day seem like a bitterly cold day. To protect against the wind, careful consideration must be given to the outside layers of clothing. Various types of nylon and newer Goretex® fabrics attempt to cut down on the wind getting through to the body. Some of these materials also prevent some of the rain or moisture from coming through to the underlying garments. If possible, the athlete tries not to get clothing wet when competing.

Figure 16.5 A Windchill Nomogram. This chart portrays the effect of the interaction of wind and cold (not precipitation) on the human body. Note that although the air temperature may be approximately at freezing, if the wind velocity is high (25–35 m.p.h.), the environmental conditions may feel *bitterly cold.*
Source: U.S.M.C. 1979.

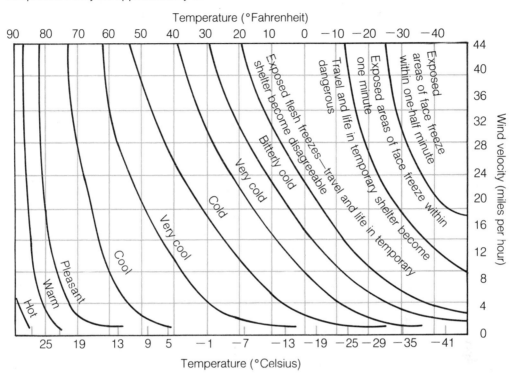

Cold and Wet

It is crucial not to get wet when out in the cold, since wet clothing conducts heat from the body nearly 240 times faster than dry clothing (USMC, 1979). Down-filled materials are very effective as insulating layers when dry, but if down gets wet, it is ineffective. The athlete must determine how much perspiration the activity is going to generate and dress in layers accordingly.

Frostbite

Because the body loses much heat through the extremities, the extremities must be very well protected. A major problem that occurs to the extremities is frostbite. Frostbite is actual freezing of body parts. Ice crystals may form on the skin, or in the tissues and fluids under the skin. Frostbite is a form of local and superficial tissue destruction.

Table 16.3 Windchill Index (equivalent in cooling power on exposed flesh)

Wind speed (mph)								Air temperature (°F)	
	35	30	25	20	15	10	5	0	−5	−10
4	35	30	25	20	15	10	5	0	−5	−10
5	32	27	22	16	11	6	0	−5	−10	−15
10	22	16	10	3	−3	−9	−15	−22	−27	−34
15	16	9	2	−5	−11	−18	−25	−31	−38	−45
20	12	4	−3	−10	−17	−24	−31	−39	−46	−53
25	8	1	−7	−15	−22	−29	−36	−44	−51	−59
30	6	−2	−10	−18	−25	−33	−41	−49	−56	−64
35	4	−4	−12	−20	−27	−35	−43	−52	−58	−67
40	3	−5	−13	−21	−29	−37	−45	−53	−60	−69
45*	2	−6	−14	−22	−30	−38	−46	−54	−62	−70

*Wind speeds greater than 40 mph have little additional cooling effect.
Example—A 30 mph wind, combined with a temperature of 30 degrees F, (−1 degree Celsius), can have the same chilling effect as a temperature of −2 degrees F, (minus19 degrees Celsius), when it is calm.
Source: U.S. Department of Commerce. National Oceanic and Atmospheric Administration.

The most prominent areas in which frostbite occurs are the nose, outer ears, cheeks, fingers, and toes. It has been reported that about 70 percent of the freezing damage in severe frostbite cases involves the toes. In less severe frostbite, the nose and fingers are usually involved. Symptoms of frostbite are a loss of sensation, a tingling sensation, or numbness. Frostbitten skin may turn grayish yellow, or white. Blisters may form.

If frostbite is suspected, the following suggestions should be followed in order.

1. Get inside to a warm shelter.
2. Carefully remove wet or frosted clothing from the suspected area.
3. Do not rub frozen region.
4. Do not warm frozen skin near warm radiator or fire.
5. Do not massage area with ice or snow.
6. Gently rewarm the frozen site with *warm water* (90° to 106°F, or 39° to 42°C).
7. Protect thawed region (do not break blisters).
8. Keep entire body warm to avoid peripheral vasoconstriction.
9. Avoid walking on frostbitten toes unless absolutely necessary.
10. Blot the skin dry, bathe in mild soapy water (not detergent or laundry soaps) and wrap individual parts with a clean towel to avoid breaking blisters.
11. Seek medical attention.

People who have had frostbite are apt to suffer it again more easily.

−15	−20	−25	−30	−35	−40	−45
−15	−20	−25	−30	−35	−40	−45
−21	−26	−31	−36	−42	−47	−52
−40	−46	−52	−58	−64	−71	−77
−51	−58	−65	−72	−78	−85	−92
−60	−67	−74	−81	−88	−95	−103
−66	−74	−81	−88	−96	−103	−110
−71	−79	−86	−93	−101	−109	−116
−74	−82	−89	−97	−105	−113	−120
−76	−84	−92	−100	−107	−115	−123
−78	−85	−93	−102	−109	−117	−125

Hypothermia

Hypothermia is cooling of the body to a rectal temperature of less than 95°F (35°C). This excessive cooling is often associated with a failure of the muscular system and also the central nervous system (the brain and spinal function). Table 16.3 shows some of the effects of hypothermia. In addition, table 16.2 shows some of the reactions that occur in the body upon prolonged exposure to cold. It is also important to note how the wind velocity interacts with cold temperatures to produce windchill factors. This is shown in table 16.3. Along the left hand column of the table the wind is indicated in miles per hour, and along the rows of the column we see what happens with increasingly colder temperatures. Study of this windchill factor table will alert the athlete to the extreme dangers of working in a very cold, windy environment. The layering system, which was suggested earlier, to protect the body against the cold and wind, is especially important in preventing hypothermia.

Proper Treatment of Hypothermia

The proper treatment of hypothermia is rapid rewarming of the body. Core temperature must be raised to near normal levels as quickly as possible. This is done by getting the victim into a warm, windless shelter. Wrapping the cold athlete in well-insulated, warm blankets helps to restore body temperature. If possible, and the athlete is conscious and able to take fluids, warm liquids should help to raise body temperature to normal. If one is out in open country with no shelter available, perhaps other athletes or colleagues may share a well-insulated sleeping bag with the hypothermic victim in an attempt to raise the body temperature. Prompt medical attention is always indicated in severe cases of hypothermia.

Practical Tips for Performing in the Cold

1. Layer clothing.
2. Cover head, nose, ears, hands, and feet.
3. Don't get wet.
4. Be well hydrated.
5. Run into the wind.
6. Get inside *fast*.

Performance at Altitude

Since the Mexico City Olympics in 1968, many athletes and medical personnel have been concerned with some of the problems of athletes when they compete at altitudes. Mexico City is approximately 7,350 feet, or 2,240 meters, above sea level. This is the point at which the air becomes rarified and the amount of oxygen is somewhat diminished.

When athletes are competing at this altitude, performance levels are generally less than those which occur at sea level. Shephard (1976) has indicated that for events lasting four minutes or longer, there was a 3 percent decrease in performance from previous Olympiads. In longer lasting events, those of up to one hour or longer, there was an 8 percent drop-off in performance.

For some competitors, particularly jumpers and sprinters, the wind resistance and the atmospheric density (air pressure per cubic liter of air) are lessened and, consequently, the athletes do not have to meet with this increased air resistance. Therefore, performances in the sprint or jumping events may equal or, in fact, exceed sea level performances, while distance runners may have had their performance diminished by nearly 24 percent in Mexico City.

Acclimatization

Unlike adjustments to heat and cold, acclimatization to altitude may be slower and contain components that require continued training and conditioning over a period of several months (Shephard, 1976). Acclimatization is a period of adjustment that the body needs to adapt itself to a rapid change in environment. Luce (1979) has noted that the most profound circulatory adaptation to altitude is the increase in red blood cell concentration. This increase mimics the changes that the athlete hopes to achieve with a blood doping transfusion. It appears that the major advantage in training at high altitudes is for performances at high altitudes. One of the things that has been emphasized throughout this text is the specificity of training concept, which requires athletes to train themselves in their practice or conditioning sessions as close to the actual competition conditions as possible. Therefore, if the athlete is expected to compete at 7,500 feet or above, it is probably worthwhile to train at this altitude for a period of weeks or months, in order to be best conditioned for the altitude. Shephard (1976) has noted that many national teams used mountain camps (at altitude) in preparation for the Munich Olympics (altitude 1700 feet) in 1972. After detailed analysis of results of performances in these Olympics after training at high altitude, it was generally conceded that there was no distinct advantage to the altitude training. This, again, emphasizes the concept of specificity of training. If the athlete is to compete at sea level, most of the training and conditioning should take place at sea level (Morris, 1983). Grover (1979) also notes that there appears to be no advantage to training at altitude for sea level contests.

Air Pollution and Athletic Performance

Air pollution must be considered an environmental stress which may adversely affect training and competition. Just as environmental stresses of wind, heat, cold, and altitude affect athletic training peak performance, so too does the stress of air pollution adversely affect performance. Virtually no area in the world is without some form of air pollution. Athletic competition in an atmosphere which is considered somewhat polluted is graphically displayed whenever a major sporting event is held in a major metropolitan area.

The Effects of Air Pollution on Physiological Performance

The late Dr. William B. McCafferty (1981) has written an excellent text on air pollution and athletic performance. In this book he notes that most research suggests that various pollutants adversely affect athletic performance. However, it is to be pointed out that there is considerable individual variation in response to different air pollutants. Of course, when people exercise, more pollutants may be brought into the body, due to the increased depth and rate of respiration, irritating the nose, mouth, and lung linings. Many of the various pollutants found in the air cause physiological responses, which may inhibit athletic performance. Some of these pollutants are carbon monoxide, sulfur pollutants, and others (McCafferty, 1981).

Practical Hints for Training in Areas of High Air Pollution

Following are several precautions that the athlete may take, if forced to exercise or work in an environment that has some sort of air pollution.

1. Negative effects of training in chronically high pollution areas may be lessened somewhat by scheduling workouts for early in the morning.
2. Prolonged, heavy exercise should be avoided when pollution levels are extreme.
3. Individuals with respiratory or cardiac ailments should avoid physical activity when pollution levels exceed recommended air quality standards.
4. Athletes should avoid training near highways or areas of heavily congested streets, if possible.

5. When competing on smoggy days, exposure may be minimized by remaining indoors as long as possible before competing outdoors. (Warm-ups and other preparations should be made indoors, if possible).
6. Smoking should be banned or curtailed at all indoor competition facilities.
7. Individuals with known heart disease should not exercise sooner than three hours following heavy exposure to carbon monoxide.
8. Attempts to adapt to air pollution by working out in heavily polluted areas are *not recommended.* ■

Summary

This chapter is concerned with environmental factors in athletic training and sports medicine. Various factors of weather that affect the athlete competing outdoors are listed. These factors are precipitation, clouds, heat, and cold. A major factor in performing outdoors in the heat is the avoidance of heatstroke, heat exhaustion, and heat cramps. Each of these medical problems is discussed and the proper treatment noted. Competing in a cold environment requires the athlete to layer themselves with clothing in order to preserve body heat. Problems that the athlete encounters in the cold, such as frostbite and hypothermia are discussed. Problems of the athlete competing at high altitudes are described. It takes the athlete several weeks to acclimatize for performances at altitudes. The effects of air pollution on physiological performances are listed. It is noted that many common pollutants, such as carbon monoxide and various sulfur pollutants, adversely affect performance.

References

Appenzeller, A., & R. Atkinson. 1981. Temperature regulation and sports. *Sports medicine.* Baltimore: Urban & Schwarzenberg.

Coote, J. H. 1975. Physiological significance of somatic afferent pathways from skeletal muscle and joints with reflex effects on the heart and circulation. *Brain Research.* 87:139.

Costill, D. L. 1979. *A scientific approach to distance running.* Los Altos: Track & Field News Press.

Editors of Runner's World Magazine. 1975. *Running with the elements.* Mountain View, CA: World Publications.

Grover, R. F. 1979. Performance at altitude. In Strauss, R. H. ed. *Sports medicine and physiology.* Philadelphia: W. B. Saunders Co.

Hanson, P. G. 1979. Heat injury in runners. *The Physician and Sportsmedicine.* 7:91.

Hanson, P. G. 1982. Coping with the elements: cold, heat, wind, rain. Paper presented at the American Medical Joggers Association Symposium, Chicago. October.

Luce, J. M. 1979. Respiratory adaption and maladaption to altitude. *The Physician and Sportsmedicine.* 7:54.

McCafferty, W. B. 1981. *Air pollution and athletic performance.* Springfield, IL: Charles C. Thomas.

Morris, A. F. 1981. The effects of heat and cold on athletes. *Potomac Valley Newsletter.* Washington, D.C.

Morris, A. F. 1983. Oxygen. In Williams, M. H. ed. *Ergogenic aids in Sport.* Champaign, IL: Human Kinetics Publishers.

Murphy, R. J. 1963. Problems of environmental heat in athletics. *Ohio Medicine Journal.* 59:799.

Murphy, R. J. 1979. Heat illness and athletics. In Strauss, R. H. ed. *Sports medicine and physiology.* Philadelphia: W. B. Saunders Co.

Nadel, E. R. 1979. *Temperature regulation.* In Strauss, R. ed. *Sports medicine and physiology.* Philadelphia: W. B. Saunders Co.

Nicholson, F. 1981. Heatstroke in athletes. *British Medical Journal.* 282:1544.

Noble, H. B., & D. Bachman. 1979. Medical aspects of distance race. *The Physician and Sportsmedicine.* 7:78.

Shephard, R. J. 1976. Environment. In Williams, J. G. P. & P. N. Sperryn. eds. *Sports medicine.* Baltimore: Williams & Wilkins.

United States Marine Corps. 1979. *Cold weather operations handbook.* Quantico, VA: USMC Development and Education Command.

The Female Athlete

Outline

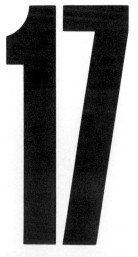

Introduction

This chapter concerns the female athlete. Early societal influences that affected the female athlete are shown. Historically, clothing styles and social mores adversely affected the female athlete. Women were initially barred from the Olympic Games. Now, women compete in many events in the Olympics. As recently as 1984, however, they were still not allowed to participate in certain events.

The biological factors affecting women's sports performance are detailed. Before puberty, there are no major differences between young boys and young girls in athletics. After puberty, there develops a marked anatomical and physiological difference between men and women. These differences are mainly in the heart and circulatory system and in body composition. There are also some major biomechanical differences between the male and female. Essentially, the female has a lower center of gravity, with more weight distributed in the lower extremities, as compared with the male athlete. The angle of the femur (lower leg), as it intersects at the hip, is slightly different in the female, and this may lead to problems in running. The female athlete has specific concerns regarding competition that the male does not have. Perhaps the major factor which must be considered is that of periodicity. In the United States, a young girl generally starts to menstruate at approximately age 12.5. From this time, until her early or mid 50s, this monthly cycle may affect practice and training schedules. However, outstanding female athletes pay minimal attention to this monthly cycle, and continue to train and compete throughout each of the phases.

Also included in this chapter is a discussion of menstrual abnormalities. These abnormalities are amenorrhea, (cessation of menstrual funotion), and dismenorrhea, (pain or discomfort at or about the time of the menstrual period). How these two factors affect the female athlete is discussed. Another section in this chapter concerns physical activity, pregnancy, and childbirth and the female athlete. Some special dietary concerns for the female athlete regarding intake of iron are listed.

Today it is quite common to see females engaged in all types of athletic competition. This was not always the case, and one has only to look at the history of the Olympic Games to note that participation for women athletes was severely limited, even up to the 1980 Games. It is the purpose of this chapter to examine the female athlete and athletic competition. Many of the topics, such as drugs, nutrition, and training, covered in other sections, relate to all performers regardless of sex. However, there are some concerns that pertain specifically to the female athlete that people in the sports medicine field should be acquainted with.

This section starts with a brief history of female involvement in sport, Then, some of the specific biological and physiological differences between the sexes are covered. Particular concerns of the female athlete, such as menstruation and athletic injuries, are discussed.

Early Societal Factors Affecting Women in Sports

Bodnar and Bodnar (1980) suggest that in the earliest of times men and women undoubtedly engaged in many of the same activities. It is believed that both males and females hunted, fished, foraged, fought, wrestled, climbed, ran, jumped, hurdled, and swam side by side, as both sexes fought for their existence. Certainly a woman was slowed periodically, during times of pregnancy, child-bearing, and child-rearing, but for the most part, women had to be strong and hardy, or they would perish.

Soon, religion, custom, and socialization began to affect and regulate certain aspects of the female's role in society. It is reported that during the Bronze Age (about 2,000 B.C.) women participated in hunting, fishing, and a type of bullfighting. The women in early Athens were secluded and not permitted to engage in physical activities. In early Rome, women were prohibited from participation in sports. Our own country has seen many changes in the role of women in our society.

During early colonial periods, women were restricted in their participation in sports and games. This model was adapted from Europe and the British Empire. With the development of the bicycle around the turn of the twentieth century, women began to wear looser clothing and to engage in more physical activities. Female athletes were participating in swimming and basketball during the early 1900s. Initially, this early sports competition was only between women from the same school or intramural type competition. The emphasis was on enjoyment at the expense of winning. This continued until the 1920s and 1930s.

Women in the Olympics

Early religion prohibited women from engaging in the Olympic Games. In fact, for many years women who were caught even watching the Games were sentenced to death. The early Olympic Games lasted from several hundred years B.C. until 394 A.D. From then until the modern Games began in 1876, there were no Olympics held.

In the 1900 Olympic Games in Paris, women were allowed to compete in golf and tennis. Then, in St. Louis in 1904, American women were again banned from competition. It seems James E. Sullivan, head of the Amateur Athletic Union (AAU) and U.S. Olympic movement, opposed women's entry to the Games. It was not until 1920 that women were formally allowed to compete again. Throughout the 1920s and 1930s the news media increased coverage of women's sporting activities and feminist activities in general. From that time on, women have competed in Olympic events, but the number of events and extent of women's participation is still not on a par with the men. As recently as 1980, women had no 5000 meter or 10,000 meter running events. The marathon for women was just added in the 1984 Olympic Games in Los Angeles.

Current Legal Advances of Women's Rights in Sports

Perhaps the most recent significant milestone was the passage of the 1972 Education Amendments Act. This federal law, referred to as Title IX, was patterned after the Civil Rights Act of 1964 and states that no person in the United States shall, on the basis of sex, be denied participation in athletic activity. The main purpose of this Act was to insure equal opportunity for women in sports participation. If athletic competition and sport are worthwhile activities, then they should be available equally to both men and women.

Other developments relate to control over collegiate sports. The National College Athletic Association (NCAA), the national governing body of men's college sports, seeks to control collegiate athletics for women. Since money and prestige are involved in these activities, these differences will have to be worked out.

Biological Factors in Women's Sports Activities

Puberty and Prepuberty Periods

Some authorities cite the biological differences between males and females as the reason why females should limit or refrain from sports participation. There is no doubt that some differences are real, however, it is believed that the differences between males and females may not lead to increased injury or to limited performance.

During the propubertal period, girls are equal to, and often are superior to, boys of the same age in physical activities requiring speed, strength, flexibility, and endurance. The physical capacity of young children is essentially equal during this period prior to puberty. Thomas (1979) notes that puberty can occur approximately two years earlier in

Women's participation in sport is growing at a fantastic rate, however, they are still limited in certain sports, such as pole vaulting and triple jumping. This will change in the future.

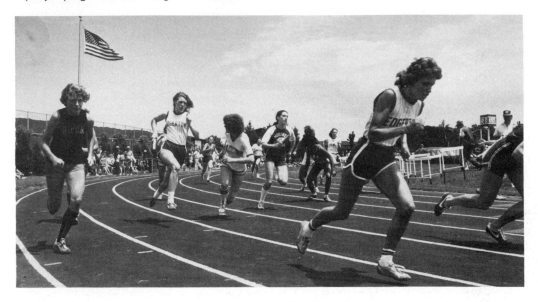

the female than in the male. Frisch (1981) cites figures that show the onset of puberty occurs at about the age of 12.5 years in young girls in the United States. The earlier puberty occurs, the earlier the epiphyses (growing areas) of the long bones close, thus preventing a further growth in height. These complex changes that take place at puberty are mediated through the endocrine system.

Wide variations—all within normal limits—in body size may exist at the time the female experiences puberty. Therefore, the maturation level of females in the eleven to fifteen year age groups is often considerably greater than for the males. This should be taken into account when programming for coeducational sports, especially those involving body contact. Even within the same sex, females may differ widely in sexual characteristics during this expanded maturation period of twelve to eighteen years.

Anatomical and Physiological Differences Between Men and Women

It was noted in the previous section that, prior to puberty, boys and girls are virtually equal in height, weight, and strength. However, in the post-pubertal period, boys are taller, heavier, and stronger than females. This added strength often makes males faster than females, so in any sport in which size, strength, and speed are crucial components, males will have an advantage over their female counterparts. A second major anatomical difference in the post-pubertal period is the amount of body fat that the individual possesses.

270

Figure 17.1 Theoretical Model of Body
Composition for a Reference Man/Woman.
Adapted from Behnke, A. R. Jr., and J. H.
Wilmore. 1974. *Evaluation and regulation of
body build and composition.* Englewood Cliffs,
NJ: Prentice Hall.

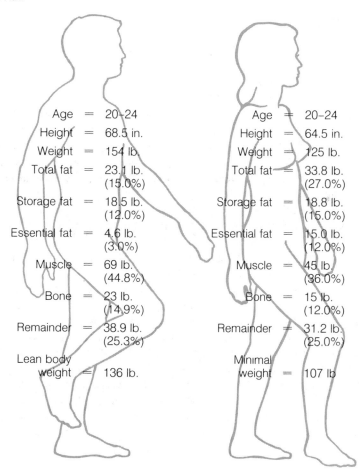

Age	=	20–24
Height	=	68.5 in.
Weight	=	154 lb.
Total fat	=	23.1 lb. (15.0%)
Storage fat	=	18.5 lb. (12.0%)
Essential fat	=	4.6 lb. (3.0%)
Muscle	=	69 lb. (44.8%)
Bone	=	23 lb. (14.9%)
Remainder	=	38.9 lb. (25.3%)
Lean body weight	=	136 lb.

Age	=	20–24
Height	=	64.5 in.
Weight	=	125 lb.
Total fat	=	33.8 lb. (27.0%)
Storage fat	=	18.8 lb. (15.0%)
Essential fat	=	15.0 lb. (12.0%)
Muscle	=	45 lb. (36.0%)
Bone	=	15 lb. (12.0%)
Remainder	=	31.2 lb. (25.0%)
Minimal weight	=	107 lb

It has been reported that body fat in boys tends to peak at around age eleven. In girls, body fat generally increases from age seven to seventeen. Figure 17.1 shows theoretical values for the average or reference man and woman.

This greater amount of adipose tissue in the female may prove to be somewhat of a handicap in certain sport activities. In other activities, such as long distance channel swimming, it may be a positive factor. In sports where the female must move her own body weight, she will be at a disadvantage compared to the male, who carries much less body fat. However, it is known that, in many sports, females have reduced their percent of body fat to extremely low levels and are most efficient.

Cardiac and Circulatory Differences

The female generally has a smaller heart than the male. A person's heart is about the size of his/her clenched fist; therefore, since a woman's fist is smaller than the male's, it might be expected that the heart is also proportionately smaller. The heart rate for the female is somewhat faster—about 6 beats per minute faster when at rest. In most species, a larger animal has a slower heart rate than a smaller animal. Elephants have slow heart rates, while birds have very rapid heart rates.

Circulatory red blood cells are more prevalent in the male. It is estimated that males have five million red blood cells per cubic millimeter, as compared to four and a half million in the female. Because of this discrepancy in red blood cells, it is estimated that the female has 8 percent less hemoglobin. Blood pressure values, both systolic and diastolic, are five to ten millimeters higher in the male.

Respiratory and Metabolic Differences

Since women tend to have smaller thoracic cavities, they breathe at a slightly faster rate than men. Women require somewhat less oxygen because of their lower metabolic rate and smaller body size. Another factor here may be the larger fat percentage in the female, since fat is more metabolically *inactive* than muscle mass. This may also contribute to the lessened metabolic rate of the female.

Vital Capacity

Vital capacity is defined as the maximal volume of air that a person can expire after a maximal inspiration. It tends to vary between the sexes, since it has a direct bearing on the body size, thoracic area, and height of the individual. The female has about a 10 percent lesser vital capacity than the male. It is important to note that training markedly increases vital capacity, and this in turn can enhance performance capabilities.

Maximal Aerobic Power

In the laboratory, we generally measure maximal oxygen uptake (VO_2 max) expressed as the maximal oxygen consumed during an all out work task. In the adult male, VO_2 max is approximately 20–30 percent higher than in the average female (over age 12). Both men and women tend to top their VO_2 max values at age eighteen, unless they are in an intensive endurance conditioning program. Body size and genetics may be contributing factors to this maximal value.

Since many determinations of VO_2 max are referenced to body size and weight, it can readily be seen that females would have lower readings when compared to males. Another factor, perhaps intruding on the VO_2 max in the female, is the reduced hemoglobin concentration. Since less O_2 can be carried throughout the system, this may be another factor limiting VO_2 max in the female. Again, percentage of body fat in the individual must be taken into account. With proper training, this maximal oxygen uptake capacity may be substantially improved (by 20–50 percent).

Metabolism

It is generally observed that the metabolic rate of the female is approximately 5 to 10 percent lower than that of the male of comparable size—assuming both have about the same body surface area. If the basal metabolic rate (resting rate) is related to actual muscle mass of the individual, then this sex difference tends to disappear. Some authors (Klafs & Arnheim, 1981) note a higher rate of calcium metabolism in the female than in the male. They point out that, since bone ossification occurs earlier in the female, this calcium ossification rate would be higher. They note also that male bones tend to be thicker and heavier. What is not taken into account here is the training, experiential, societal aspect of living which may predispose the male to more strength activities than the female. More about this in the subsequent section.

Muscular Strength Differences

In the adult, it is known that males are stronger than females. In objective testing "overall" total body strength was found to be 35 percent greater in the male. In the lower extremities (legs) females are about three quarters as strong as males. In the upper extremities (hands, arms, and shoulders) the inequality in strength is more pronounced. Some studies have

Women, generally, are not as big (in height or weight) as men and have less muscle mass.

Therefore, they are at a slight disadvantage in events which require speed, strength, and power.

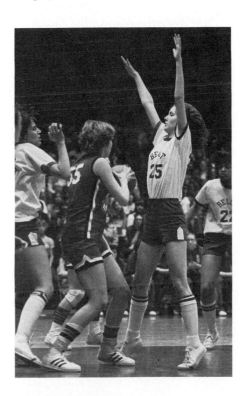

The Female Athlete

shown women to be only half as strong as males in upper body strength. Societal/cultural factors may be operating to affect these strength discrepancies. Certainly, if either sex engages in strength building activities, one can observe significant (50–100 percent) increases in body strength (Haycock, 1980).

Biomechanical Differences

Outside of the rather obvious height and weight differences, there are some fairly stable differences in biomechanical properties between males and females. The woman's pelvis is broader and shallower than the man's. This seems to make the femur attach to the pelvis at a greater degree of angle (fig. 17.2). This, in turn, tends to lower the female's center of gravity and may also make running activities slightly more difficult. It has also been reported that women's arms and legs are proportionately shorter than men's. What advantage or disadvantage this may produce is hard to evaluate. Certainly, in a sport like fencing or basketball, where reach is important, arm length may be advantageous.

Adiposity Differences

Females, as was noted earlier, have about 8–12 percent more body fat than males in the early adult years. The fat is stored in certain well-defined depots around the body. Females tend to store fat in their breasts, around the upper and inner thighs, the abdomen, and hips. It should be recalled that about 50 percent of body fat is stored subcutaneously, that is, just under the body skin layer. The other 50 percent is considered the more essential body fat, and is protective to joints and internal organs, stores fat-soluble vitamins, and performs other functions. Women generally have more subcutaneous fat than men. This greater storage of body fat may be related to her child-bearing function.

Women in certain athletic groups, such as long distance runners, gymnasts, dancers, and others who keep their body weights low, have extremely low body fat percentages. Some of these highly-trained athletes have only 10–15 percent body fat, nearly half that of their age-matched, untrained counterparts. In this instance, females can match or exceed lean body fat percentages found in males. Training and diet appear to be key elements in this body fat relationship (Marshall & Barbash, 1981).

Specific Concerns for the Female Athlete

There are several key concerns for the female athlete. The influence of the menstrual cycle on human performance is an important concern. Specific injuries to female athletes need discussion. Proper nutrition for the female athlete is essential to excellent performance. And the question of physical exercise during pregnancy and after childbirth will be discussed in subsequent sections.

Figure 17.2 Major Biomechanical Differences Between Women and Men. Note the wider hips and greater angle from thigh to lower leg in women.

Source: Marshall, J. L., and J. Barbash. 1981. The sports doctor's fitness book for women. New York: Dell.

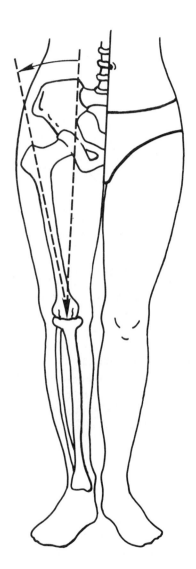
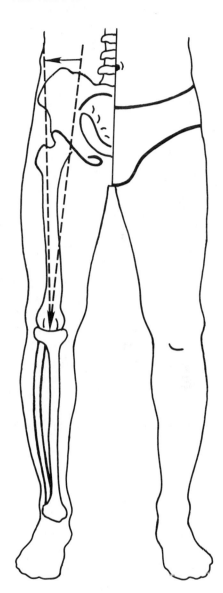

Menstrual Function and Performance

At the time of puberty, the female begins a cyclic hormonal pattern which results in the menstrual cycle. In the United States the age at menarche is approximately 12.5 years. This figure has been dropping over the past few decades. Menarche varies widely in the normal population and can begin as early as eight or nine years of age, or, in some instances, as late as seventeen to nineteen years. This monthly rhythm will continue, once started, until about the age of fifty, when about fifty percent of all women experience menopause.

Thomas (1979) notes that there is hardly a single body function or system that is not affected by the menstrual cycle. The psyche, the skin, the heat regulating system, the gastrointestinal system, may all be affected at various stages of the menstrual cycle. Much interest has been reported lately on the psychological status of women during different phases of their cycles. It must be emphasized here that the menstrual cycle is a perfectly normal, natural, human occurrence. To associate any stigma or negative views to this process would be to return to the Dark Ages.

The menstrual cycle is considered to have four phases. The cycle is based on a period of approximately 28 days. Again, some normal variability is expected in this cycle. The initial phase is considered the *menses,* the actual flow of blood and debris from the womb. This phase lasts from one to five days. The second phase is the *post-menstrual* phase—also known as the estrogenic, proliferative, or follicular phase—the buildup of the lining of the walls of the uterus. This is from day five to thirteen or fourteen. The third phase, days fifteen to twenty-eight, is the ovulation phase, also known as the luteal or progesterone phase. The final phase is the *post-ovulatory* phase—also known as the pre-menstrual phase—and may be from day fifteen to twenty-eight. Many women show considerable variability in their cycles, principally because of the differences in the duration of the pre-ovulatory phase, as opposed to the pre-menstrual phase (Caldwell, 1982).

It is not necessary to go into the complex interactions of the different hormones which seem to regulate these phases. See the references listed at the end of this section for a more detailed description of this process. Now, let us turn our attention to some specific findings on the menstrual cycle which pertain to the female athlete.

Influence of Menstrual Cycle on Athletic Performance

World class athletes do not appear to allow the menstrual cycle to influence their physical activity—either training or actual competition. This makes sense. World class athletes must train intelligently and work out nearly every day of the month. Would we expect an athlete who doesn't train for four to seven days out of each month to be competitive with another world class performer who trains for the full twenty-eight days? If a woman abstains from training during the immediate pre-menstrual days (one or two days), when she may have symptoms of discomfort, and the actual menses period (three to five days), then that would be a total of four to seven days of training lost per month. If this were the case, the athlete is missing out on one out of four days (seven of twenty-eight) per month due to menstrual complications. A good athlete does not let a normal, natural function like the menses intrude on her training or performance. Granted, occasionally one may have to take a day or two away from training, if severe cramping or other discomfort warrants, however, since one out of every seven women in competition may be in the menstrual cycle, that cannot be used as an excuse for not participating. There are other concerns for the menstrual-age female.

In studies at the 1956, 1964, and 1968 Summer Olympic Games, it was determined that female members of the United States and other Olympic teams won gold medals and set new world records during all phases of the menstrual cycle. As far as could be determined, not one female competitor abstained from any contest because of menstruation. Of course, these facts do not answer the question of selection or preselection. That is, there may have been some athletes who had menstrual problems which inhibited them from being Olympic contestants. Those women, whose menstrual cycles interfered with their training and competing, might never reach world class ability. By way of summary, it may be said that any serious competitor must build an immunity to the great number of physical and mental strains of training and competition, and one of these factors that the female athlete has to overcome is the periodicity of her menstrual cycle. This is not the case in all female athletes (Klafs and Lyon, 1978).

Cessation of Menses With Severe Training

Absence of menstruation is called *amenorrhea*. If a girl has not started her monthly cycles before age eighteen, then physicians refer to this as *primary amenorrhea*. If a young woman has menstruated for some time, and, because of some circumstances her monthly cycles cease, this is referred to as *secondary amenorrhea*.

It is known that the menstrual cycle may cease in cases of severe systemic disease or trauma of mental or physical stress, such as starvation or concentration camps. In some cases even the trauma of beginning a collegiate career may be severe enough to affect menstruation. Normalization of the menstrual cycle generally occurs when the women has the severe stress removed.

Lately, it has been reported that certain athletic groups may experience primary or secondary amenorrhea. Although it is most often noted in long distance runners, gymnasts, and dancers, amenorrhea may also occur in any female athlete who expends tremendous amounts of calories in their workouts without providing sufficient caloric intake. Several researchers have linked this amenorrhea with a low percentage of body fat in the serious female athlete. Frisch, et al (1981) notes that when the female athlete gets down near 12 to 15 percent body fat, the chance that the monthly cycles will stop is great. Performers who have been extremely active from their youth (6–8 years old) and who are extremely thin, may not have had normal periods, even though they are in their late teens. This is often found in dancers. Whether this should be a concern to the individual is open to speculation. Some gynecologists say that any girl in her mid-teens who has not menstruated should have a complete medical exam to rule out certain major body disturbances, such as cancer. Others who are familiar with the athletic female are not as concerned, and look on the thin person as one who does not have to worry about discomfort of monthly periods or the fear of pregnancy. (Of course, if she wishes to become pregnant, then monthly regularity must be established.) Dr. Frisch, of Harvard, has gone as far as to suggest, albeit with tongue in cheek, that athletics which demand a great deal of the young woman may effectively serve as birth control, provide peer approval, and enhance self-worth, all at the same time.

Certainly, the whole issue of amenorrhea deserves a careful study. Long range studies are just not available. If the female is genuinely concerned, then a complete physical is necessary. If the young woman has increased her energy expenditure a great deal, becomes very lean, and then notices her periods stop, generally she can assume that the diet and physical activity regimen are probably the reasons.

Alternatively, one must recognize that low body weight or low body fat will not always produce a cessation of menstruation. There is no cause and effect relationship here. It is more of an association. That is, as Frisch, et al (1981) note, when severe training and dietary restriction occur together and the female athlete's body fat goes below 17 percent amenorrhea is likely. Severe psychic or emotional stress, prison, starvation, etc., may also interrupt monthly cycles. And, of course, certain illnesses and diseases can curtail menstruation. The best advice to offer the young female athlete may be to seek professional guidance if any doubt exists as to why regular monthly cycles have stopped (Lutter and Cushman, 1981; Thomas, 1979).

As a sidelight to this issue is the parallel that one can draw to certain animal experimentation. In certain species of animals it is known that, if maturation can be delayed through diet and physical activity, total life span can be increased. Whether this works with humans will have to wait the test of time. Obviously, long term control experiments on humans cannot be done in this area (Morris, 1983).

Dysmenorrhea

A second condition which affects some women is discomfort or pain during the menstrual cycle. This seems to be a highly individualistic thing, affecting some women and not others. This condition of painful or discomforting menses is called *dysmenorrhea*. Other symptoms which commonly occur are pain in the lower back, lower abdominal cramps, a feeling of extreme fullness in the abdomen, headache, nausea, and even vomiting. Dysmenorrhea is poorly understood and studied because of the subjective feeling often associated with it.

There is some evidence that suggests that certain exercises and training can relieve these distressful symptoms. There may be times when dysmenorrhea may be severe enough to curtail training. If the dysmenorrhea is severe, a physician should be consulted. In rare cases, a hormonal antifertility agent could be prescribed and this may prevent ovulation and, therefore, circumvent this problem.

Oral Contraceptives

Since the 1960s there have been certain hormonal and antifertility agents available which, when prescribed for the female athlete, should prevent conception. As with any drug-taking situation, there are risk-benefit ratios. Most medical opinion seems to approve of "the pill" as an effective birth control device. However, certain side effects, such as nausea, vomiting, fluid retention, and amenorrhea have been reported. In some other cases, high blood pressure, double vision, and unusual blood clotting have also been seen (Klafs and Arnheim, 1981). Any use of these oral contraceptives should be monitored closely by the team or family physician. There seem to be no major effects of taking these drugs on athletic performance (Van Aaken, 1977).

278

Physical Activity, Pregnancy, and Childbirth Considerations

Physical Activity and Pregnancy

Pregnancy is considered a *normal, natural* human situation, and, as such, it is not to be treated with undue concern. If the woman is healthy and has been active prior to becoming pregnant, there is no reason why she cannot continue to be fairly active during the pregnancy. In fact, Jokl (1979) has noted that in the 1956 Olympic Games, three female athletes —one in the shot put, one in the discus, and one in the 100 meter race were two, three, and four months pregnant, respectively. Generally in the first three months of the pregnancy, little if any extra precautions are necessary. In the second trimester, if body weight and biomechanics should change, then activity should be reduced, and certainly the intensity of the activity may be turned down. This is not a time for experimentation with different training regimens or diets, etc. If the woman has always been active, however, then the extra physical activity should not be harmful to the developing fetus. This author knew one particularly active woman who continued to run and jog, although more slowly, right up to the day of childbirth, with no ill effects. In fact, recovery from childbirth was quicker and made easier by her excellent condition (Stifler, 1982).

Pregnancy can be considered an extra training stimulus for the female athlete. It is known that female athletes have shortened duration of labor and have fewer disorders and complications during the birth process than nonathletic women. How do older women fare in competition after having children?

Motherhood and Physical Activity

Following childbirth, many female athletes have recorded greater personal athletic achievements. The best example is that of the Dutch Olympian, Fanny Blankers-Koen, in the 1948 Olympic Games. In her seven days of competition she ran a total of eleven races, winning them all, and in the process won four gold medals. At that time she was thirty years old and the mother of two children. Other cases in the short history of women's athletics can be recalled. In the 1974 AAU women's marathon, the top two finishers were Judy Ikenberry and Marilyn Paul. Both women were mothers at the time of that marathon. As age group (Masters) competition grows, we are likely to see many more older women with children competing and excelling in sports (Morris, et al. 1982; Vaccaro et al, 1981).

Special Dietary Concerns of the Female Athlete

Prior to puberty, the nutritional concerns of the young female and male athlete are quite similar. However, at menarche, with the consequent loss of blood in the female, her need for iron becomes a concern. Because the female has less blood volume, she may have about 8 percent less hemoglobin (Klafs & Arnheim, 1981). Although blood volume may increase in the trained athlete, if that female athlete is menstruating, the average daily requirement for iron may be twice as great as her age-matched male counterpart. Pregnancy could increase this iron need even more. It is crucial that the menstruating female athlete be attuned to the special dietary need for iron, possibly as a dietary supplement. Some excellent sources of iron are listed in table 17.1. Even with iron-rich foods, some modest iron supplementation might be advisable.

Table 17.1 Selected Sources of Iron

Food*		Amount	Iron mg
Meats	Liver—Calf	3 oz	11.25
	Beef	3 oz	7.5
	Pork	3 oz	18.97
	Chicken	3 oz	9.0
	Lamb	3 oz	13.37
	Turkey, roasted	3 oz	1.5
	Pork chop	3 oz	2.7
	Hamburger	3 oz	3.0
	Beef, roast	3 oz	2.2
	Chicken	3 oz	1.3
	Bologna	3 oz	3.5
	Fish, haddock	3 oz	1.0
Eggs		1	.9
Vegetables	Kidney beans	½ cup	2.4
	Baked beans	½ cup	2.4
	Lima beans	½ cup	1.4
	Spinach	½ cup	2.0
	Mustard greens	½ cup	1.2
	Peas, green	½ cup	1.6
	Peas, split	½ cup	1.7
	Broccoli	1 stalk, medium	1.4
	Potato, baked	1 medium	1.1
Fruits	Apricots, dried	3 whole	1.2
	Raisins	1 packet (½ oz)	.5
	Prunes, stewed	½ cup	1.9
	Apple	1 medium	.4
Grains/	Bread, enriched	1 slice	.6
cereals	Bread, whole wheat	1 slice	.8
	Rice, enriched	1 cup	1.4
	Cornflakes, enriched	1 cup	.6
Other	Milk	8 oz	.1
	Cheese, cheddar	1 oz	.2
	Nuts, peanuts	½ cup	1.5
	Honey	1 tablespoon	.1
	Molasses, blackstrap	1 tablespoon	3.2

Source: United States Department of Health, Education and Welfare. 1982. Dietary intake source data. Washington, D.C.

*The iron in foods of animal sources is absorbed more efficiently than iron in foods of plant origin. Portions indicated are those most commonly used. RDA of iron for women is 18 mg per day.

Another concern that should be expressed to the female athlete is that, if she is using an intrauterine device (IUD), monthly bleeding may be more severe. This potential problem should be addressed and every precaution be made to supplement her diet, so that daily intake of iron is sufficient to meet the increased need for this important mineral. Finally, female athletes should be cautioned against being blood donors during heavy training. This loss of blood only exacerbates this problem, and could lead to iron depletion in the female athlete. In fact, Thomas (1979) notes that young males also should not be blood donors during periods of high intensity training or competition. See blood doping as a related topic.

Special Injury Concerns of the Female Athlete

As was pointed out in our injury chapter, the type of sport and the number of participants make a large contribution to the number of injuries experienced by any athletic participant group. Certainly contact sports such as football, hockey, wrestling, and boxing will have large numbers of injuries per year. When boys and girls play the same sports as young-sters, we generally find that they experience the same type of injuries.

Some early studies indicated that female athletes have a higher rate of injuries and a more severe injury index when compared to their male counterparts. It is known that faulty conditioning and improper training can lead to increased injuries. It is believed that these earlier reports of increased injuries with increased severity were primarily due to improper training programs. Not having enough strength or flexibility, or fatiguing too quickly may all lead to more injuries. Any athlete who is deficient in the areas of strength, flexibility, or endurance conditioning, is more likely to be injured. Of course, it must also be noted here that, as all athletes continue their drive toward excellence, there will be more injuries—especially of the overuse type—because the body, when pushed to the limit, will tend to break (injure) at the weakest link.

Coaches of female athletes often must give special consideration to proper support and protection for the breasts in the mature athlete. By wearing a well-fitted bra, some soreness and tenderness may be minimized in women athletes who have large or pen-dulous breasts. Clothing manufacturers are paying more attention to the needs of these female athletes and there are several sports bras on the market which provide excellent protection from excessive horizontal or vertical motion of the breasts, while not unduly restricting normal chest ventilation (Stifler, 1982). There is no conclusive evidence that not wearing a bra in athletic activity will lead to excessive sagging or stretching of breast tissues. It seems that the soundest advice is to wear what feels most comfortable, and, if that includes wearing nothing for support, then that is permissible. In contact sports, like lacrosse and field hockey, direct trauma to the breast might be expected. However, there is no relationship between the development of a malignancy and trauma to the breast. Common sense would dictate that some covering be afforded to athletes in high impact or incident positions (goalies). ■

Summary

By way of summary, there are certain biological differences between females and males. However, there is no good evidence to indicate that coaches, athletic trainers, or other officials in charge of athletics for women need to be concerned with any special rules and regulations regarding sports participation for normal, healthy girls and women. The young, pre-pubertal girl is no more at risk for injury than is the young, pre-pubertal boy.

After puberty, the young woman tends to have less strength and a greater percent of body fat than the male. She will be of shorter stature, may require more iron in her diet than the average male, and does not perform as well in speed and strength activities.

There are a number of body fluctuations which occur in the young woman with the menstrual cycle. At present there is no evidence that such variation is an overriding consideration in women's participation in sports or exercise. Further, there is no evidence that would indicate that vigorous, athletic activity, conducted in a proper and intelligent fashion, is harmful to those women athletes who subsequently will bear children. Pregnancy may be a deterrent to the competitive athlete. Certain modifications must be made during this period. Because physical activity is necessary for proper human functioning, it is essential that women, as well as men, participate in many of the opportunities which are available in sports and physical activity programs.

References

Bodnar, L. M., & T. L. Bodnar. 1980. Women, sports and the law. In Haycock, C. E. ed. *Sports medicine for the female athlete.* Oradell, NJ: Medical Economics Co.

Caldwell, F. 1982. Menstrual irregularity in athletes: the unanswered question. *The Physician and Sportsmedicine.* 10:142.

Frisch, R., et al. 1981. Delayed menarche and amenorrhea of college athletes in relation to age of onset of training. *Journal of the American Medical Association.* 246:1559.

Haycock, C. E. ed. 1980. *Sports medicine for the athletic female.* Oradell, NJ: Medical Economics Co.

Jokl, E. 1979. The athletic status of women. *American Corrective Therapy Journal.* 33:103.

Klafs, C. E., & M. J. Lyon. 1978. *The female athlete.* 2d ed. St. Louis: C. V. Mosby Co.

Klafs, C. E., & D. D. Arnheim. 1981. *Modern principles of athletic training.* St. Louis: C. V. Mosby Co.

Lutter, J. M., & S. Cushman. 1981. Medical concerns of women runners. *The Minnesota Distance Runner.* Spring.

Marshall, J. L., & H. Barbash. 1981. *The sports doctor's fitness book for women.* New York: Dell Publishing Co.

McArdle, W., F. I. Katch, & V. L. Katch. 1981. *Exercise physiology.* Philadelphia: Lea & Febiger.

Chapter 17

Morris, A. F., et al. 1982. Life quality characteristics of national class women masters long distance runners. *Annals of Sports Medicine.* 1:23.

Morris, A. F. 1983. *Physiological and psychological benefits of training.* Paper presented at Women in Sport Conference. Washington, D.C.

Stifler, J. 1982. Woman: the second wave. *The Runner.* 5:30.

Thomas, C. L. 1979. Factors important to women participants in vigorous athletics. In Straus, R. ed. *Sports medicine and physiology.* Philadelphia: W. B. Saunders.

United States Department of Health, Education and Welfare. 1982. *Dietary intake source data.* Washington, DC.

Vaccaro, P., A. F. Morris & D. H. Clarke. 1981. Physiological characteristics of masters female distance runners. *The Physician and Sportsmedicine.* 9:105.

Van Aaken, E. 1977. *Die schonungslose therapie.* Celle, Germany: Pohl-Verlag.

The Younger and Older Athlete

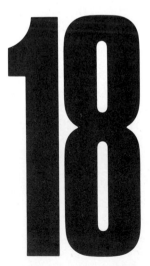

Introduction

    This chapter is concerned with the very young athlete and the older athlete. A case is made for the benefit of physical activity and sports for the young athlete. With proper coaching, officiating, levels of competition, and adult guidance, youth sports can be a very beneficial positive experience. Topics such as training and stress in kids' sports is covered. Finally, some chronic medical concerns of children in sports are given.

    In a later portion of this chapter, the older athlete in sports medicine is covered. Various effects of aging and exercise are listed. It is known that physiological alterations occur with age. However, it has also been shown that many of the physiological deteriorations which accompany aging may be related to disuse or misuse, rather than the effects of aging. The effects of a proper, intelligent, graduated program of physical activity on various physiological parameters in the older individual are covered.

The past few years have seen a rather unprecedented increase in sports participation by children. This increased participation has raised many questions from concerned parents and physicians. Parents, officials, coaches, and others who work with children, often ask pediatricians questions such as the following. "At what age should my child begin sports competition?" "Is my child too small to play football or hockey?" "Will excess running cause joint or bone injury?" "What weight should my child wrestle at?" "What sports are safe for my asthmatic child?" These questions may be asked of the primary care physician, the specialist—the pediatrician.

A Case Study of a Young Runner

By way of introduction to this area I would like to cite the case of an acquaintance of mine who also happens to be an excellent runner. I first met this young female runner in the summer of 1977 in Washington, D.C. She was about seven years old at that time, but had been running for several years. In fact, she had held the girls' marathon world record for age five and age six. Her brother, somewhat older, and her dad were also runners. Although all family members were accomplished athletes, the story of their running can be a lesson for all parents, coaches, and officials concerned with youth sports.

This family had always done things together, so when dad took up running to take off some weight and get in shape, the children naturally followed. They started at a very modest level—about a quarter of a mile the first day, but progressed gradually until they were running several miles daily. All their runs were fun. Both parents noted that all running was done without bribing or pushing their children. As the children's capacities improved, their running became extremely pleasurable and helped to sustain their interest in this new family activity. There were no hard or fast runs—only slow, long, relaxed runs. Soon, their daily mileage increased, and, as the father reported, when his daughter increased her daily mileage to over ten miles, he permitted her to run a full marathon.

The young athlete continued to set age group records as she matured. I still see her occasionally at races. She is still having fun, still running beautifully, and still setting records. She has competed in many women's races and has done remarkably well for her age. She has tremendous natural ability. A question might naturally arise that since this young woman started running before age six, will she be "burnt out" or disenchanted with running in her teens or high school years? Should her parents restrict her running? Is all this mileage (fifty-plus miles/week) too much? Both parents agree that, as long as running provides physiological and psychological benefits to their children, they will continue to allow them to run. This young runner has never been injured, to my knowledge, and always finishes her runs at a relaxed, strong pace. Certainly this activity brings her immeasurable benefits. Other people have also lauded this relaxed, easy type of sport activity for youngsters. If this schedule of activity seemed to work for the above young athlete, what other generalizations may be presented regarding other youngsters?

What is the Proper Age for Competition?

A noted physician, John D. Burrington, of Children's Hospital—Denver, suggests that, by age six, children have developed a sense of competition, and have entered a stage in their development of social comparison, where they often delight in competition. Dr. Burrington further suggests that sports for this young age group should consist of non-contact sports, such as swimming, running, and skating. Somewhat later, at age eight, some contact sports may be introduced. These sports might be soccer, baseball, wrestling, or touch football. Still later, at age ten, collision sports can be permitted. These include tackle football, and ice hockey. Of course, proper equipment, training, and trained youth sport coaches should be employed for all these activities. The emphasis must be on *fun, learning new skills* and *proper social interaction.*

As was indicated earlier, both boys and girls up to the age of puberty can be grouped together. Often, height and weight standards are a better guide to forming categories than mere age, since one 12 year old boy may be 150 lbs., while another may weigh only 75 lbs. Grouping by weight and body size is crucial, especially if the sport involves contact or collision (Gilliam et al., 1982; Sheehan, 1980; Singer, 1982, 1983; Apple & McDonald, 1981.)

The Youth Sports Examination

A thorough physical examination and detailed health history should be completed on each child before he or she is cleared for youth sport participation. Dr. Thomas Shaffer, a noted pediatric professor at Ohio State University, has produced a Youth Health Questionnaire for Sports candidates (Shaffer, 1980). A questionnaire such as the one shown in figure 18.1 should be completed prior to or during the physical exam. This pre-season exam is crucial and should cover the following major areas: cardiac and pulmonary screening, musculoskeletal examination, physical maturation, and certain information relative to the emotional state of the youngster. A measurement of physical fitness and a simple estimation of skin folds to determine body fatness should also be done. The Harvard bench step test is easily administered and yields meaningful results, while the pinch skin-fold test can help answer the question of whether it would be proper for the child to lose some weight for wrestling or some other sport. Generally, if this measurement at the triceps and below the scapula reveals over six millimeters of thickness, or is approximately the width of four pennies, then the child may be overly fat and could stand to lose some weight. If this is the case, then a suggested caloric reduction *combined* with increased physical activity programs is the best way to accomplish this. In any case, this weight loss should be *most* gradual, about *one* or *two* pounds per week. It should be pointed out that obesity may be the most common serious disease seen in American children. Also, studies at the University of Michigan have shown that many youngsters in the general population already have several risk factors of heart disease (high blood pressure, elevated fats and triglycerides) prior to their teen years.

Figure 18.1 Youth Health Questionnaire for Sports Candidates.

ATHLETIC HEALTH QUESTIONNAIRE
(To be completed by athlete, assisted by parents)

Name _____ Date of Birth _____

Home Address _____ Telephone _____

Parents' Name _____ Family Physician _____

School _____ Grade _____

Have you:

1. Had any injuries requiring medical attention?	No	Yes
2. Had any head or neck injuries?	No	Yes
3. Had any convulsions?	No	Yes
4. Had any illness lasting more than a week?	No	Yes
5. Been taking any medication recently?	No	Yes
6. Had any surgical operation?	No	Yes
7. Been in a hospital (except for tonsillectomy)?	No	Yes
8. Had rheumatic fever?	No	Yes
9. Had any chronic illness (blood disease, epilepsy, diabetes)?	No	Yes
10. Been recently or are you now under a physician's care?	No	Yes
11. Any allergies or drug reactions?	No	Yes
12. Ever been told not to participate in any particular sport for health reasons?	No	Yes

Explain any "yes" answers.

_____

_____

_____

Have you had a polio immunization? _____

Have you had a tetanus toxoid and booster? _____

Training Children for Sports

Children differ from adults in both magnitude and duration of their cardiovascular responses to exercise. Nevertheless, if one has observed children playing in any schoolyard, one can note their tremendous capacity for sustained physical activity. If gradual training principles, which were suggested in earlier sections, are followed, increases in performances of an endurance nature will follow. There is some disagreement as to whether early athletic training will improve adult capabilities. Some scientists suggest that training prior to adolescence increases adult capacities. Other studies with twins showed that there was little, if any, effect on ultimate performance, if the person had been trained in childhood. One fact is apparently clear. The youngster who is taught proper skills for a sport activity is more proficient in that activity as an adult. So it is, perhaps, in this area of skill development that youth sport coaches should place their emphasis in training.

Stress in Children's Sports

Nearly everyone connected with youth sports notes that it is important to consider the youngsters' emotions foremost in the organization and conduction of youth sports. I concur in this. Even at the outset, during the routine physical examination, the pediatrician should begin to form an opinion regarding the young athlete's psychological or emotional characteristics. Does the physician detect *excessive* shyness, uncooperativeness, compulsiveness, hypochondriasis, or accident-proneness, among other traits? Such information may be passed on to a team leader or coach who may be able to bring about some modifications, or be better able to deal with the emotional outbursts of their young athletes. The understanding coach, with a genuine concern for the emotional well-being of the young athlete, is a necessary prerequisite for youth sports.

There have been several studies which have addressed the question of stress in youth sports and, generally, these have found that if the coach does not overemphasize winning, the youngsters are not placed in a stressful situation. A 1981 research study from the University of Illinois, by Julie Simon, compared stress and anxiety in three groups of school activities: (1) required school activities (academic test, physical education class, softball game); (2) non-required non-sport activities (band solo competition, band group competition); and (3) non-school sport activities (baseball, football, basketball, etc.). In an attempt to assess anxiety levels, a ten item questionnaire was given to all youngsters immediately before each activity started. Children were asked to rate whether they were nervous, calm, etc.

Findings for this study are shown in figure 18.2. It can be seen that non-required (band) activities were most stressful to these youngsters. Sports were next stressful, but only slightly higher than required school activities. Figure 18.3 shows non-sport and sport evaluative activities. Again, it may be seen that, when properly conducted, youth sport activities may not be stressful to the youngsters. Simon concluded that all youth sport coaches should adhere to the following suggestions in an attempt to *minimize* the stressfulness of the youth sport athletic situation.

288

Figure 18.2 Anxiety Levels In School Children in Three Types of Evaluative Activities.

Source: Simon, J. 1981. Stress in kids' sports. *Sports Line*. University of Illinois. 3:5.

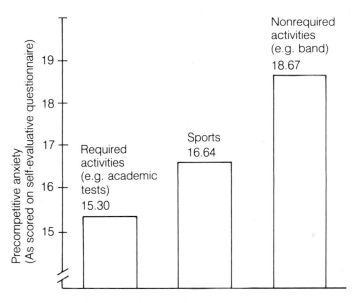

Figure 18.3 Comparative Anxiety Levels In School Children in Sport and Nonsport Activities.

Source: Simon, J. 1981. Stress in kids' sports. *Sports Line*. University of Illinois. 3:5.

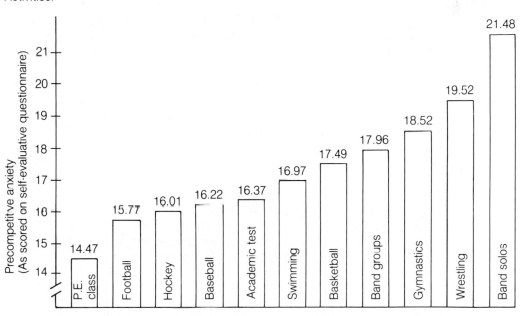

1. Coaches and parents should emphasize effort—trying hard and doing one's best—not emphasize winning at all costs.
2. Reassure young athletes that their worth as human beings is not affected by winning or losing. It is only a game.
3. Teach youngsters to concentrate on the game or contest and not on people in the audience.
4. Try to reduce uncertainty in the game. Young athletes are uncertain about being a starter, about playing, about the outcome of the contest. In a close match-up the coach may not be able to control the latter, but the coach can reduce uncertainty of participation by telling all the athletes that they will play each game, thereby emphasizing participation, not winning.

There is some uncertainty in all of life, sports included. The good youth sports coach tries to control as much of this uncertainty for the young athlete as possible, and therefore, helps the youngster to maximize enjoyment of the sport activity.

Self Esteem in Children

Morris, Vaccaro, and Clarke (1979) took measures of locus of control and self-esteem in twenty age group male swimmers, aged seven to seventeen years, who each had nearly five years of swimming competition under their belts. Locus of control is a concept which is discussed in another section, but essentially is the way in which an individual perceives reinforcement received. An internal person believes that the rewards received are due mostly to hard work and personal effort. An external person feels that reinforcements are largely due to luck, fate, or chance. It was shown in the study that these young swimmers were more internal and had higher self-esteem measures when contrasted to age-matched controls. It appeared that the young swimmers seemed to have a more realistic view of the world and a more positive self-attitude than their peers. At present we do not know if these young swimmers were more internally oriented and high in self-esteem when they came to the sport or whether the conditions of practice/training and competition tended to encourage personal self-motivation. We would like to think it was the latter.

A final study, by Dr. W. Mark Shipman, a psychiatrist and director of the San Diego Center for Children, has shown that increasing physical activity, specifically by running, brought about a marked decrease in day-to-day aggressiveness in children who were classified as having emotional problems. These children, aged six to thirteen years, were diagnosed as having behavioral and emotional problems and were often on medication to control aggressive tendencies to disrupt class, throw supplies, or punch other students. After a specific twelve-week program, marked improvement was shown in the running group.

The studies have shown that a properly organized and conducted program of sport or physical activity can aid a child to better self-understanding and more emotional self-control without being unduly stressful. Specific guidelines which tend to emphasize individual effort, not winning, seem to lead to better youth sport activities.

Some Chronic Medical Concerns of Children

Every physician, coach, parent, or other interested person should be concerned with special medical situations which may occur with children (Thornton, 1974). Some of these are listed in this section.

Asthma

Millions of people suffer, to some degree, with exercise-induced asthma. A certain type of broncho-spasm (uncontrolled smooth muscle contracting of airway passages) may occur in some children. Typically, the child with this condition experiences dizziness, wheezing, and pain upon beginning exercise or five to fifteen minutes into the exercise bout. There are medications that can help this condition. Swimming may be suggested to the child who has this problem, because the warm, moist air surrounding pools seems to help. Other sports, like cycling, fencing, and gymnastics, might be suggested to these affected children.

Diabetes

With certain precautions, children with diabetes can compete successfully in all areas of sports. Strenuous exercise lowers insulin requirements, therefore the child may require additional small snacks of carbohydrates. Expert consultation with a physician who understands caloric requirements of different sporting activities is a must here.

Seizures

Some children have a problem with seizures. If the seizures occur as a result of a previous head injury or accident, obviously, contact sports should be avoided. Some control is gained with medication. Again, expert medical advice is necessary.

Missing Organs

Finally, the young athlete with one eye or one kidney should be dissuaded from contact or collision sports. There are a large number of other sports that could be of interest to an individual with this type of condition.

Guidelines for Participation by Children in Sports

By way of summarizing this area on youth sport activities, it may be said that, if youth sports are safe and enjoyable then they will be a profitable human activity. Why should we delay participation in this wholesome activity until a certain age? Dr. George Sheehan, a noted cardiologist and runner and the father of twelve children, has pointed out that if running or another sport activity is good for the child physically, it is even better for him psychologically (Sheehan, 1983). The child can get the same improvement in self-image and self-esteem that the adult achieves from sport and fitness. Sport and physical activity can give any child the opportunity to do something of value. They can feel good about themselves. Remember that each of us wants to feel good about something for ourselves. Children want no less.

Some special guidelines and rules for children's participation in sports have been developed by the U.S. Department of Health and Human Services (1980).

Bill of Rights for Young Athletes

1. Right to the opportunity to participate in sports regardless of ability level.
2. Right to participate at a level that is commensurate with each child's developmental level.
3. Right to have qualified adult leadership.
4. Right to participate in safe and healthy environments.
5. Right of each child to share in the leadership and decision-making of their sport participation.
6. Right to play as a child and not as an adult.
7. Right to proper preparation for participation in the sport.
8. Right to an equal opportunity to strive for success.
9. Right to be treated with dignity by all involved.
10. Right to have fun through sport.

The Older Athlete and Sports Medicine

Aging and Exercise

Several years ago, one of the leading scientists in the field of physical education, Dr. H. Harrison Clarke, of the University of Oregon, devoted an entire issue of The Physical Fitness Research Digest to the topic of exercise and aging. After first describing the nature of physical fitness, Dr. Clarke went on to note certain physiological changes that occur with age. These age-affected physiological processes are detailed in the following section.

Physiological Alterations With Age

Heart Rate

Unless affected by continued exercise, there is little change in the resting heart rate during the adult life. Maximal heart rate tends to fall slightly over the life span of the individual.

Blood Pressure

The average values for blood pressure for young adults is 120/72 for men; for women it is slightly lower. Both systolic and diastolic pressures tend to increase by 10 to 15 millimeters over the span of adult life.

Cardiac Output

The cardiac output (heart rate times the stroke volume), or the amount of blood put out of the heart with a single contraction, tends to decrease with advancing years. Since maximum heart rate decreases and heart size also tends to decrease, therefore decreasing stroke volume, one could expect the cardiac output to diminish.

Respiratory Efficiency

A decline in respiratory efficiency occurs in adults as they age. This is partly influenced by a decrease in elasticity of the lungs, less flexibility of the chest, and decreased aerobic capacity, among other things.

Aerobic Power

Maximum aerobic power, as measured in milliliters per kilogram per minute, shows a progressive loss from age twenty to sixty. Experts think this is due to an increase in body weight (fat) as well as previously mentioned factors.

Anaerobic Power

Capacity for anaerobic, or fast-paced, work seems to decline in older people. The accumulation of lactate in the blood stream appears greater in older men after a standard work task. The ability to tolerate this increased lactate also appears to diminsh.

Bones

Generally, it may be said that bones become less resilient, more porous and brittle, and increasingly fragile with advancing age. Whether this is due to a decreased activity level, hormonal changes (in the female), or a loss of bone marrow to produce new bone cells is not exactly known.

Flexibility

With disuse, bone cartilage lining the ends of long bones or lying between the bones of the spine, etc. tends to become harder and calcify. This leads to decreased elasticity and less flexibility in the human skeleton.

Muscular Strength

Using grip strength tests, it has been found that peak strength in men can be reached at approximately age seventeen. This level may be maintained until about age forty-five, if the man is active, and then tends to decline for the next twenty years. A similar pattern was found for women, except that peak strength may occur earlier, at about the time of puberty. However, there are some exceptions to these findings, since it is noted that men who are into weight training throughout their forties and fifties can maintain their body strength at near maximum levels.

Muscular and Cardiovascular Endurance

It is assumed that, as one ages, one loses about 5 percent of their maximum muscular and cardiovascular endurance per decade. This rate of slow down may be retarded if the person is extremely active. We now have examples of men in their fifth decade of life running the marathon in two hours and twenty minutes and women in their sixth decade running it in under two hours and fifty minutes. These are remarkable achievements for these master athletes.

Trainability of Older Athletes

If one examines the short histories of masters' level age group swimming, track and field, and road running competition, one can see the remarkable training levels that can be achieved with intelligent, gradual, physiological training. Masters' swimming competition for people aged twenty-five up to eighty, ninety, and one hundred, was started by Dr. Random J. Arthur in the early 1970s. This swimming competition for adults attracts thousands of older people each year and their performance times are outstanding, even when compared to top collegiate records.

A similar program was started in the sport of athletics (track and field and road racing). Now, hundreds of thousands of older people from many countries turn out to race marathons in New York, Boston, Washington, Chicago, Honolulu, and London. With proper training, these older athletes can attain remarkable fitness levels, as well as derive the immense gratification of competition, the camaraderie of the sport, and the sense of satisfaction that comes with giving a superb physical effort (Vaccaro, et al. 1981; Morris, et al. 1982).

Dr. H. deVries, of the University of Southern California, has spent several decades studying the trainability of older people, and has come up with interesting and informative figures regarding these individuals. In summary, Dr. deVries (1980) and others (Kasch and Kulberg, 1981; Kasch, 1981) note that the trainability of the older individual is roughly equal to that of the young adult when expressed on a relative basis.

Benefits of Exercise for Older Adults

This last section looks at age and exercise. Some physiological alterations that accompany advancing age are noted. Essentially, all physical systems, especially the neuro-muscular system, begin to deteriorate with age. If the individual remains physically active, several important health benefits can be realized. These physiological benefits include: (1) improved O_2 transport and aerobic capacity, (2) lowered blood pressure and blood fats, (3) improved breathing capacity, (4) improved joint mobility, (5) a lessening of detrimental osteoporotic changes, and (6) a tranquilizer effect that tends to reduce neuromuscular tension and anxiety (deVries, 1980).

As a final sidelight to this section on age and physical activity, Dr. Robert F. Allen has put together a personal life-expectancy quiz, based on certain specific personal facts and life-style activities of an individual. This life-expectancy quiz is shown in figure 18.4.

294

Figure 18.4 Life Expectancy Quiz. This is one of many health questionnaires now used by doctors, medical centers and insurance groups. While quizzes can hardly be precise, they do give a more realistic picture of probable longevity than old-fashioned actuarial tables, which relied almost exclusively on the subject's heredity patterns and medical history. Current computations try to measure risk in relation to environment, stress, and general behavior, though statisticians and experts do not always agree on how to weigh the components. A high salary may not be as detrimental to longevity—because of competitive stress—as many quizzes suggest. On the other hand, marriage or living together, usually assumed to increase one's chances of living longer, may actually increase stress, especially for notably embattled partners. National average life spans: 70.5 for white males, 65.3 for all other males: 78.1 for white females, 74 for all other females.

Source: Allen, R. F. 1981. *Lifegain: the exciting new program that will change your health and your life.* New York: Appleton, Century, Crofts.

PERSONAL FACTS:

Start with Age 72

If you are male **subtract 3.**
If female, **add 4.**
If you live in an urban area with a population over 2 million, **subtract 2.**
If you live in a town under 10,000, or on a farm, **add 2.**
If any grandparent lived to 85, **add 2.**
If all four grandparents lived to 80, **add 6.**
If either parent died of a stroke or heart attack before the age of 50, **subtract 4.**
If any parent, brother or sister under 50 has (or had) cancer or a heart condition, or has had diabetes since childhood, **subtract 3.**
Do you earn over $50,000 a year? **Subtract 2.**
If you finished college, **add 1.** If you have a graduate or professional degree, **add 2 more.**
If you are 65 or over and still working, **add 3.**
If you live with a spouse or friend, **add 5.** If not, **subtract 1** for every ten years alone since age 25.

LIFE-STYLE STATUS:

If you work behind a desk, **subtract 3.**
If your work requires regular, heavy physical labor, **add 3.**
If you exercise strenuously (tennis, running, swimming, etc.) five times a week for at least a half-hour, **add 4.** Two or three times a week, **add 2.**
Do you sleep more than ten hours each night? **Subtract 4.**
Are you intense, aggressive, easily angered? **Subtract 3.**
Are you easygoing and relaxed? **Add 3.**
Are you happy? **Add 1.** Unhappy? **Subtract 2.**
Have you had a speeding ticket in the past year? **Subtract 1.**

Do you smoke more than two packs a day? **Subtract 6.** One to two packs? **Subtract 6.** One-half to one? **Subtract 3.**
Do you drink the equivalent of 1½ oz. of liquor a day? **Subtract 1.**
Are you overweight 50 lbs. or more? **Subtract 8.** By 30 to 50 lbs.? **Subtract 4.** By 10 to 30 lbs.? **Subtract 2.**
If you are a man over 40 and have annual checkups, **add 2.**
If you are a woman and see a gynecologist once a year, **add 2.**

RUNNING TOTAL ADD UP YOUR SCORE TO GET YOUR LIFE EXPECTANCY

AGE ADJUSTMENT:

If you are between 30 and 40, **add 2.**
If you are between 40 and 50, **add 3.**
If you are between 50 and 70, **add 4.**
If you are over 70, **add 5.**

295

After studying the figure for a short time, it can be seen how engaging in physical activity, controlling one's body weight, and proper diet, rest, and relaxation, may aid in one's life-expectancy score. This re-emphasizes the risk index that was introduced in an earlier chapter. ■

Summary

This chapter considers athletes at two ends of the age spectrum. The young athlete and the older athlete are considered in detail. One of the positive factors that affects youth in sport is increased self-esteem. Certain physiological aspects of the young child, such as asthma, diabetes, and seizures affect the choice of sport. If the youngsters have a proper pre-season examination, they should benefit from both the training and competitive aspects of the sport. In youth athletics, *fun* and the *development of motor skills* should be stressed. Coaches and parents should work together to make sure that fun is an element of all aspects of training and conditioning for sport, as well as the competitive phase of the youngster's sport activities. Proper supervision, officiating, and conduct of activities should be paramount at all times in sports for children.

The second part of the chapter considers the older athlete. Many sports, such as swimming, track and field, and skiing, now have age group competition. Some of these athletes are performing extremely well in their fifth, sixth, seventh, and eighth decades of life. Some of the physiological alterations that accompany age are listed. Maximum heart rate declines over the life of each individual. Certain changes in blood pressure and cardiac output indicate reduced efficiency in the older athlete. Bones become more brittle and less resilient with age, especially in the person with diminished physical activity. Flexibility will also diminish with a lessening of physical activity. Some studies have shown the value of training in the older age group. These decreases in performance over the lifetime of an individual may be retarded somewhat with a proper endurance training regime.

A life expectancy quiz is given in this chapter. The emphasis in the life expectancy quiz is that people who pay particular attention to diet and nutrition, rest and relaxation, and physical activity, may significantly improve their chances of a longer, more productive life. Obvious detrimental risk factors, such as smoking, poor diet, alcohol consumption, increases in blood pressure, and the stress to which the individual is exposed, may all contribute to an exacerbation of the aging process.

References

Allen, R. F. 1981. *Lifegain: the exciting new program that will change your health and your life.* New York: Appleton, Century, Crofts.

Apple, D. F., & A. McDonald. 1981. Long-distance running and the immature skeleton. *Contemporary Orthopaedics.* 3:929.

deVries, H. 1980. *Physiology of exercise* 3d ed. Dubuque, IA: Wm. C. Brown.

Gilliam, T. B., et al. 1982. Exercise programs for children: a way to prevent heart disease. *The Physician and Sportsmedicine.* 10:101, 105, 108.

Kasch, F. W. 1981. Physiological changes with swimming and running during two years of training. *Scandinavian Journal of Sports Sciences.* 3:23.

Kasch, F. W., & J. Kulberg. 1981. Physiological variables during 15 years of endurance exercise. *Scandinavian Journal of Sports Sciences.* 3:59.

Morris, A. F., P. Vaccaro, & D. H. Clark. 1979. Psychological characteristics of age-group competitive swimmers. *Perceptual and Motor Skills.* 48:1265.

Morris, A. F., et al. 1982. Life quality characteristics of national class women masters long distance runners. *Annals of Sports Medicine.* 1:23.

Shaffer, T. E. 1980. The young athlete: new guidelines in sports medicine. *Pediatric Consult.* 1:1.

Sheehan, G. 1980. *This running life.* New York: Simon & Schuster.

Sheehan, G. 1983. Children running? Why not? *The Physician and Sportsmedicine.* 11:51.

Simon, J. 1981. Stress in kids' sports. *Sports Line.* Office of Youth Sports, Department of Physical Education, University of Illinois, Urbana-Champaign. 3:5.

Singer, K. M. 1982. Upper extremity injuries in young athletes. *Sportsmedicine Digest.* 4:1.

Thornton, M. L. 1974. Pediatric concerns about competitive preadolescent sports. *Journal of the American Medical Association.* 227:418.

United States Department of Health and Human Services. 1980. Children and youth in action: physical activities and sports. Washington, D.C.

Vaccaro, P., G. M. Drummer, & D. H. Clarke. 1981. Physiological characteristics of female masters swimmers. *The Physician and Sportsmedicine.* 9:75.

Psychology of Sports

Outline

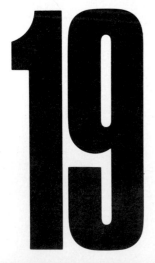

Introduction

When we refer to top world class athletes, we note that they have a tough mental makeup, in addition to a tough physical makeup. This chapter on the psychology of sports looks at certain aspects of mental functioning in top flight athletes. Such topics as anxiety, attention, and arousal and how these concepts affect athletic performance, are covered. A small section on motivation in sports is included. Other sections on the psychology of competition and the psychology of winning and losing are delineated.

The topic of aggression in sports is covered as well. Aggression is necessary in many combative or contact type sports. This leads into a discussion of the athletic personality.

Final topics covered in this chapter include life quality and sports participation, locus of control as it relates to sports participation, and the injury aspect of sports. It is pointed out that individuals with a certain psychological makeup appear not to become injured as often as other individuals, or recover from injuries at a much quicker rate, depending on their perceived control in particular situations.

If one examines the winning times in the individual sports of swimming and running in the most recent Olympics, one observes that the differences between first and fifth places may have been only hundredths of a second. Certainly, physiology may account for some of these differences, but can one always ascribe a physiological factor or factors to the difference between the winner and the runners-up? Often, factors of the mind or psychological behavior may account for such differences.

Authors have written, since the earliest of times, that the human being is composed of a mind and a body, and that these two entities are indivisible. However, when it comes to human athletic performance, many theories for understanding and controlling this human behavior are based upon *intuition* rather than on rational, empirical, scientific knowledge (Singer, 1975; Kroll, 1975).

Many sports fans, athletic trainers, coaches, and athletes believe that psychological factors are an essential ingredient for athletic success. Unfortunately, much of this thinking is opinion and cannot be substantiated by hard scientific evidence. In fact, some researchers in sport psychology often note that the area of psychology of sport is an investigative field that is somewhat "soft". Sport psychology investigators can pose excellent questions, but often the methodology for answering these difficult questions is lacking. Nevertheless, the purpose of this chapter is to present some of the most important topics in sport psychology and the relevant information that has been discovered on each of them.

These topics are presented in no particular order and they are chosen from a listing of important areas compiled by prominent workers in this field. Sport psychology has been defined as psychology applied to sports and athletic situations. Taken in the context of sports medicine, this definition is expanded to include psychology of athletic injuries and rehabilitation.

Dr. Robert Singer (1981) has divided the field of sport psychology into five major areas. These areas are: (1) developmental psychology, including motor development, (2) personal and clinical psychology, including personality and motivation, (3) learning and training, including skill acquisition and performance, (4) social psychology, including social learning theories, and (5) psychometrics, including diagnosis and measurement of individual and group differences.

Examining other authors in psychology of sport, one finds (Straub, 1978) topics to include: motivation, aggression, anxiety, social involvement, personality, leadership, and team cohesion. A text by Fisher (1976) includes the following major sections: affiliation and sport, motivation, aggression, and personality. Kroll (1975) includes: competitive spirit, anxiety, aggression and guilt, sportsmanship, and learning and teaching strategies in athletics. From these lists, one can see several topics appearing over and over again. The topics of aggression, anxiety, motivation, personality, and social facilitation are given consideration in this chapter.

It must be realized that there are several excellent texts in this area (Singer, 1981; Martens, 1975; Morgan, 1972; Fisher, 1976; Suinn, 1980) and many summary articles. Of necessity, the topics listed here will be treated in summary fashion. Those who wish more detail are referred to the reading list at the end of this section.

Anxiety, Attention, Arousal, Activation, and Athletic Performance

Anxiety and athletic performance is a complex area. Definitions and descriptions of concepts in this field are difficult, at best, and even experts in this field of sport psychology do not agree on various concepts. Added to this befuddled area are some similar adjacent psychological concepts, such as attention, arousal activation, and how these factors relate to athletic performance. Techniques for measuring these psychological constructs are often vague and specific to the situation. One researcher has compared it to trying to catch minnows with a whaling net. Nevertheless, what is presented here is a brief description of major concepts in the area of anxiety and human athletic performance and a short discussion of how some allied concepts of attention, arousal and activation relate to anxiety and sports.

Anxiety is defined as a fear, real or imagined, about an upcoming event, which may lead the individual to behave irrationally. Sometimes anxiety is justified. If, as you are crossing the street, a bus is coming toward you, you may feel certain anxiety (fear). This is normal and probably causes you to react and move quickly to safety. However, another person could be paralyzed with fear and not react rationally in the above situation, with disastrous consequences. Sometimes this occurs in sport situations, such as the young Little Leaguer, who fears an opposing fastball pitcher and fails to react and move away from a stray pitch. Many similar examples in sporting situations could be given, however, we will now turn our attention toward the two major types of anxiety—state and trait anxiety—which are discussed in the literature.

State anxiety refers to a tendency of an individual to become anxious or fearful in certain arousing situations. *Trait anxiety* is a tendency of a person to maintain a high level of arousal across situations of varying intensity. Extremes of either state or trait anxiety will most likely lead to poor athletic performance. This concept has been in the psychological literature for some time and is referred to as the Yerkes-Dodson Law (Oxendine, 1980).

This law, which was based on studies with experimental animals, states that, if arousal is very low or very high, performance will be adversely affected. There is an optimal level of arousal which will lead to highest performance. To state this in other terms, there is an inverted U relationship between arousal and performance. (See fig. 19.1.) Unfortunately, human athletic performance is much more complicated than that pictured in the figure.

Some researchers (Oxendine, 1980; Fisher, 1976) have reported that one must also consider whether the athletic performance being studied involves complex, fine muscle movements of coordination necessitating extreme concentration (a concert pianist) or gross motor movements (sprinting, weight lifting, or jumping). Still other factors may be age, maturation, and skill level of the athlete. Certainly, all these factors are important in considering anxiety as it relates to sports performance.

300

Figure 19.1 The Yerkes-Dodson Law. If arousal is very low *(a)* or very high *(b)*, performance will suffer. Conversely, if arousal is optimum, then performance will also be at the peak *(c)*.

Source: Oxendine, J. B. 1980. Emotional arousal and motor performance. In R. M. Suinn. *Psychology in sports.* Minneapolis: Burgess.

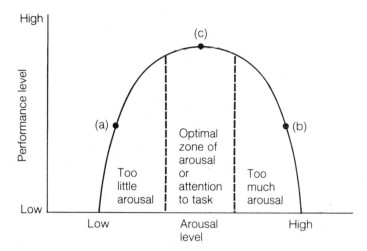

It is necessary to focus the athlete's attention on the task at hand, but a wise coach or team official will not attempt to do too much "psyching up" because this may result in a "psyching out" of highly anxious participants. There is some evidence in football players that high anxiety players may need to be calmed down rather than further aroused prior to playing (Langer, 1966). If the coach were to give a pep talk in the mold of Knute Rockne or Vince Lombardi, the inspirational "psych up" message may not affect the level of anxiety in highly skilled players, but may adversely affect somewhat unskilled players, leading to poor performance.

Some sport psychologists have suggested an alternate strategy of demotivating the athlete to calm him or her down before crucial athletic events (Kroll, 1970; Straub, 1978). Psychological techniques, such as using various relaxation strategies, appear to calm the athlete so that they are at optimal levels of anxiety and arousal prior to the contest.

Autogenic training, yoga, transcendental meditation, and various progressive relaxation techniques may be used to relax and demotivate a super-charged, overly anxious competitor. Successful coaches have noted that they must plan the pre-event period very carefully (sometimes as much as a day or two before competition) in order to insure optimal activation and arousal levels in their players. Several long distance runners have informed me that, if they occupy the entire pre-event period, on the day of the event, with meaningful, but time-consuming activities, they do not have the time to become anxious about the upcoming event. It must be remembered that each athlete is an individual person and a relaxation or de-activating strategy for one performer may not work for another.

One person may need the quiet and solitude of a church prior to competition, while another may need loud, stimulating music. Coaches and athletic trainers should seek to understand all the different personality types in their athletes so as to promote the best pre-event preparation possible.

This topic of the athletic personality is another important consideration in the area of sport psychology and is discussed in the next section.

Motivation in Sports

It has been said that motivation and sport performance are nearly synonymous terms (Fisher, 1976). Any discussion of the top flight athlete involves references to that athlete's persistence and dedication to the sport. What motivates a young gymnast to work out two to four hours per day, while still in junior high school? Also, what motivates Hill, the British Marathon champion, to continue his consecutive daily running record of over one dozen years? Do certain people have needs that must be satisfied and expressed in sport? Why do some athletes risk death (race car drivers) and injury in athletics? Can factors, such as motivation, influence which athlete will be number one and which will be losers? These are all important questions that various sport psychologists (Fisher, 1976; Straub, 1978; Singer, 1981) have sought answers to. Unfortunately, like other topics in sport psychology, much confusion and personal bias exist in this area. Outlined below is a brief description of some concepts in motivating the athlete for sports along with a short discussion of some of the more factual information in this area. Some definitions are presented first.

Motivation is operationally defined as consisting of physiological processes, social determinants, psychological needs, motives, incentives, and emotional influences, which can all impact on a person's behavior (Fisher, 1976). The complexity of motivation can be seen from this definition. The nature of motivation can be drawn from three aspects of behavior—activating, directing, and sustaining (Fisher, 1976).

The activating component of motivation involves descriptive words, such as arousal, stress, and tension. The second and third components of motivation—directing and sustaining—consider *drives, needs, incentives,* and *motives.* A *drive* may lead an individual to behave in a manner that sustains an organic need (a drive for food to satisfy a need for food). *Incentives* are somewhat more subjective and may represent behaviors which have been learned or rewarded. Incentives may be positive or negative. For many athletes, winning or doing well in a sport activity represents a positive incentive. Continued losing or extremely poor performances might be negative incentives and lead the individual athlete to withdraw from competition. A final term under consideration is *motives.* Motives are described as rather stable components of behavior that predispose an athlete to behave in a predictable fashion. Readiness to aggress may be considered an example of a motive. Fisher (1976) summarizes these terms by noting that drives initiate action to satisfy needs, but the incentives and motives actually determine the specific behavior that results.

Now that these basic terms are understood, one can see how activation and perception affect motivation. One can measure a person's heart rate and galvanic skin response to get at a person's level of activation. This arousal level affects a person's performance. Several other factors may influence motivation in sport. Some of them were reviewed by Singer (1981), who noted that personal variables, societal variables, activity dimensions, and situational variables are all necessary in order to predict or explain human athletic performance. Personal variables include self-image, need to achieve, and aspiration level. Examples of societal variables are cultural or social expectancies impacting on the athlete. What impact do the opinions of the coach, parent, or peer group have on the athlete? Cultural influences may be life styles or activity preferences because of geographic location (ice hockey in Canada, for example). Added to personal and societal variables is the dimension of the activity itself. Is it a complex sport? Football is an example. Running may be a more simplistic sport. What are the demands in terms of speed, strength, power, or endurance? How relevant and meaningful is the activity to the athlete? Finally, one must evaluate the situational variables of the athletic event. Is it an important (championship) event? Are friendly or unfriendly spectators present? (Roberts, 1982)

A final consideration in understanding how motivation and human athletic performance are related is to consider *intrinsic* versus *extrinsic* motivation. Intrinsic motivation is when the activity, itself, supplies the reward as in the feeling of accomplishment after a person completes a well-run race. Extrinsic motivation is displayed when one sees the activity as a means to an end. To extend the above example, extrinsic motivation would be when the runner is running the race to satisfy the race sponsor and to receive possible under-the-table payments and not really running the race for the joy of effort, etc. Many athletes in professional sports today participate mostly for the extrinsic rewards that they receive. Even in many amateur situations, where the athlete *should* be competing for more intrinsic rewards, various extrinsic rewards can creep into the athletic situation. Several authors (Walker, 1980; Sheehan, 1980) stress the importance of self-motivation and a striving for excellence through the sport experience. This concept will be further developed in the succeeding section.

Physical Activity and Sex

There are at least two ways of approaching this question. First, a consideration is whether being fit affects sexual activity, and a second concern revolves around how sexual activity, immediately before a game or contest, affects the performer? Unfortunately, there is nearly no information on the second question, and only indirect evidence relating to the first.

How Exercise Affects Sex

Dr. Gabe Mirkin (1978) has a good section on this topic in his text. Unfortunately, only part of the story is told. Mirkin notes that, when a person is fit, they tend to be a better sexual partner, and they also tend to enjoy sex more. This makes sense. If a part of the sexual act is physical, then being in good physical shape should help each partner. Sexual intercourse has been shown to increase the body's need for oxygen. Though it is only a slight elevation, it may be an effort for someone who is extremely unfit. Sexual relations have been compared to the energy expenditure of walking up a flight of stairs, and, unfortunately, some people become breathless with just this little exertion. Mirkin goes on to describe the ideal love act as "one in which both partners stimulate each other with ever-increasing intensity until climax." He further notes that, when both partners are physically fit, they participate in lovemaking longer, and with more intensity.

Another aspect to this question of how fitness aids sexual performance is the relationship that a fit body has to self-confidence and self-esteem. Some sexual counselors note that the most important organ of sexual functioning is the human brain. If a person is extremely fit and feels good about his or her body, then they are almost certain to have extra confidence and self-assurance about their sexual performance. This is the indirect connection between fitness and sexual functioning that was noted earlier.

Sex and Athletic Performance

There is much heresay concerning this topic, but very few published reports of a scientific nature on this topic. Dr. Warren Johnson, formerly a professor at the University of Maryland and a leading pioneer in sex education, reported that sexual activity has no effect on muscular performance in men. Many authorities point out that, after sexual activity, both partners experience feelings of relief, happiness, sadness, or guilt in varying degrees. These emotional responses run the gamut of human feelings. Human sexual response and feelings are highly individual. Therefore, it may be said with confidence that, if the athlete is accustomed to certain sexual activity on the night or day prior to an event, then this normal, natural activity would not be detrimental. If, however, the athlete believed that any sexual activity the night before the contest would be detrimental, then it may well be for that athlete. In this situation the mind set can influence the body to a large degree.

As a final note in this area, there are reported cases where runners performed outstanding times in races very shortly after sexual relations. Mirkin reports one athlete set a world record in a dash and another ran a sub-four-minute mile. If the fit athlete has time to adequately prepare for the athletic competition, including proper warmup routines, then the energy expenditure in any lovemaking should not detract from athletic performance. In summary, if time permits the lovemaking and still allows adequate preparation for the event, *and the athlete is not emotionally disturbed* by the sexual activity, then performance is not affected.

The Psychology of Competition

Dr. Stuart H. Walker, a pediatrician and international sailboat racer, has written an excellent book on the psychology of winning (Walker, 1980). In this treatise, Dr. Walker makes the case for understanding the psychology of the athlete in competition. As he explains, the "psychological factors of athletic competition are far more important and are the major determinants of success and failure in athletic performance" (Walker, 1980). In this monograph, Walker attempts to explain why winners win and why losers lose.

Walker begins by noting that competition is a necessary and vital component of human life. Other authors have also commented on this crucial aspect of the human condition. Walker further elaborates on this theme of competing by saying that all athletes, whenever they enter their sports, enter a unique world where challenge, risk, and uncertainty exist. The athlete, by entering the competition, makes a statement regarding his own preparation and ability for the sport, usually in the presence of others. There are few other human activities whereby one can find this opportunity to put oneself on the line and risk the uncertainty of the outcome of the game or contest. In many other aspects of the real world the outcome of a performance may be etched in shades of gray. But, in the athletic world, it is rather clear. You either won or lost. You either performed up to your ability, or not. You were either prepared, or you were not. Playing and competing serve a useful function in life.

Both Sheehan (1980) and Walker (1980) note that the athlete is like a child. The child seeks uncertainty, challenges, risks—always looking for a sense of adventure. Playing games may serve as a release to the child. The child often plays the game seriously, but spontaneously. There is a certain innocence in children's sport activities (if not overly organized by adults) that is a joy to watch. Children strive for victory in whatever way they can. They are not content in doing simple easy tasks. Their games involve risk, daring, excitement, and fun. The child is able to relax while playing sports, and enjoy the adventure, the struggle, and the challenge. Make the contest easy, leading to simple victory, and the child becomes dull and disinterested. Adults can learn something from this. The message may be that a contest that has a dead certain outcome may be a dull and uninteresting affair. Children do not like dull games.

Several sport philosophers make the point that the struggle is worth more than the victory (Walker, 1980; Sheehan, 1980). If the win was the final thing and one had won a world or Olympic title, then one would quit. But we know that good athletes don't quit. The true athlete continues to seek the challenge, the uncertainty, the risks of the contest. It has been noted that no Olympic champion in the marathon event has won the prestigious Boston Marathon. Yet, several have tried. Why? Because it is there. Walker (1980) makes an insightful comment about winning and competence that many coaches and athletes fail to recognize. This concept states that the best athletes are those who strive to understand themselves and improve control of themselves. If this happens, then they will attain competence and hence, control of their game. This increased competence in their performance leads to more creativity and risk-taking in practice, training, and conditioning, and ultimately more fun and adventure in their chosen sport. Figure 19.2 portrays this relationship.

The Psychology of Losing

Perhaps a comment is necessary concerning losing in sports. Some coaches and athletes have placed such a great emphasis on winning that one may logically ask what can be done concerning losing games and contests. Walker (1980) provides us with an insightful answer. It goes like this. Winning should be the object of the game or contest. One should try to win. But when one loses, all is not lost, if, during the contest the athlete has sought

Figure 19.2 Proposed athletic growth cycle for the new jogger or runner. Athlete starts cycle at the top (1) and begins running/ training. This training leads to improvements (2) and perhaps a time trial or race (3). Goals may be met as a result of the race and more competence gained (4). As a result of the competition, increased self-confidence and self-esteem, the individual may come to the top of the proposed growth cycle. Once back at the top, the cycle begins again. Injury or lack of motivation will disrupt the cycle.

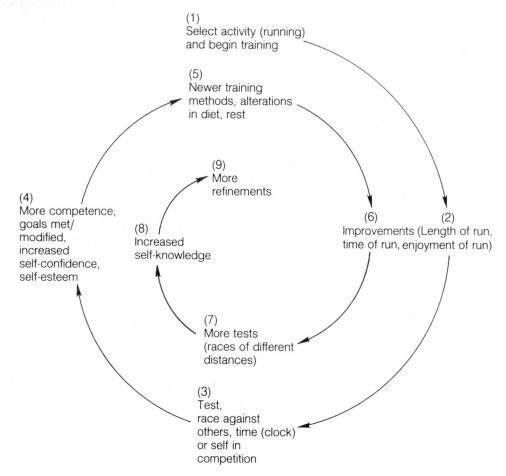

(1)
Select activity (running)
and begin training

(5)
Newer training
methods, alterations
in diet, rest

(9)
More
refinements

(4)
More competence,
goals met/
modified,
increased
self-confidence,
self-esteem

(8)
Increased
self-knowledge

(6)
Improvements (Length of run,
time of run, enjoyment of run)

(2)

(7)
More tests
(races of different
distances)

(3)
Test,
race against
others, time (clock)
or self in
competition

his or her own particular level of competence and has enjoyed striving toward it. Then, the ultimate victor is the person who has participated. The person who has sought to risk, has sought to gain more self knowledge. Walker maintains that losing, viewed in this manner, does not have to make the athlete feel a failure, or embarrassed. The losing athlete does not feel the need to surrender, to cheat, or deliberately harm an opponent. This losing athlete realizes that in every defeat there is some learning. A message regarding future competence is gained. Different solutions, strategies, and decisions will have to be made in practice and training. More adjustments will have to be made. Every attempt at competition is significant, because it can provide a learning experience. The true athlete never gives up, never accepts defeat. The athlete accepts a loss as a learning experience for tomorrow's preparation. The truly mature competitor realizes that absolute, complete mastery over the sport may never come, and if it does, then only fleetingly, so continued effort must be maintained. In this way, temporary failure (losing) might be expected, but ultimately improvement and winning will be attained. The reward for this increased competence will consist of mostly inner satisfaction and a mastery of self. This, in the end, is the ultimate attainment.

Aggression

One of the major topics for discussion in sports psychology is **aggression.** In nearly every text on sport psychology or conference on the subject, a significant part of the dialogue is on aggression in sport. Aggression is defined as an *intent* to inflict harm (damage or pain) on the opposition (VanDyke, 1980). If the aggression is severe, it is often referred to as violence. Another aspect of this definition is to realize that, if one person beats another in sport, then some form of harm or damage has been inflicted. It may be only minimal, but nevertheless, some small amount of aggression has been perpetrated. More regarding this train of thought will follow.

There are, generally, two major theories regarding human aggression. In one school of thought, Lorenz (1966) speculates that aggression is a normal, natural impulse in the human being. Further, this theory holds that aggressive energy can build within a human being and must be released or purged from time to time. If this happens, the organism does not suffer undue physiological or psychological harm. This group of theoreticians conceive of sport as being beneficial in that it allows an opportunity for humans to release their pent-up aggressive energies in a positive, controlled, socially accepted manner. An extension of this view is that the competitive sport milieu is an appropriate arena for athletes to compete aggressively for power, dominance, and mastery. This view of aggression is a cathartic view in that sports serve as a release of normal, aggressive tensions, which build up naturally in the human.

An opposite view of human aggression is the social learning position forwarded by Berkowitz (1969). This second view of aggressive athletic behavior holds that aggression is learned and is not innate. Extending this social learning theory of aggression reasons that, since aggression is learned in the process of socialization, sport may reinforce aggression by reinforcing the intent to harm or injure a perceived opponent. This group of psychologists warns us that sports may reward and foster aggressive behavior in the athlete. This social learning view of aggression is obviously opposite from the cathartic view of aggression. How can it be that several outstanding thinkers have formulated such opposing views concerning aggression? Like other cases in scientific thinking, it may be that, where two opposing theories are forwarded, each side may have merit and elements from both positions may be correct. Sports may, in some veins, serve as a cathartic experience, while in other ways, a sporting experience may lead to a fostering of more aggressive behavior. To better understand this new idea on aggression, let's examine a subdivision of the aggression definition.

Some authors further explain reactive aggression as specific, initiated behavior toward another person with specific intent to do bodily harm. In this refined definition, *intent* is a major component, and often anger and purposeful injury against an opponent are involved. Taken from a humanistic point of view, this *reactive aggression,* involving *intent to harm* or *inflict injury* against an opponent, cannot be condoned in any sporting situation. Obviously, sportsmanlike conduct is dismissed in this view of aggression, and an attitude of winning at all costs is encouraged.

In a somewhat different view of human aggression, the term *instrumental aggression* is favored by more enlightened sports officials. Instrumental aggression is defined as a "striving to attain a goal" (Fisher, 1976). Thus, instrumental aggression is used by an athlete as a tool to gain something important, like a victory, and not prompted by an "intent to harm" the opponent. In sum, a person who practices instrumental aggression is goal-oriented and sees the opponent as someone also interested in pursuing that same goal, while the reactive aggressive individual may indeed be intending to hurt an opponent. The reactive aggressive person may think that the only way victory may be achieved is to truly injure the opponent. Very often, this reactive aggressive individual displays unsportsmanlike conduct, and feels guilty later because of purposeful, intentional acts of questionable sportsmanship displayed during the competition. The instrumental-oriented person may not feel guilty after a contest since their striving was toward a *goal* or accomplishment.

Parents, athletic coaches, and officials should understand these two areas of human aggressive behavior, and try to plan for the most positive outcome of the sporting contests. If aggression can be directed in this positive fashion, there can be more winners and fewer losers in sport. Since aggression is so intertwined in a person's physiology and psychology, structuring athletic events in such a manner so as to insure positive benefits should make sports a wholesome activity for all individuals.

The Athletic Personality

In perhaps no other area in sports psychology is there as much confusion present as the area of the athletic personality. The leading texts in sport psychology (Straub, 1978; Fisher, 1976; Morgan, 1972; Suinn, 1980) have included major sections in personality dynamics of the athlete, testifying to its importance. Why has so much controversy existed in this area? Why are important questions in sport personality often answered with philosophical speculation or personal anecdotes? A major factor for this confusion may be the lack of an adequate definition of personality itself.

Somatotype and Personality

Early researchers in the field defined personality from a biophysical standpoint. A prime example of this is William H. Sheldon, M.D., who wrote several texts on the behavior-physique relationship. Another group of personality researchers defined personality from a social learning theory aspect. This view holds that behavior varies as situations vary, hence, behavior is situation specific. It must be realized that each individual's past experiences

experiences are dissimilar, and each situation is somewhat unique, so the personality response could be expected to be slightly different in varying situations. A final personality theory describes a person's behavior as a combination of traits. Once an athlete's traits are identified, behavior in a certain athletic situation might be predicted.

Based upon these views of personality, sport psychologists have tried to answer questions like the following (Fisher, 1976):

Do successful athletes and athletic teams fit a specific personality profile?
Can athletic participation influence personality?
Do individual sport athletes display certain kinds of personality, while team athletes display others?
Does personality influence athletic performance, or even choice of sport?
Can participation in sport alter sex-role orientation in males and females?

All of the above questions can legitimately be raised by coaches and athletes. Unfortunately, little specific information can be reported from scientific research in this area. Why is this so?

Kroll (1970), has said that sport psychologists have borrowed instruments for analyzing personality from traditional psychologists and therefore, these tests may not be genuine to the athletic situation. Kroll further notes that sport psychologists must first develop testing instruments specific to particular sports, and then, perhaps, developments regarding the athletic personality might be forthcoming. Professor Kroll (1970) has done many studies on wrestlers and finds that this wrestling experience promotes a tough and aggressive profile in these individuals. In another study by Kroll (1953) it was found that, for beginning wrestlers, strength is a key component, but that later wrestling success is evidenced by increasing skill levels. This concept of the changing importance of ability components is significant for many coaches and suggests that athletes have to be coached differently at different stages of their development.

Morgan (1972), who has written extensively in the area of the athletic personality, believes that some useful information can be gleaned from studying athletic personalities. Working with elite oarsmen, wrestlers, and long distance runners, Morgan has characterized these exceptional athletes as normal in every respect with regard to personality traits. In several studies he has shown an iceberg profile for these top athletes. That is, elite performers in rowing, long distance running, and wrestling show high positive attributes on psychological vigor, and lower values on scales of trait anxiety, depression, tension, fatigue, and confusion. This represents significant positive mental health characteristics in these top class performers. Morgan further notes that, when psychological data such as gathered above, is used in conjunction with physiological and other data (coaches' input, past ability records), this serves to enhance prediction of successful performers.

Martens (1975), a prolific researcher in the area of psychology of sports, notes that much personality research in this area involves either a study of traits, or, at the opposite extreme, an examination of the situation. Dr. Martens suggests an interactional model whereby the sport psychologist must examine the personality traits of the athlete *together* with the specific sporting situation. This would be difficult to do, but it may more adequately explain the complex issue of the athletic personality.

Table 19.1 Self-Description Test

1. I feel most of the time _____ , _____ , and _____ .

calm	contented	tense	reticent
anxious	relaxed	impetous	energetic
cheerful	confident	complacent	self-conscious

2. When I study or work, I seem to be _____ , _____ , and
_____ .

efficient	placid	leisurely	determined
enthusiastic	sluggish	meticulous	thoughtful
reflective	competitive	precise	cooperative

3. Socially, I am _____ , _____ , and _____ .

outgoing	gentle-tempered	affected	shy
affable	considerate	soft-tempered	talkative
tolerant	awkward	argumentative	hot-tempered

4. I am rather _____ , _____ , and _____ .

active	introspective	suspicious	serious
warm	forgiving	cool	soft-hearted
domineering	courageous	sympathetic	enterprising

5. Other people consider me rather _____ , _____ , and _____ .

generous	dominant	reckless	kind
adventurous	optimistic	detached	cautious
withdrawn	affectionate	sensitive	dependent

6. Underline one word out of the three in each of the following lines which most closely describes the way you are.

a) assertive, released, tense
b) hot-tempered, cool, warm
c) withdrawn, sociable, active

d) confident, tactful, kind
e) dependent, dominant, detached
f) enterprising, affable, anxious

Source: Cortes, J. B., and F. M. Gatti. 1970. Physique and propensity. *Psychology Today.* 4: 42–44.

To amplify the interesting theory put forth by Sheldon (1951) regarding somatotype (physique or body type), personality, and temperament, the following comments are in order. Sheldon attempted to develop a typing system for human behavior based upon physical and psychological constitution. He examined the nearly nude photographs of college males in front, back, and side views. From this analysis, he isolated three body types: endomorphy (roundness or fatness), mesomorphy (muscularity), and ectomorphy (extreme thinness or linearity). Each of these components was rated on a seven point scale. A scale score of seven on mesomorphy indicates extreme muscle definition and development, while a 1 or 2 indicates little prominence of this trait.

In addition to this physical assessment, Sheldon studied psychological traits in these same persons. He found that there appeared to be three major temperament clusters which appeared to coincide with the physical traits. His three temperament components were viscerotonia (being relaxed and social), somatotonia (being assertive and motoric), and cerebrotonia (being tense and socially restrained). These three temperament components were correlated to endomorphy, mesomorphy, and ectomorphy, respectively. It is important to recall here that correlational values do not imply *causation,* but merely association with another variable. Other authors (Sheehan, 1978; Cortes & Gatti, 1970) have suggested a similar relationship between temperament, personality, and physical characteristics. In fact, Cortes and Gatti have suggested that there is a short (pencil and paper) inventory that can ascertain propensity toward one type of personality characteristic. See tables 19.1 and 19.2.

Table 19.2. Key to Self-Description Test

Endomorphic	Mesomorphic	Ectomorphic
dependent	dominant	detached
calm	cheerful	tense
relaxed	confident	anxious
complacent	energetic	reticent
contented	impetuous	self-conscious
sluggish	efficient	meticulous
placid	enthusiastic	reflective
leisurely	competitive	precise
cooperative	determined	thoughtful
affable	outgoing	considerate
tolerant	argumentative	shy
affected	talkative	awkward
warm	active	cool
forgiving	domineering	suspicious
sympathetic	courageous	introspective
soft-hearted	enterprising	serious
generous	adventurous	cautious
affectionate	reckless	tactful
kind	assertive	sensitive
sociable	optimistic	withdrawn
soft-tempered	hot-tempered	gentle-tempered

Source: Cortes, J. B., and F. M. Gatti. 1970. Physique and propensity. *Psychology Today.* 4:42.

Count the number of adjectives that you selected in each of the three categories. For example, if your totals are 10, 6, and 5, you have predominantly endomorphic traits; a 6, 10, 5 means you are high in mesomorphic traits.

Sheehan has further suggested that certain somatotypes gravitate to certain sports. He describes himself as an ectomorph with chickenlike bones, introverted, and with the temperament of a cerebrotonic person. Others he knows are aggressive, assertive, and fit in more combative, muscular type sports (football, wrestling). Sheehan further indicates that people should pick their friends on physique and temperament, rather than risk disappointment with people who have opposing viewpoints and mannerisms (Sheehan, 1978)!

Life Quality and Sports Participation

One final area of sports psychology that is interesting to study involves the aspect of **life quality.** It is often said now that the generations of the 60s, 70s, and 80s are becoming extremely interested in life quality. Life quality has been defined as "the degree to which an individual or a society is able to satisfy its perceived psychological and physiological needs" (Dalkey, Lewis & Snyder, 1972). A psychologist, Pflaum (1973), defined life quality as "the degree to which the environment is perceived as facilitating or retarding one's functioning."

The term, life quality, has been seen to surpass older terms, such as happiness or welfare of the individual. The term, life quality, itself denotes a positive connotation because of reference to the term, quality. There have been several life quality paper and pencil inventories used to evaluate a person's state. We have used these inventories in some of our studies at the University of Maryland.

Morris and Husman (1978) examined the life quality changes in a group of college students who were participating in an endurance conditioning class of about fifteen weeks duration. This class stressed aerobic training involving long distance running activities. A control class of students, enrolled in a history of sports class, who were not engaged in any planned regular physical activity served as controls. The life quality inventories were administered to both groups at the beginning and at the end of this fifteen week period. Results revealed that the endurance conditioning class made significant improvements in the construct of life quality. Morris and Husman (1978) suggested that the endurance trained students, perhaps, gained some new found self-esteem, self-respect, and self-confidence as a result of this vigorous training program. Similar results have also been reported by other researchers, who have used aerobic activities to improve self concepts in certain groups of individuals who had displayed mild symptoms of anxiety or depression (Glasser, 1976, and Kostrubala, 1976).

The relationship between the psyche and the body is a difficult one to explain. Early writers from Greece and Rome indicated that the mind and body were of an indivisible nature. Some recent scientists have continued to try to explore this interesting relationship and their findings are very important. Some of these concepts are discussed in this chapter.

Social Learning Theory, Attribution Theory, and Locus of Control

It has been indicated earlier that the athlete's personality and motivation play a crucial part in the total preparation and in the sport performance itself. There is a particular aspect of social learning theory that involves locus of control. This concept was first developed by Rotter (1966) and it examines the way a person perceives the reinforcement or outcomes from certain situations. Rotter's concept revolves around an internal or external personality orientation. As one reevaluates the outcomes of a particular happening, one can ascribe them to luck, fate, chance, or powerful outside factors, which would be external orientations. Conversely, one may ascribe the outcomes of competition to the internal factors of individual effort, dedication, perseverance, and just plain hard work. Obviously, other factors are involved when one analyzes any situation. Factors, such as difficulty of the task and the ability level of the participant are also crucial elements in the locus of control construct. The variables of luck or fate, degree of effort of the athlete, difficulty of the task and ability level of the athlete, may be said to interact in what is known as the **attribution theory** (Weiner, 1974). (See fig. 19.3.) The locus of control dimension considers internal factors such as ability and effort, while the external factors are luck and task difficulty. Weiner (1974) notes that a stability dimension also exists and that ability and task difficulty tend to remain fairly stable, while effort and luck seem relatively unstable.

Figure 19.3 illustrates these interrelationships. In any case, most individuals do not fall at either end of the locus of control spectrum. A person is not always internal, nor completely external. Most people fluctuate along this continuum throughout life. However, some general comments can be made regarding this locus of control (LOC) personality construct. It has been found that many younger children are external. This might seem to be inherently logical, since very young children are dependent on their parents for many of life's necessities. As people mature past adolescence, they become more internal, responsible for their own actions and potential reinforcements. At the other end of the age spectrum, many older individuals become external again, since many older people on fixed incomes, without many relatives or friends close by, and often with health related problems, may feel that they are dependent on the external world and that they have lost some control over their individual lives. Dr. Wayne Dyer (1976), a psychologist who has written many popular self-help books, indicates that about 75 percent of the adult American population seem to be external in most of their life situations.

This LOC construct has been studied in athletic situations and some interesting findings have been reported. Duke, Johnson, and Nowicki (1977) found six to fourteen year old children to become more internal following an eight-week summer sports fitness camp. These children experienced an increase in the ability to control what happened to them during this fitness experience. Perhaps even at this young age, these campers saw that their efforts lead directly to increased fitness levels, and this translated into more positive internal orientation.

Figure 19.3 Weiner's Classification System for Attribution Theory and Motivation in Sports. Weiner theorizes that success and failure are based upon four main elements: luck, ability, degree of effort and task difficulty, which fall into four dimensions.

Source: Weiner, B. 1974. *Achievement motivation and attribution theory.* Morristown, N.J.: General Learning Press.

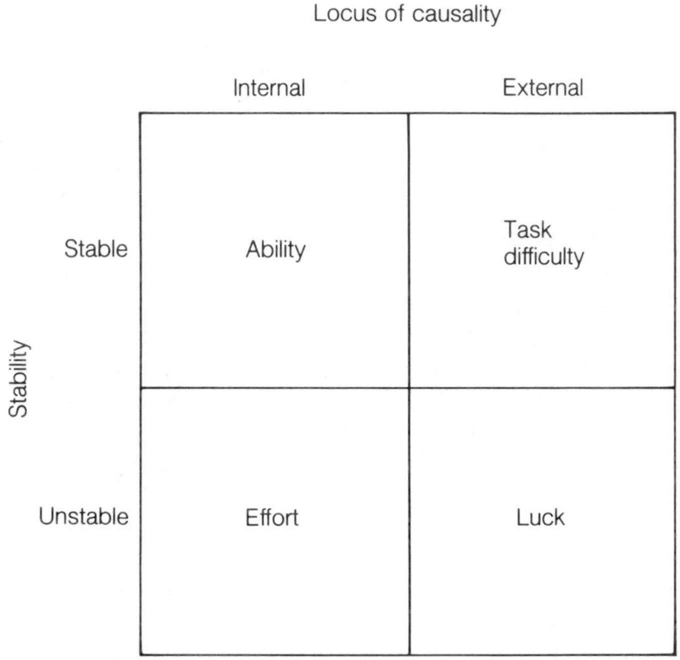

Locus of causality

	Internal	External
Stable	Ability	Task difficulty
Unstable	Effort	Luck

Stability

In another study (Morris, Clarke and Vaccaro, 1979) it was found that young, age group swimmers were more internal than other age matched controls. Morris (1980) in a paper presented to a medical group, indicated that women national class master long distance runners were also more internally inclined than other age matched controls. Unfortunately, these types of studies are descriptive, and in no way tell us whether these various athletic subgroups were internal when they came to their sport, or whether the long, arduous training and conditioning made these athletes more internal. Could it be that athletes realize, as they train and become more competent, that they control more of their destiny in the sporting situation? Does increased competition and the increased competence that Walker (1980) notes in his text on winning enable the athlete to move toward the internal end of this LOC continuum? Is the internal personality orientation necessarily better than the external orientation? No value judgments are being rendered here, except to note that, if one adopted more of the external orientation, ascribing more of the sport experience to the external factors of fate, luck, or chance, then these athletes might not be willing to put in the long, arduous, practice sessions necessary to become a champion.

The internally oriented person, more often than not, points to internal factors as responsible for their success. The internal athlete will make remarks to the extent that they were well-prepared for the game, that their training, conditioning, and game plans were well-conceived, wise and appropriate to their opponent.

On the other hand, the external athlete often looks to external factors to explain unsuccessful outcomes. These athletes often say that the field conditions were wet, too windy, too cold, too hot, the sun was in their eyes, the wind shifted on them, etc. These are all external conditions that, in most cases, affected both competing individuals and teams equally. Again, it is important to remember that the athlete is probably never truly 100 percent internal or external in personality orientation, however, most athletes seem to adopt one or the other LOC personality orientation. Might this be related to athletic rehabilitation? Some evidence for a certain personality orientation has been suggested as being a positive factor in rehabilitation after injury.

Some other sports medicine texts (Ryan, 1962; O'Donohue, 1976, and Hirata, 1968) have indicated that the athlete who works most intelligently in the post-injury phase will perhaps return to the activity sooner than the athlete who merely waits for "the doctor to make them well again." This concept is portrayed on a statement over the door of a training room of one of the Atlantic Coast Conference schools. It reads, "The greatest single factor in returning the athlete to activity is the fierce desire on the part of the injured athlete to work to get well." This quote places a great deal of the burden of rehabilitation squarely on the athlete's shoulders. The team doctor and athletic trainers assist in diagnosing and initial treatment of the injury, but once a rehabilitation program is established, the biggest single factor becomes the athlete's fierce desire to get well and return to the sport.

A recent report, by orthopedic specialists (Wise, Jackson, and Rocchio, 1979) from California, studied post-operative recovery in a group of athletes who had undergone surgery on their knees. A personality test, the Minnesota Multiphasic Personality Inventory (MMPI), was given to the athletes before and after the surgery. Based upon the results of this psychological testing, the speed and degree of recovery were noted for each individual athlete. It was found that the most rapid and thorough recovery was made by athletes who had scored highly on the MMPI personality test. This type of study is related to the LOC concept of personality, in that it indicates that internally oriented athletes feel that they may be more intimately responsible for their own recovery. We can all think of some athletes who fit this internal mold, while there are other athletes who display mostly external orientations. Some people also believe that significant outside influences, like parents, coaches, and teammates can create a positive environment whereby athletes are encouraged toward a particular LOC orientation.

I have had personal experiences with the LOC personality outlook, while associated with a medical school in Atlanta. While working with stroke patients (people who were partially paralyzed because of a reduced or temporary lack of blood supply to the brain) in our rehabilitation center, we administered LOC inventories to them to try to determine their locus of control after this serious neurological damage. Naturally, one would expect that LOC would be affected. However, in our preliminary findings, we noted that those people who had a more internal personality orientation felt more in charge of their rehabilitation programs and were likely to make more rapid and total progress than other patients who adopted the attitude that a terrible event had happened to them; and now their physician must make them well. After working with these stroke patients over many months, the staff was able to predict which personality type patients would be more successful with particular rehabilitation programs, irrespective of the initial damage which had been done to the nervous system.

In summary, it is suggested here that athletes are often "the captain of their soul and the master of their fate" when it comes to training and preparation for sports activity, and also when it comes to adhering to and mastering a rehabilitation program which has been set out for them after an injury. The locus of control (LOC) personality construct, indicating whether a person holds an internal or external orientation, may be crucial in predicting athletic success. It is further suggested that important members of the athletic environment (coaches, parents, teammates) may subconsciously or overtly influence the athlete to adopt a particular LOC orientation which may lead to greater athletic success. ■

Summary

Psychology of sports, and how it affects the athlete, are discussed in this chapter. Various topics, such as anxiety, attention, arousal, and activation, as they relate to athletic performance, are given. Anxiety may be defined as a fear, real or imagined, that confronts athletes as they are about to perform in competition. Athletes must understand how this anxiety may affect performance, attempt to control it, and have it function for them in a positive sense.

Motivation is operationally defined in this chapter as consisting of physiological processes, social determinants, psychological needs, motives, incentives, and emotional influences, which can all impact on the athlete's behavior. The complexity of this subject of motivation can be seen from the above definition. Intrinsic and extrinsic aspects of motivation are listed. Intrinsic rewards tend to be incentives that the athletes gain for themselves, in terms of inner emotional satisfaction received from participation in the event. Extrinsic rewards are more material and worldly in nature, and may consist of payment or contracts that the athlete receives, as a result of participation in the sport.

The psychology of competition is detailed. Dr. Shepard Walker has indicated that psychological factors may be far more important determinants of success and failure in athletic performance than physiological factors. He notes that the athlete who has a compelling desire and motivation to excel in the sport is often the person who wins the particular event. He details, in a rather elegant manner, the psychology of competition and the effects that winning and losing have on the athlete. A comment is made on the psychology of losing. If the athletes have performed up to their capabilities, then there is no need to feel that there was a defeat in the performance.

A proposed growth cycle for an athlete, such as a runner, is given. In this growth cycle, the athlete aims for improvement through proper training and conditioning. Often, this leads to improvement in performance, in terms of times and records established for a certain event. Fine tuning of the cycle involves newer modifications to diet, rest, and additional refinements to training, which can lead to increased performances. In any case, there should be increased self-knowledge within the athlete. It is this self-knowledge and understanding of the individual which may be a most significant aspect of individual participation in sport.

The topic of aggression is dealt with in this chapter. The two theories of aggression—instrumental and reactive aggression—are noted. Reactive aggression involves the *intent to harm* or inflict injury on an opponent. This cannot be condoned in any sporting situation. The second type of aggression, instrumental aggression, is more favored by coaches and enlightened and educated athletes. Instrumental aggression can be defined as *striving to attain a goal,* in which the athlete attempts to compete against himself or herself with the aim of achieving a better performance. There is no intent to harm the opponent. Whenever there is a prize to be won, some concern has to be given to these various factors of instrumental and reactive aggression.

In a final section of this chapter the athletic personality is described. Several researchers have attempted to define specific personality traits of the athlete. Some of these researchers have been successful in assigning certain characteristics to particular groups of athletes. Somewhat related to this area is the question of somatotype, or body type, and how it relates to athletic participation.

An aspect of sport psychology that is given some attention in this chapter is attribution theory and locus of control. Locus of control is defined as the outlook that athletes adopt when they evaluate their performance or the outcome of a particular event. Internal locus of control athletes credit effort and ability (internal factors) to their performance on the task. External LOC athletes tend to favor luck and task difficulty, or other factors which are external, such as the weather, the lighting, environment, etc., as possible reasons why they were not successful in a given athletic event.

This locus of control construct is important because it relates to the attitudes which the athletes adopt toward their environment. Some studies have indicated that a more successful performer begins to ascribe more training and performance attributes to internal characteristics. The relationship between locus of control and rehabilitation after injury is also significant. Some medical doctors have indicated that the athlete who works with an intelligent rehabilitation program in the post-injury phase can perhaps return to normal activities sooner than the athlete who merely waits "for the doctor to make them well again." The influence of this internal locus of control personality outlook, as it affects the rehabilitation process, is important.

References

Berkowitz, L. 1969. Simple views of aggression: an essay review. *American Scientist.* 57:372–383.

Cortoo, J. D., & F. M. Gatti. 1970. Physique and propensity. *Psychology Today.* 4:42–44.

Dalkey, N. C., R. Lewis, & D. Snyder. 1972. *Studies in the quality of life.* Boston: D. C. Heath.

Duke, M., T. C. Johnson, & S. Nowicki. 1977. Effects of sports fitness camp experience on locus of control orientation in children ages 6–14. *Research Quarterly.* 48:280.

Dyer, W. W. 1976. *Your erroneous zones.* New York: Funk & Wagnalls.

Fisher, A. C. 1976. *Psychology of sport.* Palo Alto: Mayfield.

Glasser, W. 1976. *Positive addiction.* New York: Harper & Row.

Hirata, I. 1968. *The doctor and the athlete.* Philadelphia: J. B. Lippincott.

Kostrubala, T. 1976. *The joy of running.* Philadelphia: J. B. Lippincott.

Kroll, W. 1953. *An anthropometrical study of some big ten varsity wrestlers.* Masters thesis, University of Illinois, Urbana-Champaign.

Kroll, W. 1970. Current strategies and problems in personality assessment of athletes. In L. Smith, ed. *Psychology of motor learning.* Chicago: The Athletic Institute.

Kroll, W. 1975. Psychology of coaching. Lecture notes, University of Massachusetts. Spring.

Langer, P. 1966. Varsity football performance. *Perceptual and Motor Skills.* 23:1191–99.

Lorenz, K. 1966. *On aggression.* New York: Harcourt, Brace & World.

Martens, R. 1975. *Social psychology in physical activity.* New York: Harper and Row.

Mirkin, G., & M. Hoffman. 1978. *The sports medicine book.* Boston: Little Brown & Co.

Morgan, W. 1972. Sport psychology. In Robert N. Singer, ed. *The psychomotor domain: movement behavior.* Philadelphia: Lea & Febiger.

Morris, A. F. 1980. Psychological and life quality characteristics of national class women long distance runners. Paper presented at the Boston Marathon Medical Seminar. April.

Morris, A. F., D. H. Clarke, & P. Vaccaro. 1979. Psychological characteristics in age group competitive swimmers. *Perceptual and Motor Skills,* 48:1265–66.

Morris, A. F., & B. F. Husman. 1978. Life quality changes following an endurance conditioning program. *American Corrective Therapy Journal.* 32:3–6.

O'Donohue, D. H. 1976. *Treatment of injuries to athletes.* 3d ed. Philadelphia: W. B Saunders.

Oxendine, J. B. 1980. Emotional arousal and motor performance. In R. M. Suinn, *Psychology in sports.* Minneapolis: Burgess.

Pflaum, H. J. 1973. *Development of a life quality inventory.* Doctoral dissertation, University of Maryland, College Park, MD.

Roberts, G. C. 1982. Achievement motivation in sport. *Exercise and Sport Science Reviews.* New York: Academic Press. 10:236.

Rotter, J. B. 1966. Generalized expectancies for internal versus external control of reinforcement. *Psychological Monographs.* 80.

Ryan, A. J. 1962. *Medical care of the athlete.* New York: McGraw-Hill.

Sheehan, G. 1978. *Running and being.* New York: Simon & Schuster.

Sheehan, G. 1980. *This running life.* New York: Simon & Schuster.

Sheldon, W., J. S. Stevens, & W. B. Tucker. 1951. *Varieties of human physique.* New York: Harper & Row.

Singer, R. N. 1975. Sports psychology. *American Corrective Therapy Journal.* 29:115–20.

Singer, R. N. 1981. Sport psychology: waves of the future. *The Physician and Sportsmedicine.* 9:153–56.

Straub, W. F., ed. 1978. *Sport psychology: an analysis of athlete behavior.* Ithaca, New York: Mouvement Publications.

Suinn, R. M., ed. 1980. *Psychology in sports.* Minneapolis: Burgess Publishing Co.

Chapter 19

VanDyke, R. 1980. Aggression in sport. *Quest.* 32:201–208.

Walker, S. H. 1980. *Winning: the psychology of competition.* New York: W. W. Norton.

Weiner, B. 1974. *Achievement motivation and attribution theory.* Morristown, NJ: General Learning Press.

Wise, A., D. W. Jackson, & P. Rocchio. 1979. Preoperative psychologic testing as a predictor of success in knee surgery. *American Journal of Sports Medicine.* 2:287–92.

Appendix 1: Proper and Improper Weight Loss Programs

Millions of individuals are involved in weight reduction programs. With the number of undesirable weight loss programs available and a general misconception by many about weight loss, the need for guidelines for proper weight loss programs is apparent.

Based on the existing evidence concerning the effects of weight loss on health status, physiologic processes, and body composition parameters, the American College of Sports Medicine makes the following statements and recommendations for weight loss programs.

For the purposes of this position statement, body weight will be represented by two components, fat and fat-free (water, electrolytes, minerals, glycogen stores, muscular tissue, bone, etc.):

1. Prolonged fasting and diet programs that severely restrict caloric intake are scientifically undesirable and can be medically dangerous.
2. Fasting and diet programs that severely restrict caloric intake result in the loss of large amounts of water, electrolytes, minerals, glycogen stores, and other fat-free tissue (including proteins within fat-free tissues), with minimal amounts of fat loss.
3. Mild calorie restriction (500–1000 kcal less than the usual daily intake) results in a smaller loss of water, electrolytes, minerals, and other fat-free tissue, and is less likely to cause malnutrition.
4. Dynamic exercise of large muscles helps to maintain fat-free tissue, including muscle mass and bone density, and results in losses of body weight. Weight loss resulting from an increase in energy expenditure is primarily in the form of fat weight.
5. A nutritionally sound diet resulting in mild calorie restriction coupled with an endurance exercise program along with behavioral modification of existing eating

American College of Sports Medicine. 1983. Position Statement on Proper and Improper Weight Loss Programs.

habits is recommended for weight reduction. The rate of sustained weight loss should not exceed 1 kg (2 lb) per week.

6. To maintain proper weight control and optimal body fat levels, a lifetime commitment to proper eating habits and regular physical activity is required.

Research Background for the Position Statement

Each year millions of individuals undertake weight loss programs for a variety of reasons. It is well known that obesity is associated with a number of health-related problems (3,4,57). These problems include impairment of cardiac function due to an increase in the work of the heart (2) and to left ventricular dysfunction (1,40); hypertension (6,22,80); diabetes (83,97); renal disease (95); gall bladder disease (55,72); respiratory dysfunction (19); joint diseases and gout (90); endometrial cancer (15); abnormal plasma lipid and lipoprotein concentrations (56,74); problems in the administration of anesthetics during surgery (93); and impairment of physical working capacity (49). As a result, weight reduction is frequently advised by physicians for medical reasons. In addition, there are a vast number of individuals who are on weight reduction programs for aesthetic reasons.

It is estimated that 60–70 million American adults and at least 10 million American teenagers are overfat (49). Because millions of Americans have adopted unsupervised weight loss programs, it is the opinion of the American College of Sports Medicine that guidelines are needed for safe and effective weight loss programs. This position statement deals with desirable and undesirable weight loss programs. Desirable weight loss programs are defined as those that are nutritionally sound and result in maximal losses in fat weight and minimal losses of fat-free tissue. Undesirable weight loss programs are defined as those that are not nutritionally sound, that result in large losses of fat-free tissue, that pose potential serious medical complications, and that cannot be followed for long-term weight maintenance.

Therefore, a desirable weight loss program is one that:

1. Provides a caloric intake not lower than 1200 kcal $\cdot$ d^{-1} for normal adults in order to get a proper blend of foods to meet nutritional requirements. (Note: this requirement may change for children, older individuals, athletes, etc.).
2. Includes foods acceptable to the dieter from the viewpoints of socio-cultural background, usual habits, taste, cost, and ease in acquisition and preparation.
3. Provides a negative caloric balance (not to exceed 500–1000 kcal $\cdot$ d^{-1} lower than recommended), resulting in gradual weight loss without metabolic derangements. Maximal weight loss should be 1 kg $\cdot$ wk^{-1}.
4. Includes the use of behavior modification techniques to identify and eliminate dieting habits that contribute to improper nutrition.
5. Includes an endurance exercise program of at least 3 d/wk, 20–30 min in duration, at a minimum intensity of 60% of maximum heart rate (refer to ACSM Position Statement on the Recommended Quantity and Quality of Exercise for Developing and Maintaining Fitness in Healthy Adults, *Med. Sci. Sports* 10:vii, 1978).
6. Provides that the new eating and physical activity habits can be continued for life in order to maintain the achieved lower body weight.

1. Since the early work of Keys et al. (50) and Bloom (16), which indicated that marked reduction in caloric intake or fasting (starvation or semistarvation) rapidly reduced body weight, numerous fasting, modified fasting, and fad diet and weight loss programs have emerged. While these programs promise and generally cause rapid weight loss, they are associated with significant medical risks.

The medical risks associated with these types of diet and weight loss programs are numerous. Blood glucose concentrations have been shown to be markedly reduced in obese subjects who undergo fasting (18,32,74,84). Further, in obese non-diabetic subjects, fasting may result in impairment of glucose tolerance (10,52). Ketonuria begins within a few hours after fasting or low-carbohydrate diets are begun (53) and hyperuricemia is common among subjects who fast to reduce body weight (18). Fasting also results in high serum uric acid levels with decreased urinary output (59). Fasting and low-calorie diets also result in urinary nitrogen loss and a significant decrease in fat-free tissue (7,11, 17,42,101; see section 2). In comparison to ingestion of a normal diet, fasting substantially elevates urinary excretion of potassium (10,32,37,52,53,78). This, coupled with the aforementioned nitrogen loss, suggests that the potassium loss is due to a loss of lean tissue (78). Other electrolytes, including sodium (32,53), calcium (30,84), magnesium (30,84), and phosphate (84) have been shown to be elevated in urine during prolonged fasting. Reductions in blood volume and body fluids are also common with fasting and fad diets (18). This can be associated with weakness and fainting (32). Congestive heart failure and sudden death have been reported in subjects who fasted (48,79,80) or markedly restricted their caloric intake (79). Myocardial atrophy appears to contribute to sudden death (79). Sudden death may also occur during refeeding (25,79). Untreated fasting has also been reported to reduce serum iron binding capacity, resulting in anemia (47,73,89). Liver glycogen levels are depleted with fasting (38,60,63) and liver function (29,31,37,75,76,92) and gastrointestinal tract abnormalities (13,32,53,65,85,91) are associated with fasting. While fasting and calorically restricted diets have been shown to lower serum cholesterol levels (88,96), a large portion of the cholesterol reduction is a result of lowered HDL-cholesterol levels (88,96). Other risks associated with fasting and low-calorie diets include lactic acidosis (12,26), alopecia (73), hypoalaninemia (34), edema (23,78), anuria (101), hypotension (18,32,78), elevated serum bilirubin (8,9), nausea and vomiting (53), alterations in thyroxine metabolism (71,91), impaired serum triglyceride removal and production (86), and death (25,37,48,61,80).

2. The major objective of any weight reduction program is to lose body fat while maintaining fat-free tissue. The vast majority of research reveals that starvation and low-calorie diets result in large losses of water, electrolytes, and other fat-free tissue. One of the best controlled experiments was conducted from 1944 to 1946 at the Laboratory of Physiological Hygiene at the University of Minnesota (50). In this study subjects had their base-line caloric intake cut by 45% and body weight and body composition changes were followed for 24 wk. During the first 12 wk of semistarvation, body weight declined by 25.4 lb (11.5 kg) with only an 11.6-lb (5.3 kg) decline in body fat. During the second 12-wk period, body weight declined an additional 9.1 lb (4.1 kg) with only a 6.1-lb (2.8 kg) decrease in body fat. These data clearly demonstrate that fat-free tissue significantly contributes to weight loss from semistarvation. Similar results have been reported by several other investigators. Buskirk et al. (20) reported that the 13.5-kg weight loss in six subjects on a low-calorie mixed diet averaged 76% fat and 24% fat-free tissue. Similarly, Passmore

323

et al. (64) reported results of 78% of weight loss (15.3 kg) as fat and 22% as fat-free tissue in seven women who consumed a 400-kcal $\cdot$ d^{-1} diet for 45 d. Yang and Van Itallie (101) followed weight loss and body composition changes for the first 5 d of a weight loss program involving subjects consuming either an 800-kcal mixed diet, an 800-kcal ketogenic diet, or undergoing starvation. Subjects on the mixed diet lost 1.3 kg of weight (59% fat loss, 3.4% protein loss, 37.6% water loss), subjects on the ketogenic diet lost 2.3 kg of weight (33.2% fat, 3.8% protein, 63.0% water), and subjects on starvation regimens lost 3.8 kg of weight (32.3% fat, 6.5% protein, 61.2% water). Grande (41) and Grande et al. (43) reported similar findings with a 1000-kcal carbohydrate diet. It was further reported that water restriction combined with 1000-kcal $\cdot$ d^{-1} of carbohydrate resulted in greater water loss and less fat loss.

Recently, there has been renewed speculation about the efficacy of the very-low-calorie diet (VLCD). Krotkiewski and associates (51) studied the effects on body weight and body composition after 3 wk on the so-called Cambridge diet. Two groups of obese middle-aged women were studied. One group had a VLCD only, while the second group had a VLCD combined with a 55-min/d, 3-d/wk exercise program. The VLCD-only group lost 6.2 kg in 3 wk, of which only 2.6 kg was fat loss, while the VLCD-plus-exercise group lost 6.8 kg in 3 wk with only a 1.9-kg body fat loss. Thus it can be seen that VLCD results in undesirable losses of body fat, and the addition of the normally protective effect of chronic exercise to VLCD does not reduce the catabolism of fat-free tissue. Further, with VLCD, a large reduction (29%) in HDL-cholesterol is seen (94).

3. Even mild calorie restriction (reduction of 500–1000 kcal $\cdot$ d^{-1} from base-line caloric intake), when used alone as a tool for weight loss, results in the loss of moderate amounts of water and other fat-free tissue. In a study by Goldman et al. (39), 15 female subjects consumed a low-calorie mixed diet for 7–8 wk. Weight loss during this period averaged 6.43 kg (0.85 kg $\cdot$ wk^{-1}), 88.6% of which was fat. The remaining 11.4% represented water and other fat-free tissue. Zuti and Golding (102) examined the effect of 500 kcal $\cdot$ d^{-1} calorie restriction on body composition changes in adult females. Over a 16-wk period the women lost approximately 5.2 kg; however, 1.1 kg of the weight loss (21%) was due to a loss of water and other fat-free tissue. More recently, Weltman et al. (96) examined the effects of 500 kcal $\cdot$ d^{-1} calorie restriction (from base-line levels) on body composition changes in sedentary middle-aged males. Over a 10-wk period subjects lost 5.95 kg, 4.03 kg (68%) of which was fat loss and 1.92 kg (32%) was loss of water and other fat-free tissue. Further, with calorie restriction only, these subjects exhibited a decrease in HDL-cholesterol. In the same study, the two other groups who exercised and/or dieted and exercised were able to maintain their HDL-cholesterol levels. Similar results for females have been presented by Thompson et al. (88). It should be noted that the decrease seen in HDL-cholesterol with weight loss may be an acute effect. There are data that indicate that stable weight loss has a beneficial effect on HDL-cholesterol (21,24,46,88).

Further, an additional problem associated with calorie restriction alone for effective weight loss is the fact that it is associated with a reduction in basal metabolic rate (5). Apparently exercise combined with calorie restriction can counter this response (14).

4. There are several studies that indicate that exercise helps maintain fat-free tissue while promoting fat loss. Total body weight and fat weight are generally reduced with endurance training programs (70) while fat-free weight remains constant (36,54,69,70,98) or increases slightly (62,96,102). Programs conducted at least 3 d/wk (66–69, 98), of at

least 20-min duration (58,69,98) and of sufficient intensity and duration to expend at least 300 kcal per exercise session have been suggested as a threshold level for total body weight and fat weight reduction (27,44,69,70). Increasing caloric expenditure above 300 kcal per exercise session and increasing the frequency of exercise sessions will enhance fat weight loss while sparing fat-free tissue (54,102). Leon et al. (54) had six obese male subjects walk vigorously for 90 min, 5 d/wk for 16 wk. Work output progressed weekly to an energy expenditure of 1000–1200 kcal/session. At the end of 16 wk, subjects averaged 5.7 kg of weight loss with a 5.9-kg loss of fat weight and a 0.2-kg gain in fat-free tissue. Similarly, Zuti and Golding (102) followed the progress of adult women who expended 500 kcal/exercise session 5 d/wk for 16 wk of exercise. At the end of 16 wk the women lost 5.8 kg of fat and gained 0.9 kg of fat-free tissue.

5. Review of the literature cited above strongly indicates that optimal body composition changes occur with a combination of calorie restriction (while on a well-balanced diet) plus exercise. This combination promotes loss of fat weight while sparing fat-free tissue. Data of Zuti and Golding (102) and Weltman et al. (96) support this contention. Calorie restriction of 500 $kcal \cdot d^{-1}$ combined with 3–5 d of exercise requiring 300–500 kcal per exercise session results in favorable changes in body composition (96,102). Therefore, the optimal rate of weight loss should be between 0.45–1 kg (1–2 lb) per wk. This seems especially relevant in light of the data which indicates that rapid weight loss due to low caloric intake can be assoicated with sudden death (79). In order to institute a desirable pattern of calorie restriction plus exercise, behavior modification techniques should be incorporated to identify and eliminate habits contributing to obesity and/or over-fatness (28,33,35,81,87,99,100).

6. The problem with losing weight is that, although many individuals succeed in doing so, they invariably put the weight on again (45). The goal of an effective weight loss regimen is not merely to lose weight. Weight control requires a lifelong commitment, an understanding of our eating habits and a willingness to change them. Frequent exercise is necessary, and accomplishment must be reinforced to sustain motivation. Crash dieting and other promised weight loss cures are ineffective (45).

References

1. Alexander, J. K. and J. R. Pettigrove. Obesity and congestive heart failure. *Geriatrics* 22:101–108, 1967.
2. Alexander, J. K. and K. L. Peterson. Cardiovascular effects of weight reduction. *Circulation* 45:310–318, 1972.
3. Angel, A. Pathophysiologic changes in obesity. *Can. Med. Assoc. J.* 119:1401–1406, 1978.
4. Angel, A. and D. A. K. Roncari. Medical complications of obesity. *Can. Med. Assoc. J.* 119:1408–1411, 1978.
5. Appelbaum, M., J. Bostsarron, and D. Lacatis. Effect of caloric restriction and excessive caloric intake on energy expenditure. *Am. J. Clin. Nutr.* 24:1405–1409, 1971.
6. Bachman, L., V. Freschuss, D. Hallberg, and A. Melcher. Cardiovascular function in extreme obesity. *Acta Med. Scand.* 193:437–446, 1972.
7. Ball, M. F., J. J. Canary, and L. H. Kyle. Comparative effects of caloric restrictions and total starvation on body composition in obesity. *Ann. Intern. Med.* 67:60–67, 1967.
8. Barrett, P. V. D. Hyperbilirubinemia of fasting. *JAMA* 217:1349–1353, 1971.
9. Barrett, P. V. D. The effect of diet and fasting on the serum bilirubin concentration in the rat. *Gastroenterology* 60:572–576, 1971.
10. Beck, P., J. J. T. Koumans, C. A. Winterling, M. F. Stein, W. H. Daughaday, and D. M. Kipnis. Studies of insulin and growth hormone secretion in human obesity. *J. Lab. Clin. Med.* 64:654–667, 1964.

11. Benoit, F. L., R. L. Martin, and R. H. Watten. Changes in body composition during weight reduction in obesity. *Ann. Intern. Med.* 63:604–612, 1965.
12. Berger, H. Fatal lactic acidosis during "crash" reducing diet. *N.Y. State J. Med.* 67:2258–2263, 1967.
13. Billich, C., G. Bray, T. F. Gallagher, A. V. Hoffbrand, and R. Levitan. Absorptive capacity of the jejunum of obese and lean subjects; effect of fasting. *Arch. Intern. Med.* 130:377–387, 1972.
14. Bjorntorp, P. L. Sjostrom, and L. Sullivan. The role of physical exercise in the management of obesity. In: *The Treatment of Obesity,* J. F. Munro (Ed.). Lancaster, England: MTP Press, 1979.
15. Blitzer, P. H., E. C. Blitzer, and A. A. Rimm. Association between teenage obesity and cancer in 56,111 women. *Prev. Med.* 5:20–31, 1976.
16. Bloom, W. L. Fasting as an introduction to the treatment of obesity. *Metabolism* 8:214–220, 1959.
17. Bolinger, R. E., B. P. Lukert, R. W. Brown, L. Guevera, and R. Steinberg. Metabolic balances of obese subjects during fasting. *Arch. Intern. Med.* 118:3–8, 1966.
18. Bray, G. A., M. B. Davidson, and E. J. Drenick. Obesity: a serious symptom. *Ann. Intern. Med.* 77:779–805, 1972.
19. Burwell, C. S., E. D. Robin, R. D. Whaley, and A. G. Bickelmann. Extreme obesity associated with alveolar hypoventilation—a Pickwickian syndrome. *Am. J. Med.* 21:811–818, 1956.
20. Buskirk, E. R., R. H. Thompson, L. Lutwak, and G. D. Whedon. Energy balance of obese patients during weight reduction: influence of diet restriction and exercise. *Ann. NY Acad. Sci.* 110:918–940, 1963.
21. Caggiula, A. W., G. Christakis, M. Ferrand, et al. The multiple risk factors intervention trial. IV Intervention on blood lipids. *Prev. Med.* 10:443–475, 1981.
22. Chaing, B. M., L. V. Perlman, and F. H. Epstein. Overweight and hypertension: a review. *Circulation* 39:403–421, 1969.
23. Collison, D. R. Total fasting for up to 249 days. *Lancet* 1:112, 1967.
24. Contaldo, F., P. Strazullo, A. Postiglione, et al. Plasma high density lipoprotein in severe obesity after stable weight loss. *Atherosclerosis* 37:163–167, 1980.
25. Cruickshank, E. K. Protein malnutrition. In: Proceedings of a conference in Jamaica (1953), J. C. Waterlow (Ed.). Cambridge: University Press, 1955, p. 107.
26. Cubberley, P. T., S. A. Polster, and C. L. Shulman. Lactic acidosis and death after the treatment of obesity of fasting. *N. Engl. J. Med.* 272:628–633, 1965.
27. Cureton, T. K. *The Physiological Effects of Exercise Programs Upon Adults.* Springfield, IL: C. Thomas Company, 1969.
28. Dahlkoetter, J., E. J. Callahan, and J. Linton. Obesity and the unbalanced energy equation: exercise versus eating habit change. *J. Consult. Clin. Psychol.* 47:898–905, 1979.
29. Drenick, E. J. The relation of BSP retention during prolonged fasts to changes in plasma volume. *Metabolism* 17:522–527, 1968.
30. Drenick, E. J., I. F. Hunt, and M. E. Swendseid. Magnesium depletion during prolonged fasting in obese males. *J. Clin. Endoctrinol. Metab.* 29:1341–1348, 1969.
31. Drenick, E. J., F. Simmons, and J. F. Murphy. Effect on hepatic morphology of treatment of obesity by fasting, reducing diets and small-bowel bypass. *N. Engl. J. Med.* 282:829–834, 1970.
32. Drenick, E. J., M. E. Swendseid, W. H. Blahd, and S. G. Tuttle. Prolonged starvation as treatment for severe obesity. *JAMA* 187:100–105, 1964.
33. Epstein, L. H. and R. R. Wing. Aerobic exercise and weight. *Addict. Behav.* 5:371–388, 1980.
34. Felig, P., O. E. Owen, J. Wahren, and G. F. Cahill, Jr. Amino acid metabolism during prolonged starvation. *J. Clin. Invest.* 48:584–594, 1969.
35. Ferguson, J. *Learning to Eat: Behavior Modification for Weight Control.* Palo Alto, CA: Bull Publishing, 1975.
36. Franklin, B., E. Buskirk, J. Hodgson, H. Gahagan, J. Kollias, and J. Mendez. Effects of physical conditioning on cardiorespiratory function, body composition and serum lipids in relatively normal-weight and obese middle-aged women. *Int. J. Obesity* 3:97–109, 1979.
37. Garnett, E. S., J. Ford, D. L. Barnard, R. A. Goodbody, and M. A. Woodehouse. Gross fragmentation of cardiac myofibrils after therapeutic starvation for obesity. *Lancet* 1:914, 1969.
38. Garrow, J. S. *Energy Balance and Obesity in Man.* New York: American Elsevier, 1974.
39. Goldman, R. F., B. Bullen, and C. Seltzer. Changes in specific gravity and body fat in overweight female adolescents as a result of weight reduction. *Ann. NY Acad. Sci.* 110:913–917, 1963.
40. Gordon, T. and W. B. Kannel. The effects of overweight on cardiovascular disease. *Geriatrics* 28:80–88, 1973.
41. Grande, F. Nutrition and energy balance in body composition studies In: *Techniques for Measuring Body Composition.* J. Brozek and A. Henschel (Eds.). Washington, DC: National Academy of Sciences—National Research Council, 1961. (Reprinted by the Office of Technical Services, U.S. Department of Commerce, Washington, DC as U.S. Government Research Report AD286, 1963, 560.)

42. Grande, F. Energy balance and body composition changes. *Ann. Intern. Med.* 68:467–480, 1968.
43. Grande, F., H. L. Taylor, J. T. Anderson, E. Buskirk, and A. Keys. Water exchange in men on a restricted water intake and a low calorie carbohydrate diet accompanied by physical work. *J. Appl. Physiol.* 12:202–210, 1958.
44. Gwinup, G. Effect of exercise alone on the weight of obese women. *Arch. Intern. Med.* 135:676–680, 1975.
45. Hafen, B. A. *Nutrition, Food and Weight Control.* Boston: Allyn and Bacon, 1981, pp. 271–289.
46. Hulley, S. B., R. Cohen, and G. Widdowson. Plasma high-density lipoprotein cholesterol level: influence of risk factor intervention. *JAMA* 238:2269–2271, 1977.
47. Jagenburg, R. and A. Svanborg. Self-induced protein-calorie malnutrition in a healthy adult male. *Acta Med. Scand.* 183:67–71, 1968.
48. Kahan, A. Death during therapeutic starvation. *Lancet* 1:1378–1379, 1968.
49. Katch, F. I. and W. B. McArdle. *Nutrition, Weight Control and Exercise.* Boston: Houghton Mifflin, 1977.
50. Keys, A., J. Brozek, A. Henshel, O. Mickelson, and H. L. Taylor. *The Biology of Human Starvation.* Minneapolis: University of Minnesota Press, 1950.
51. Krotkiewski, M., L. Toss, P. Bjorntorp, and G. Holm. The effect of a very-low-calorie diet with and without chronic exercise on thyroid and sex hormones, plasma proteins, oxygen uptake, insulin and c peptide concentrations in obese women. *Int. J. Obes.* 5:287–293, 1981.
52. Laszlo, J., R. F. Klein, and M. D. Bogdonoff. Prolonged starvation in obese patients, in vitro and in vivo effects. *Clin. Res.* 9:183, 1961. (Abstract)
53. Lawlor, T. and D. G. Wells, Metabolic hazards of fasting. *Am. J. Clin. Nutr.* 22:1142–1149, 1969.
54. Leon, A. S., J. Conrad, D. M. Hunninghake, and R. Serfass. Effects of a vigorous walking program on body composition, and carbohydrate and lipid metabolism of obese young men. *Am. J. Clin. Nutr.* 32:1776–1787, 1979.
55. Mabee, F. M., P. Meyer, L. DenBesten, and E. E. Mason. The mechanism of increased gallstone formation on obese human subjects. *Surgery* 79:460–468, 1978.
56. Matter, S., A. Weltman, and B. A. Stamford. Body fat content and serum lipid levels. *J. Am. Diet. Assoc.* 77:149–152, 1980.
57. McArdle, W. D., F. I. Katch, and V. L. Katch. *Exercise Physiology: Energy, Nutrition and Human Performance.* Philadelphia: Lea and Febiger, 1981.
58. Milesis, C. A., M. L. Pollock, M. D. Bah, J. J. Ayres, A. Ward, and A. C. Linnerud. Effects of different durations of training on cardiorespiratory function, body composition and serum lipids. *Res. Q.* 47:716–725, 1976.
59. Murphy, R. and K. H. Shipman. Hyperuricemia during total fasting. *Arch. Intern. Med.* 112:954–959, 1963.
60. Nilsson, L. H. and E. Hultman. Total starvation or a carbohydrate-poor diet followed by carbohydrate refeeding. *Scand J. Clin. Lab. Invest.* 32:325–330, 1973.
61. Norbury, F. B. Contraindication of long term tasting. *JAMA* 188:88, 1964.
62. O'Hara, W., C. Allen, and R. J. Shepard. Loss of body weight and fat during exercise in a cold chamber. *Eur. J. Appl. Physiol.* 37:205–218, 1977.
63. Oyama, J., J. A. Thomas, and R. L. Brant. Effect of starvation on glucose tolerance and serum insulin-like activity of Osborne-Mendel rats. *Diabetes* 12:332–334, 1963.
64. Passmore, R., J. A. Strong, and F. J. Ritchie. The chemical composition of the tissue lost by obese patients on a reducing regimen. *Br. J. Nutr.* 12:113–122, 1958.
65. Pittman, F. E. Primary malabsorption following extreme attempts to lose weight. *Gut* 7:154–158, 1966.
66. Pollock, M. L., T. K. Cureton, and L. Greninger. Effects of frequency of training on working capacity, cardiovascular function and body composition of adult men. *Med. Sci. Sports* 1:70–74, 1969.
67. Pollock, M. L., J. Tiffany, L. Gettman, R. Janeway, and H. Lofland. Effects of frequency of training on serum lipids, cardiovascular function and body composition. In: *Exercise and Fitness.* B. D. Franks (Ed.). Chicago: *Athletic Institute,* 1969, pp. 161–178.
68. Pollock, M. L., J. Broida, Z. Kendrick, H. S. Miller, Jr., R. Janeway, and A. C. Linnerud. Effects of training two days per week at different intensities on middle aged men. *Med. Sci. Sports* 4:192–197, 1972
69. Pollock, M. L. The quantification of endurance training programs. *Exercise and Sports Sciences Reviews,* J. Wilmore (Ed.), New York: Academic Press, 1973, pp. 155–188.
70. Pollock, M. L. and A. Jackson. Body composition: measurement and changes resulting from physical training. In: *Proceedings National College Physical Education Association for Men and Women,* 1977, pp. 123–137.
71. Portnay, G. I., J. T. O'Brian, J. Bush, et al. The effect of starvation on the concentration and binding of thyroxine and triiodothyronine in serum and on the response to TRH. *J. Clin. Endocrinol. Metab.* 39:191–194, 1974.
72. Rimm, A. A., L. H. Werner, R. Bernstein, and B. VanYserloo. Disease and obesity in 73,532 women. *Obesity Bariatric Med.* 1:77–84, 1972.

73. Rooth, G. and S. Carlstrom. Therapeutic fasting. *Acta Med. Scand.* 187:455–463, 1970.
74. Rossner, S. and D. Hallberg. Serum lipoproteins in massive obesity. *Acta Med. Scand.* 204:103–110, 1978.
75. Rozental, P., C. Biara, H. Spencer, and H. J. Zimmerman. Liver morphology and function tests in obesity and during starvation. *Am. J. Dig. Dis.* 12:198–208, 1967.
76. Runcie, J. Urinary sodium and potassium excretion in fasting obese subjects. *Br. Med. J.* 3:432–435, 1970.
77. Runcie, J. and T. J. Thomson. Total fasting, hyperuricemia and gout. *Postgrad. Med. J.* 45:251–254, 1969.
78. Runcie, J. and T. J. Thomson. Prolonged starvation—a dangerous procedure? *Br. Med. J.* 3:432–435, 1970.
79. Sours, H. E., V. P. Frattali, C. D. Brand, et al. Sudden death associated with very low calorie weight reduction regimens. *Am. J. Clin. Nutr.* 34:453–461, 1981.
80. Spencer, I. O. B. Death during therapeutic starvation for obesity. *Lancet* 2:679–680, 1968.
81. Stalonas, P. M., W. G. Johnson, and M. Christ. Behavior modification for obesity: the evaluation of exercise, contingency, management, and program behavior. *J. Consult. Clin. Psychol.* 46:463–467, 1978.
82. Stamler, R., J. Stamler, W. F. Riedlinger, G. Algera, and R. H. Roberts, Weight and blood pressure. Findings in hypertension screening of 1 million Americans. *JAMA* 240:1607–1610, 1978.
83. Stein, J. S., and J. Hirsch. Obesity and pancreatic function. In: *Handbook of Physiology, Section I. Endocrinology,* Vol. 1, D. Steener and N. Frankel (Eds.). Washington, DC: American Physiological Society, 1972.
84. Stewart, W. K. and L. W. Fleming. Features of a successful therapeutic fast of 382 days duration. *Postgrad. Med. J.* 49:203–209, 1973.
85. Stewart, J. S., D. L. Pollock, A. V. Hoffbrand, D. L. Mollin, and C. C. Booth. A study of proximal and distal intestinal structure and absorptive function in idiopathic steatorrhea. *Q.J. Med.* 36:425–444, 1967.
86. Streja, D. A., E. B. Marliss, and G. Steiner. The effects of prolonged fasting on plasma triglyceride kinetics in man. *Metabolism* 26:505–516, 1977.
87. Stuart, R. B. and B. Davis. *Slim Chance in a Fat World. Behavioral Control of Obesity.* Champagin, IL: Research Press, 1972.
88. Thompson, P. D., R. W. Jeffrey, R. R. Wing, and P. D. Wood. Unexpected decrease in plasma high density lipoprotein cholesterol with weight loss. *Am. J. Clin. Nutr.* 32:2016–2021, 1979.
89. Thomson, T. J., J. Runcie, and V. Miller. Treatment of obesity by total fasting up to 249 days. *Lancet* 2:992–996, 1966.
90. Thorn, G. W., M. M. Wintrobe, R. D. Adams, E. Braunwald, K. J. Isselbacher, and R. G. Petersdorf. *Harrison's Principles of Internal Medicine,* 8th Edition. New York: McGraw-Hill, 1977.
91. Vegenakis, A. G., A. Burger, G. I. Portnay, et al. Diversion of peripheral thyroxine metabolism from activating to inactivating pathways during complete fasting. *J. Clin. Endocrinol. Metab.* 41:191–194, 1975.
92. Verdy, M. B.S.P. retention during total fasting. *Metabolism* 15:769, 1966.
93. Warner, W. A. and L. P. Garrett. The obese patient and anesthesia. *JAMA* 205:102–103, 1968.
94. Wechsler, J. G., V. Hutt, H. Wenzel, H. Klor, and H. Ditschuneit. Lipids and lipoproteins during a very-low calorie diet. *Int. J. Obes.* 5:325–331, 1981.
95. Weisinger, J. R., A. Seeman, M. G. Herrera, J. P. Assal, J. S. Soeldner, and R. E. Gleason. The nephrotic syndrome: a complication of massive obesity. *Ann. Intern. Med.* 80:332–341, 1974.
96. Weltman, A., S. Matter, and B. A. Stamford. Caloric restriction and/or mild exericse: effects on serum lipids and body composition. *Am. J. Clin. Nutr.* 33:1002–1009, 1980.
97. West, K. *Epidemiology of Diabetes and its Vascular Lesions.* New York: Elsevier, 1978.
98. Wilmore, J. H., J. Royce, R. N. Girandola, F. I. Katch, and V. L. Katch. Body composition changes with a 20 week jogging program. *Med. Sci. Sports* 2:113–117, 1970.
99. Wilson, G. T. Behavior modification and the treatment of obesity. In: *Obesity,* A. J. Stunkard (Ed.). Philadelphia: W. B. Saunders, 1980.
100. Wooley, S. C., O. W. Wooley, and S. R. Dyrenforth. Theoretical, practical and social issues on behavioral treatments of obesity. *J. Appl. Behav. Anal.* 12:3–25, 1979.
101. Yang, M. and T. B. Van Itallie. Metabolic responses of obese subjects to starvation and low calorie ketogenic and nonketogenic diets. *J. Clin. Invest.* 58:722–730, 1976.
102. Zuti, W. B. and L. A. Golding. Comparing diet and exercise as weight reduction tools. *Phys. Sportsmed.* 4 (1):49–53, 1976.

Appendix 2:
The Use of Alcohol in Sports

Based upon a comprehensive analysis of the available research relative to the effects of alcohol upon human physical performance, it is the position of the American College of Sports Medicine that:

1. The acute ingestion of alcohol can exert a deleterious effect upon a wide variety of psychomotor skills such as reaction time, hand-eye coordination, accuracy, balance, and complex coordination.
2. Acute ingestion of alcohol will not substantially influence metabolic or physiological functions essential to physical performance such as energy metabolism, maximal oxygen consumption (Vo_2max), heart rate, stroke volume, cardiac output, muscle blood flow, arteriovenous oxygen difference, or respiratory dynamics. Alcohol consumption may impair body temperature regulation during prolonged exercise in a cold environment.
3. Acute alcohol ingestion will not improve and may decrease strength, power, local muscular endurance, speed, and cardiovascular endurance.
4. Alcohol is the most abused drug in the United States and is a major contributing factor to accidents and their consequences. Also, it has been documented widely that prolonged excessive alcohol consumption can elicit pathological changes in the liver, heart, brain, and muscle, which can lead to disability and death.
5. Serious and continuing efforts should be made to educate athletes, coaches, health and physical educators, physicians, trainers, the sports media, and the general public regarding the effects of acute alcohol ingestion upon human physical performance and on the potential acute and chronic problems of excessive alcohol consumption.

American College of Sports Medicine. 1982. Position Statement on The Use of Alcohol in Sports.

Research Background for the Position Statement

This position statement is concerned primarily with the effects of acute alcohol ingestion upon physical performance and is based upon a comprehensive review of the pertinent international literature. When interpreting these results, several precautions should be kept in mind. First, there are varying reactions to alcohol ingestion, not only among individuals, but also within an individual depending upon the circumstances. Second, it is virtually impossible to conduct double-blind placebo research with alcohol because subjects can always tell when alcohol has been consumed. Nevertheless, the results cited below provide us with some valid general conclusions relative to the effects of alcohol on physical performance. In most of the research studies, a small dose consisted of 1.5–2.0 ounces (45–60 ml) of alcohol, equivalent to a blood alcohol level (BAL) of 0.04–0.05 in the average-size male. A moderate dose was equivalent to 3–4 ounces (90–120 ml), or a BAL of about 0.10. Few studies employed a large dose, with a BAL of 0.15.

1. Athletes may consume alcohol to improve psychological function, but it is psychomotor performance that deteriorates most. A consistent finding is the impairment of information processing. In sports involving rapid reactions to changing stimuli, performance will be affected most adversely. Research has shown that small to moderate amounts of alcohol will impair reaction time (8,25,26,34–36,42) hand-eye coordination (8,9,14,40), accuracy (36,39), balance (3), and complex coordination or gross motor skills (4,8,22,36,41). Thus, while Coopersmith (10) suggests that alcohol may improve self-confidence, the available research reveals a deterioration in psychomotor performance.

2. Many studies have been conducted relative to the effects of acute alcohol ingestion upon metabolic and physiological functions important to physical performance. Alcohol ingestion exerts no beneficial influence relative to energy sources for exercise. Muscle glycogen at rest was significantly lower after alcohol compared to control (30). However, in exercise at 50% maximal oxygen uptake (Vo_2max), total glycogen depleted in the leg muscles was not affected by alcohol (30). Moreover, Juhlin-Dannfelt et al. (29) have shown that although alcohol does not impair lipolysis or free fatty acid (FFA) utilization during exercise, it may decrease splanchnic glucose output, decrease the potential contribution from liver gluconeogenesis, elicit a greater decline in bood glucose levels leading to hypoglycemia, and decrease the leg muscle uptake of glucose during the latter stages of a 3-h run. Other studies (17,19) have supported the theory concerning the hypoglycemic effect of alcohol during both moderate and prolonged exhaustive exercise in a cold environment. These studies also noted a significant loss of body heat and a resultant drop in body temperature and suggested alcohol may impair temperature regulation. These changes may impair endurance capacity.

    In one study (5), alcohol has been shown to increase oxygen uptake significantly during submaximal work and simultaneously to decrease mechanical efficiency, but this finding has not been confirmed by others (6,15,33,44). Alcohol appears to have no effect on maximal or near-maximal Vo_2 (5–7,44).

The effects of alcohol on cardiovascular-respiratory parameters associated with oxygen uptake are variable at submaximal exercise intensities and are negligible at maximal levels. Alcohol has been shown by some investigators to increase submaximal exercise hart rate (5,20,23) and cardiac output (5), but these heart rate findings have not been confirmed by others (6,15,33,36,44). Alcohol had no effect on stroke volume (5), pulmonary ventilation (5,15), or muscle blood flow (16,30) at submaximal levels of exercise, but did decrease peripheral vascular resistance (5). During maximal exercise, alcohol ingestion elicited no significant effect upon heart rate (5–7), stroke volume and cardiac output, arteriovenous oxygen difference, mean arterial pressure and peripheral vascular resistance, or peak lactate (5), but did significantly reduce tidal volume resulting in a lowered pulmonary ventilation (5).

In summary, alcohol appears to have little or no beneficial effect on the metabolic and phsyiological responses to exercise. Further, in those studies reporting significant effects, the change appears to be detrimental to performance.

3. The effects of alcohol on tests of fitness components are variable. It has been shown that alcohol ingestion may decrease dynamic muscular strength (24), isometric grip strength (36), dynamometer strength (37), power (20) and ergographic muscular output (28). Other studies (13,20,24,27,43) reported no effect of alcohol upon muscular strength. Local muscular endurance was also unaffected by alcohol ingestion (43). Small doses of alcohol exerted no effect upon bicycle ergometer exercise tasks simulating a 100-m dash or a 1500-m run, but larger doses had a deleterious effect (2). Other research has shown that alcohol has no significant effect upon physical performance capacity (15,16), exercise time at maximal levels (5), or exercise time to exhaustion (7).

Thus, alcohol ingestion will not improve muscular work capacity and may lead to decreased performance levels.

4. Alcohol is the most abused drug in the United States (11). There are an estimated 10 million adult problem drinkers and an additional 3.3 million in the 14–17 age range. Alcohol is significantly involved in all types of accidents— motor vehicle, home, industrial, and recreational. Most significantly, half of all traffic fatalities and one-third of all traffic injuries are alcohol related. Although alcohol abuse is associated with pathological conditions such as generalized skeletal myopathy, cardiomyopathy, pharyngeal and esophageal cancer, and brain damage, its most prominent effect is liver damage (11,31,32).

5. Because alcohol has not been shown to help improve physical performance capacity, but may lead to decreased ability in certain events, it is important for all those associated with the conduct of sports to educate athletes against its use in conjunction with athletic contests. Moreover, the other dangers inherent in alcohol abuse mandate that concomitantly we educate our youth to make intelligent choices regarding alcohol consumption. Anstie's rule, or limit (1), may be used as a reasonable guideline to moderate, safe drinking for adults (12). In essence, no more than 0.5 ounces of pure alcohol per 23 kg body weight should be consumed in any one day. This would be the equivalent of three bottles of 4.5% beer, three 4-ounce glasses of 14% wine, or three ounces of 50% whiskey for a 68-kg person.

References

1. Anstie, F. E. *On the Uses of Wine in Health and Disease.* London: MacMillan, 1877, pp. 5–6.
2. Asmussen, E. and O. Boje. The effects of alcohol and some drugs on the capacity for work. *Acta Physiol. Scand.* 15:109–118, 1948.
3. Begbie, G. The effects of alcohol and of varying amounts of visual information on a balancing test. *Ergonomics* 9:325–333, 1966.
4. Belgrave, B., K. Bird, G. Chesher, D. Jackson, K. Lubbe, G. Starmer, and R. Teo. The effect of cannabidiol, alone and in combination with ethanol, on human performance. *Psychopharmacology* 64:243–246, 1979.
5. Blomqvist, G., B. Saltin, and J. Mitchell. Acute effects of ethanol ingestion on the response to submaximal and maximal exercise in man. *Circulation* 42:463–470, 1970.
6. Bobo, W. Effects of alcohol upon maximum oxygen uptake, lung ventilation, and heart rate. *Res. Q.* 43:1–6, 1972.
7. Bond, V. Effect of alcohol on cardiorespiratory function. In: *Abstracts: Research Papers of 1979 AAHPER Convention.* Washington, DC: AAHPER, 1979, p. 24.
8. Carpenter, J. Effects of alcohol on some psychological processes. *Q.J. Stud. Alcohol* 23:274–314, 1962.
9. Collins, W., D. Schroeder, R. Gilson, and F. Guedry. Effects of alcohol ingestion on tracking performance during angular acceleration. *J. Appl. Psychol.* 55:559–563, 1971.
10. Coopersmith, S. The effects of alcohol on reaction to affective stimuli. *Q.J. Stud. Alcohol* 25:459–475, 1964.
11. Department of Health, Education, and Welfare. Third special report to the U.S. Congress on alcohol and health. *NIAAA Information and Feature Service.* DHEW Publication No. (ADM) 78–151, November 30, 1978, pp. 1–4.
12. *Dorland's Illustrated Medical Dictionary,* 24th Edition. Philadelphia: W. B. Saunders, 1974, p. 1370.
13. Enzer, N., E. Simonson, and G. Ballard. The effect of small doses of alcohol on the central nervous system. *Am. J. Clin. Pathol.* 14:333–341, 1944.
14. Forney, R., F. Hughes, and W. Greatbatch. Measurement of attentive motor performance after alcohol. *Percept. Mot. Skills* 19:151–154, 1964.
15. Garlind, T., L. Goldberg, K. Graf, E. Perman, T. Strandell, and G. Strom. Effect of ethanol on circulatory, metabolic, and neurohumoral function during muscular work in man. *Acta Pharmacol. et Toxicol.* 17:106–114, 1960.
16. Graf, K. and G. Strom. Effect of ethanol ingestion on arm blood flow in healthy young men at rest and during work. *Acta Pharmacol. et Toxicol.* 17:115–120, 1960.
17. Graham. T. Thermal and glycemic responses during mild exercise in $+ 5$ to $- 15°C$ environments following alcohol ingestion. *Aviat. Space Environ. Med.* 52:517–522, 1981.
18. Graham, T. and J. Dalton. Effect of alcohol on man's response to mild physical activity in a cold environment. *Aviat. Space Environ. Med.* 51:793–796, 1980.
19. Haight, J. and W. Keatinge. Failure of thermoregulation in the cold during hypoglycemia induced by exercise and ethanol. *J. Physiol. (Lond.)* 229:87–97, 1973.
20. Hebbelinck, M. The effects of a moderate dose of alcohol on a series of functions of physical performance in man. *Arch. Int. Pharmacod.* 120:402–405, 1959.
21. Hebbellinck, M. The effect of a moderate dose of ethyl alcohol on human respiratory gas exchange during rest and muscular exercise. *Arch. Int. Pharmacod.* 126:214–218, 1960.
22. Hebbelinck, M. *Spierarbeid en Ethylalkohol.* Brussels: Arsica Uitgaven, N.V., 1961, pp. 81–84.
23. Hebbelinck, M. The effects of a small dose of ethyl alcohol on certain basic components of human physical performance. The effect on cardiac rate during muscular work. *Arch. Int. Pharmacod.* 140:61–67, 1962.
24. Hebbelinck, M. The effects of a small dose of ethyl alcohol on certain basic components of human physical performance. *Arch. Int. Pharmacod.* 143:247–257, 1963.
25. Huntley, M. Effects of alcohol, uncertainty and novelty upon response selection. *Psychopharmacologia* 39:259–266, 1974.
26. Huntley, M. Influences of alcohol and S-R uncertainty upon spatial localization time. *Psychopharmacologia* 27:131–140, 1972.
27. Ikai, M. and A. Steinhaus. Some factors modifying the expression of human strength. *J. Appl. Physiol.* 16:157–161, 1961.
28. Jellinek, E. Effect of small amounts of alcohol on psychological functions. In Yale University Center for Alcohol Studies. *Alcohol, Science and Society.* New Haven, CT: Yale University, 1954, pp. 83–94.
29. Juhlin-Dannfelt, A. G. Ahlborg, L. Hagenfeldt, L. Jorfeldt, and P. Felig. Influence of ethanol on splanchnic and skeletal muscle substrate turnover during prolonged exeircse in man. *Am. J. Physiol.* 233:EI95-E202, 1977.

30. Juhlin-Dannfelt, A. L. Jorfeldt, L. Hagenfeldt, and B. Hulten. Influence of ethanol on non-esterified fatty acid and carbohydrate metabolism during exercise in man. *Clin. Soc. Mol. Med.* 53:205–214, 1977.
31. Lieber, C. S. Liver injury and adaptation in alcoholism. *N. Engl. J. Med.* 288:356–362, 1973.
32. Lieber, C. S. The metabolism of alcohol. *Sci. Am.* 234 (March):25–33, 1976.
33. Mazess, R., E. Picon-Reategui, and R. Thomas. Effects of alcohol and altitude on man during rest and work. *Aerospace Med.* 39:403–406, 1968.
34. Moskowitz, H. and M. Burns. Effect of alcohol on the psychological refractory period. *Q.J. Stud. Alcohol* 32:782–790, 1971.
35. Moskowitz, H. and S. Roth. Effect of alcohol on response latency in object naming. *Q.J. Stud. Alcohol* 32:969–975, 1971.
36. Nelson, D. Effects of ethyl alcohol on the performance of selected gross motor tests. *Res. Q.* 30:312–320, 1959.
37. Pihkanen, T. Neurological and physiological studies on distilled and brewed beverages. *Ann. Med. Exp. Biol. Fenn.* 35:Suppl. 9, 1–152, 1957.
38. Riff, D., A. Jain, and J. Doyle. Acute hemodynamic effects of ethanol on normal human volunteers. *Am. Heart J.* 78:592–597, 1969.
39. Rundell, O. and H. Williams. Alcohol and speed-accuracy tradeoff. *Hum. Factors* 21:433–443, 1979.
40. Sidell, F. and J. Pless. Ethyl alcohol blood levels and performance decrements after oral administration to man. *Psychopharmacologia* 19:246–261, 1971.
41. Tang, P. and R. Rosenstein. Influence of alcohol and Dramamine, alone and in combination, on psychomotor performance. *Aerospace Med.* 39:818–821, 1967.
42. Tharp, V., O. Rundell, B. Lester and H. Williams. Alcohol and information processing. *Psychopharmacologia* 40:33–52, 1974.
43. Williams, M. H. Effect of selected doses of alcohol on fatigue parameters of the forearm flexor muscles. *Res. Q.* 40:832–840, 1969.
44. Williams, M. H. Effect of small and moderate doses of alcohol on exercise heart rate and oxygen consumption. *Res. Q.* 43:94–104, 1972.

Appendix 3: The Recommended Quantity and Quality of Exercise for Developing and Maintaining Fitness in Healthy Adults

Increasing numbers of persons are becoming involved in endurance training activities and thus, the need for guidelines for exercise prescription is apparent.

Based on the existing evidence concerning exercise prescription for healthy adults and the need for guidelines, the American College of Sports Medicine makes the following recommendations for the quantity and quality of training for developing and maintaining cardiorespiratory fitness and body composition in the healthy adult:

1. Frequency of training: 3 to 5 days per week.
2. Intensity of training: 60% to 90% of maximum heart rate reserve or, 50% to 85% of maximum oxygen uptake (Vo_2max).
3. Duration of training: 15 to 60 minutes of continuous aerobic activity. Duration is dependent on the intensity of the activity, thus lower intensity activity should be conducted over a longer period of time. Because of the importance of the "total fitness" effect and the fact that it is more readily attained in longer duration programs, and because of the potential hazards and compliance problems associated with high intensity activity, lower to moderate intensity activity of longer duration is recommended for the non athletic adult.
4. Mode of activity: Any activity that uses large muscle groups, that can be maintained continuously, and is rhythmical and aerobic in nature, e.g. running-jogging, walking-hiking, swimming, skating, bicycling, rowing, cross-country skiing, rope skipping, and various endurance game activities.

The American College of Sports Medicine. 1978. Position Statement on The Recommended Quantity and Quality of Exercise for Developing and Maintaining Fitness in Healthy Adults.

335

Rationale and Research Background

The questions, "How much exercise is enough and what type of exercise is best for developing and maintaining fitness?", are frequently asked. It is recognized that the term 'physical fitness' is composed of a wide variety of variables included in the broad categories of cardiovascular-respiratory fitness, physique and structure, motor function, and many histochemical and biochemical factors. It is also recognized that the adaptive response to training is complex and includes peripheral, central, structural, and functional factors. Although many such variables and their adaptive response to training have been documented, the lack of sufficient in-depth and comparative data relative to frequency, intensity, and duration of training make them inadequate to use as comparative models. Thus, in respect to the above questions, fitness will be limited to changes in VO_2max, total body mass, fat weight (FW), and lean body weight (LBW) factors.

Exercise prescription is based upon the frequency, intensity, and duration of training, the mode of activity (aerobic in nature, e.g. listed under No. 4 above), and the initial level of fitness. In evaluating these factors, the following observations have been derived from studies conducted with endurance training programs.

1. Improvement in Vo_2max is directly related to frequency (2,23,32,58,59,65,77,79), intensity (2,10,13,26,33,37,42,56,77), and duration (3,14,29,49,56,77,86) of training. Depending upon the quantity and quality of training, improvement in Vo_2max ranges from 5% to 25% (4,13,27,31,35,36,43,45,52,53,62,71,77,78,82,86). Although changes in Vo_2max greater than 25% have been shown, they are usually associated with large total body mass and FW loss, or a low initial level of fitness. Also, as a result of leg fatigue or a lack of motivation, persons with low initial fitness may have spuriously low initial Vo_2max values.

2. The amount of improvement in Vo_2max tends to plateau when frequency of training is increased above 3 days per week (23,62,65). For the non-athlete, there is not enough information available at this time to speculate on the value of added improvement found in programs that are conducted more than 5 days per week. Participation of less than two days per week does not show an adequate change in Vo_2max (24,56,62).

3. Total body mass and FW are generally reduced with endurance training programs (67), while LBW remains constant (62,67,87) or increases slightly (54). Programs that are conducted at least 3 days per week (58,59,61,62,87), of at least 20 minutes duration (48,62,87) and of sufficient intensity and duration to expend approximately 300 kilocalories (Kcal) per exercise session are suggested as a threshold level for total body mass and FW loss (12,29,62,67). An expenditure of 200 Kcal per session has also been shown to be useful in weight reduction if the exercise frequency is at least 4 days per week (80). Programs with less participation generally show little or no change in body composition (19,25,42,62,67,84,85,87). Significant increases in Vo_2max have been shown with 10 to 15 minutes of high intensity training (34,49,56,62,77,78), thus, if total body mass and FW reduction is not a consideration, then short duration, high intensity programs may be recommended for healthy, low risk (cardiovascular disease) persons.

336

4. The minimal threshold level for improvement in Vo_2max is approximately 60% of the maximum heart rate reserve (50% of Vo_2max) (33,37). Maximum heart rate reserve represents the percent difference between resting and maximum heart rate, added to the resting heart rate. The technique as described by Karvonen, Kentala, and Mustala (37), was validated by Davis and Convertino (14), and represents a heart rate of approximately 130 to 135 beats/minute for young persons. As a result of the aging curve for maximum heart rate, the absolute heart rate value (threshold level) is inversely related to age, and can be as low as 100 to 120 beats/minute for older persons. Initial level of fitness is another important consideration in prescribing exercise (10,40,46,75,77). The person with a low fitness level can get a significant training effect with a sustained training heart rate as low as 100 to 120 beats/minute, while persons of higher fitness levels need a higher threshold of stimulation (26).

5. Intensity and duration of training are interrelated with the total amount of work accomplished being an important factor in improvement in fitness (2,7,12,40,61,62,76,78). Although more comprehensive inquiry is necessary, present evidence suggests that when exercise is performed above the minimal threshold of intensity, the total amount of work accomplished is the important factor in fitness development (2,7,12,61,62,76,79) and maintenance (68). That is, improvement will be similar for activities performed at a lower intensity-longer duration compared to higher intensity-shorter duration if the total energy cost of the activities is equal.

   If frequency, intensity, and duration of training are similar (total Kcal expenditure), the training result appears to be independent of the mode of aerobic activity (56,60,62,64). Therefore, a variety of endurance activities, e.g. listed above, may be used to derive the same training effect.

6. In order to maintain the training effect, exercise must be continued on a regular basis (2,6,11,21,44,73,74). A significant reduction in working capacity occurs after two weeks of detraining (73) with participants returning to near pretraining levels of fitness after 10 weeks (21) to 8 months of detraining (44). Fifty percent reduction in improvement of cardiorespiratory fitness has been shown after 4 to 12 weeks of detraining (21,41,73). More investigation is necessary to evaluate the rate of increase and decrease of fitness with varying training loads and reduction in training in relation to level of fitness, age, and length of time in training. Also, more information is needed to better identify the minimal level of work necessary to maintain fitness.

7. Endurance activities that require running and jumping generally cause significantly more debilitating injuries to beginning exercisers than other non-weight bearing activities (42,55,69). One study showed that beginning joggers had increased foot, leg, and knee injuries when training was performed more than 3 days per week and longer 30 minutes duration per exercise session (69). Thus, caution should be taken when recommending the type of activity and exercise prescription for the beginning exercise. Also, the increase of orthopedic injuries as related to overuse (marathon training) with chronic jogger-runners is apparent. Thus, there is a need for more inquiry into the effect that different types of activities and the quantity and quality of training has on short-term and long-term participation.

8. Most of the information concerning training described in this position statement has been conducted on men. The lack of information on women is apparent, but the available evidence indicates that women tend to adapt to endurance training in the same manner as men (8,22,89).

9. Age in itself does not appear to be a deterrent to endurance training. Although some earlier studies showed a lower training effect with middle-aged or elderly participants (4,17,34,83,86), more recent study shows the relative change in Vo_2max to be similar to younger age groups (3,52,66,75,86). Although more investigation is necessary concerning the rate of improvement in Vo_2max with age, at present it appears that elderly participants need longer periods of time to adapt to training (17,66). Earlier studies showing moderate to no improvement in Vo_2max were conducted over a short time-span (4) or exercise was conducted at a moderate to low Kcal expenditure (17), thus making the interpretation of the results difficult.

   Although Vo_2max decreases with age, and total body mass and FW increase with age, evidence suggests that this trend can be altered with endurance training (9,12,38,39,62). Also, 5 to 10 year follow-up studies where participants continued their training at a similar level showed maintenance of fitness (39,70). A study of older competitive runners showed decreases in Vo_2max from the fourth to seventh decade of life, but also showed reductions in their training load (63). More inquiry into the relationship of long-term training (quantity and quality) for both competitors and non-competitors and physiological function with increasing age, is necessary before more definitive statements can be made.

10. An activity such as weight training should not be considered as a means of training for developing Vo_2max, but has significant value for increasing muscular strength and endurance, and LBW (16,24,47,49,88). Recent studies evaluating circuit weight training (weight training conducted almost continuously with moderate weights, using 10 to 15 repetitions per exercise session with 15 to 30 seconds rest between bouts of activity) showed little to no improvements in working capacity and Vo_2max (1,24,90).

Despite an abundance of information available concerning the training of the human organism, the lack of standardization of testing protocols and procedures, methodology in relation to training procedures and experimental design, a preciseness in the documentation and reporting of the quantity and quality of training prescribed, make interpretation difficult (62,67). Interpretation and comparison of results are also dependent on the initial level of fitness (18,74–76,81), length of time of the training experiment (20,57,58,61,62), and specificity of the testing and training (64). For example, data from training studies using subjects with varied levels of Vo_2max, total body mass and FW have found changes to occur in relation to their initial values (5,15,48,50,51), i.e., the lower the initial Vo_2max the larger the percent of improvement found, and the higher the FW the greater the reduction. Also, data evaluating trainability with age, comparison of the different magnitudes and quantities of effort, and comparison of the trainability of men and women may have been influenced by the initial fitness levels.

In view of the fact that improvement in the fitness variables discussed in this position statement continue over many months of training (12,38,39,62), it is reasonable to believe that short-term studies conducted over a few weeks have certain limitations. Middle-aged sedentary and older participants may take several weeks to adapt to the initial rigors of training, and thus need a longer adaptation period to get the full benefit from a program. How long a training experiment should be conducted is difficult to determine, but 15 to 20 weeks may be a good minimum standard. For example, two investigations conducted with middle-aged men who jogged either 2 or 4 days per week found both groups to improve in Vo_2max. Mid-test results of the 16 and 20 week programs showed no difference between groups, while subsequent final testing found the 4 day per week group to improve significantly more (58,59). In a similar study with young college men, no differences in Vo_2max were found among groups after 7 and 13 weeks of interval training (20). These latter findings and those of other investigators point to the limitations in interpreting results from investigations conducted over a short time-span (62,67).

In summary, frequency, intensity and duration of training have been found to be effective stimuli for producing a training effect. In general, the lower the stimuli, the lower the training effect (2,12,13,27,35,46,77,78,90), and the greater the stimuli, the greater the effect (2,12,13,27,58,77,78). It has also been shown that endurance training less than two days per week, less than 50% of maximum oxygen uptake, and less than 10 minutes per day is inadequate for developing and maintaining fitness for healthy adults.

References

1. Allen, T. E., R. J. Byrd and D. P. Smith. Hemodynamic consequences of circuit weight training. *Res. Q.* 43:299–306, 1976.
2. American College of Sports Medicine. *Guidelines for Graded Exercise Testing and Exercise Prescription.* Philadelphia: Lea and Febiger, 1976.
3. Barry, A. J., J. W. Daly, E. D. R. Pruett, J. R. Steinmetz, H. F. Page, N. C. Birkhead and K. Rodahl. The effects of physical conditioning on older individuals. I. Work capacity, circulatory-respiratory function, and work electrocardiogram. *J. Gerontol.* 21:182–191, 1966.
4. Bensetad, A. M. Trainability of old men. *Acta Med. Scandinav.* 178:321–327, 1965.
5. Boileau, R. A., E. R. Buskirk, D. H. Horstman, J. Mendez and W. C. Nicholas. Body composition changes in obese and lean men during physical conditioning. *Med. Sci. Sports* 3:183–189, 1971.
6. Brynteson, P. and W. E. Sinning. The effects of training frequencies on the retension of cardiovascular fitness. *Med. Sci. Sports* 5:29–33, 1973.
7. Burke, E. J. and B. D. Franks. Changes in Vo_2max resulting from bicycle training at different intensities holding total mechanical work constant. *Res. Q.* 46:31–37, 1975.
8. Burke, E. J. Physiological effects of similar training programs in males and females. *Res. Q.* 48:510–517, 1977.
9. Carter, J. E. L. and W. H. Phillips. Structural changes in exercising middle-aged males during a 2-year period. *J. Appl. Physiol.* 27:787–794, 1969.
10. Crews, T. R. and J. A. Roberts. Effects of interaction of frequency and intensity of training. *Res. Q.* 47:48–55, 1976.
11. Cureton, T. K. and E. E. Phillips. Physical fitness changes in middle-aged men attributable to equal eight-week periods of training, non-training and retraining. *J. Sports Med. Phys. Fitness* 4:1–7, 1964.
12. Cureton, T. K. *The Physiological Effects of Exercise Programs upon Adults.* Springfield: C. Thomas Company, 1969.
13. Davies, C. T. M. and A. V. Knibbs. The training stimulus, the effects of intensity, duration and frequency of effort on maximum aerobic power output. *Int. Z. Angew. Physiol.* 29:299–305, 1971.

14. Davis, J. A. and V. A. Convertino. A comparison of heart rate methods for predicting endurance training intensity. *Med. Sci. Sports* 7:295–298, 1975.
15. Dempsey, J. A. Anthropometrical observations on obese and non-obese young men undergoing a program of vigorous physical exercise. *Res. Q.* 35:275–287, 1964.
16. Delorme, T. L. Restoration of muscle power by heavy resistance exercise. *J. Bone and Joint Surgery* 27:645–667, 1945.
17. DeVries, H. A. Physiological effects of an exercise training regimen upon men aged 52 to 88. *J. Gerontol.* 24:325–336, 1970.
18. Ekblom, B., P. O. Astrand, B. Saltin, J. Sternberg and B. Wallstrom. Effect of training on circulatory response to exercise. *J. Appl. Physiol.* 24:518–528, 1968.
19. Flint, M. M., B. L. Drinkwater and S. M. Horvath. Effects of training on women's response to submaximal exercise. *Med. Sci. Sports* 6:89–94, 1974.
20. Fox, E. L., R. L. Bartels, C. E. Billings, R. O'Brien, R. Bason and D. K. Mathews. Frequency and duration of interval training programs and changes in aerobic power. *J. Appl. Physiol.* 38:481–484, 1975.
21. Fringer, M. N. and A. G. Stull. Changes in cardiorespiratory parameters during periods of training and detraining in young female adults. *Med. Sci. Sports* 6:20–25, 1974.
22. Getchell, L. H. and J. C. Moore. Physical training: comparative responses of middle-aged adults. *Arch. Phys. Med. Rehab.* 56:250–254, 1975.
23. Gettman, L. R., M. L. Pollock, J. L. Durstine, A. Ward, J. Ayres and A. C. Linnerud. Physiological responses of men to 1, 3, and 5 day per week training programs. *Res. Q.* 47:638–646, 1976.
24. Gettman, L. R., J. Ayres, M. L. Pollock, J. L. Durstine and W. Grantham. Physiological effects of circuit strength training and jogging on adult men. *Arch. Phys. Med. Rehab.*, In press.
25. Girandola, R. N. Body composition changes in women: Effects of high and low exercise intensity. *Arch. Phys. Med. Rehab.* 57:297–300, 1976.
26. Gledhill, N. and R. B. Eynon. The intensity of training. In: A. W. Taylor and M. L. Howell (editors). *Training Scientific Basis and Application.* Springfield: Charles C. Thomas, pp. 97–102, 1972.
27. Golding, L. Effects of physical training upon total serum cholesterol levels. *Res. Q.* 32:499–505, 1961.
28. Goode, R. C., A. Virgin, T. T. Romet, P. Crawford, J. Duffin, T. Pallandi and Z. Woch. Effects of a short period of physical activity in adolescent boys and girls. *Canad. J. Appl. Sports Sci.* 1:241–250, 1976.
29. Gwinup, G. Effect of exercise alone on the weight of obese women. *Arch. Int. Med.* 135:676–680, 1975.
30. Hanson, J. S., B. S. Tabakin, A. M. Levy and W. Nedde. Long-term physical training and cardiovascular dynamics in middle-aged men. *Circulation* 38:783–799, 1968.
31. Hartley, L. H., G. Grimby, A. Kilbom, J. J. Nilsson, I. Astrand, J. Bjure, B. Ekblom and B. Saltin. Physical training in sedentary middle-aged and older men. *Scand. J. Clin. Lab. Invest.* 24:335–344, 1969.
32. Hill, J. S. The effects of frequency in exercise on cardiorespiratory fitness of adult men. M. S. Thesis, Univ. of Western Ontario, London, 1969.
33. Hollmann, W. and H. Venrath. Experimentelle Untersuchungen zur bedentung aines trainings unterhalb und oberhalb der dauerbeltz stungsgranze. In: Korbs (editor). *Carl Diem Festschrift.* W. u. a. Frankfurt/ Wein, 1962.
34. Hollmann, W. Changes in the capacity for maximal and continuous effort in relation to age. *Int. Res. Sport Phys. Ed.*, (E. Jokl and E. Simon, editors). Springfield: C. C. Thomas Co., 1964.
35. Huibregtse, W. H., H. H. Hartley, L. R. Jones, W. D. Doolittle and T. L. Criblez. Improvement of aerobic work capacity following non-strenuous exercise. *Arch. Env. Health,* 27:12–15, 1973.
36. Ismail, A. H., D. Corrigan and D. F. McLeod. Effect of an eight-month exercise program on selected physiological, biochemical, and audiological variables in adult men. *Brit. J. Sports Med.* 7:230–240, 1973.
37. Karvonen, M., K. Kentala and O. Mustala. The effects of training heart rate: a longitudinal study. *Ann. Med. Exptl. Biol. Fenn.* 35:307–315, 1957.
38. Kasch, F. W., W. H. Phillips, J. E. L. Carter and J. L. Boyer. Cardiovascular changes in middle-aged men during two years of training. *J. Appl. Physiol.* 314:53–57, 1972.
39. Kasch, F. W. and J. P. Wallace. Physiological variables during 10 years of endurance exercise. *Med. Sci. Sports* 8:5–8, 1976.
40. Kearney, J. T., A. G. Stull, J. L. Ewing and J. W. Strein. Cardiorespiratory responses of sedentary college women as a function of training intensity. *J. Appl. Physiol.* 41:822–825, 1976.
41. Kendrick, Z. B., M. L. Pollock, T. N. Hickman and H. S. Miller. Effects of training and detraining on cardiovascular efficiency. *Amer. Corr. Ther. J.* 25:79–83, 1971.
42. Kilbom, A., L. Hartley, B. Saltin, J. Bjure, G. Grimby and I. Astrand. Physical training in sedentary middle-aged and older men. *Scand. J. Clin. Lab. Invest.* 24:315–322, 1969.
43. Knehr, C. A., D. B. Dill and W. Neufeld. Training and its effect on man at rest and at work. *Amer. J. Physiol.* 136:148–156, 1942.
44. Knuttgen, H. G., L. O. Nordesjo, B. Ollander and B. Saltin. Physical conditioning through interval training with young male adults. *Med. Sci. Sports* 5:220–226, 1973.

45. Mann, G. V., L. H. Garrett, A. Farhi, H. Murray, T. F. Billings, F. Shute and S. E. Schwarten. Exercise to prevent coronary heart disease. *Amer. J. Med.* 46:12–27, 1969.

46. Marigold, E. A. The effect of training at predetermined heart rate levels for sedentary college women. *Med. Sci. Sports* 6:14–19, 1974.

47. Mayhew, J. L. and P. M. Gross. Body composition changes in young women with high resistance weight training. *Res. Q.* 45:433–439, 1974.

48. Milesis, C. A., M.L. Pollock, M. D. Bah, J. J. Ayres, A. Ward and A. C. Linnerud. Effects of different durations of training on cardiorespiratory function, body composition and serum lipids. *Res. Q.* 47:716–725, 1976.

49. Misner, J. E., R. A. Boileau, B. H. Massey and J. H. Mayhew. Alterations in body composition of adult men during selected physical training programs. *J. Amer. Geriatr. Soc.* 22:33–38, 1974.

50. Moody, D. L., J. Kollias and E. R. Buskirk. The effect of a moderate exercise program on body weight and skinfold thickness in overweight college women. *Med. Sci. Sports* 1:75–80, 1969.

51. Moody, D. L., J. H. Wilmore, R. N. Girandola and J. P. Royce. The effects of a jogging program on the body composition of normal and obese high school girls. *Med. Sci. Sports* 4:210–213, 1972.

52. Myrhe, L., S. Robinson, A. Brown and F. Pyke. Paper presented to the American College of Sports Medicine, Albuquerque, New Mexico, 1970.

53. Naughton, J. and F. Nagle. Peak oxygen intake during physical fitness and program for middle-aged men. *JAMA* 191:899–901, 1965.

54. O'Hara, W., C. Allen and R. J. Shephard. Loss of body weight and fat during exercise in a cold chamber. *Europ. J. Appl. Physiol.* 37:205–218, 1977.

55. Oja, P., P. Teraslinna, T. Partaner and R. Karava. Feasibility of an 18 months' physical training program for middle-aged men and its effect on physical fitness. *Am. J. Public Health* 64:459–465, 1975.

56. Olree, H. D., B. Corbin, J. Penrod and C. Smith. Methods of achieving and maintaining physical fitness for prolonged space flight. Final Progress Rep. to NASA, Grant No. NGR-04-002-004, 1969.

57. Oscai, L. B., T. Williams and B. Hertig. Effects of exercise on blood volume. *J. Appl. Physiol.* 24:622–624, 1968.

58. Pollock, M. L., T. K. Cureton and L. Greninger. Effects of frequency of training on working capacity, cardiovascular function, and body composition of adult men. *Med. Sci. Sports* 1:70–74, 1969.

59. Pollock, M. L., J. Tiffany, L. Gettman, R. Janeway and H. Lofland. Effects of frequency of training on serum lipids, cardiovascular function, and body composition. In: *Exercise and Fitness* (B. D. Franks, ed.), Chicago: Athletic Institute, 1969, pp. 161–178.

60. Pollock, M. L., H. Miller, R. Janeway, A. C. Linnerud, B. Robertson and R. Valentino. Effects of walking on body composition and cardiovascular function of middle-aged men. *J. Appl. Physiol.* 30:126–130, 1971.

61. Pollock, M. L., J. Broida, Z. Kendrick, H. S. Miller, R. Janeway and A. C. Linnerud. Effects of training two days per week at different intensities on middle-aged men. *Med. Sci. Sports* 4:192–197, 1972.

62. Pollock, M. L. The quantification of endurance training programs. *Exercise and Sport Sciences Reviews*, (J. Wilmore, editor). New York: Academic Press, pp. 155–188, 1973.

63. Pollock, M. L., H. S. Miller, Jr. and J. Wilmore. Physiological characteristics of champion American track athletes 40 to 70 years of age. *J. Gerontol.* 29:645–649, 1974.

64. Pollock, M. L., J. Dimmick, H. S. Miller, Z. Kendrick and A. C. Linnerud. Effects of mode of training on cardiovascular function and body composition of middle-aged men. *Med. Sci. Sports* 7:139–145, 1975.

65. Pollock, M. L., H. S. Miller, A. C. Linnerud and K. H. Cooper. Frequency of training as a determinant for improvement in cardiovascular function and body composition of middle-aged men. *Arch. Phys. Med. Rehab.* 56:141–145, 1975.

66. Pollock, M. L., G. A. Dawson, H. S. Miller, Jr., A. Ward, D. Cooper, W. Headly, A. C. Linnerud and M. M. Nomeir. Physiologic response of men 49 to 65 years of age to endurance training. *J. Amer. Geriatr. Soc.* 24:97–104, 1976.

67. Pollock, M. L. and A. Jackson. Body composition: measurement and changes resulting from physical training. Proceedings National College Physical Education Association for Men and Women, pp. 125–137, January, 1977.

68. Pollock, M. L., J. Ayres and A. Ward. Cardiorespiratory fitness. Response to differing intensities and durations of training. *Arch. Phys. Med. Rehab.* 58:467–473, 1977.

69. Pollock, M. L., L. R. Gettman, C. A. Milesis, M. D. Bah, J. L. Durstine and R. B. Johnson. Effects of frequency and duration of training on attrition and incidence of injury. *Med. Sci. Sports* 9:31–36, 1977.

70. Pollock, M. L., H. S. Miller and P. M. Ribisl. Body composition and cardiorespiratory fitness in former athletes. *Phys. Sports Med.,* In press, 1978.

71. Ribisl, P. M. Effects of training upon the maximal oxygen uptake of middle-aged men. *Int. Z. Angew. Physiol.* 26:272–278, 1969.

72. Robinson, S. and P. M. Harmon. Lactic acid mechanism and certain properties of blood in relation to training. *Amer. J. Physiol.* 132:757–769, 1941.

73. Roskamm. H. Optimum patterns of exercise for healthy adults. *Canad. Med. Ass. J.* 96:895–899, 1967.

74. Saltin, B., G. Blomqvist, J. Mitchell, R. L. Johnson, K. Wildenthal and C. B. Chapman. Response to exercise after bed rest and after training. *Circulation* 37 and 38, Suppl. 7, 1–78, 1968.
75. Saltin, B., L. Hartley, A. Kilbom and I. Astrand. Physical training in sedentary middle-aged and older men. *Scand. J. Clin. Lab. Invest.* 24:323–334, 1969.
76. Sharkey, B. J. Intensity and duration of training and the development of cardiorespiratory endurance. *Med. Sci. Sports* 2:197–202, 1970.
77. Shephard, R. J. Intensity, duration, and frequency of exercise as determinants of the response to a training regime. *Int. Z. Angew, Physiol.* 26:272–278, 1969.
78. Shephard, R. J. Future research on the quantifying of endurance training. *J. Human Ergology* 3:163–181, 1975.
79. Sidney, K. H., R. B. Eynon and D. A. Cunningham. Effect of frequency of training of exercise upon physical working performance and selected variables representative of cardiorespiratory fitness. In: *Training Scientific Basis and Application* (A. W. Taylor, ed.) Springfield: C. C. Thomas, Co., pp. 144–188, 1972.
80. Sidney, K. H., R. J. Shephard and J. Harrison. Endurance training and body composition of the elderly. *Amer. J. Clin. Nutr.* 30:326–333, 1977.
81. Siegel, W., G. Blomqvist and J. H. Mitchell. Effects of a quantitated physical training program on middle-aged sedentary males. *Circulation* 41:19, 1970.
82. Skinner, J., J. Holloszy and T. Cureton. Effects of a program of endurance exercise on physical work capacity and anthropometric measurements of fifteen middle-aged men. *Amer. J. Cardiol.* 14:747–752, 1964.
83. Skinner, J. The cardiovascular system with aging and exercise. In: Brunner, D. and E. Jokl (editors). *Physical Activity and Aging.* Baltimore: University Park Press, 1970, pp. 100–108.
84. Smith, D. P. and F. W. Stransky. The effect of training and detraining on the body composition and cardiovascular response of young women to exercise. *J. Sports Med.* 16:112–120, 1976.
85. Terjung, R. L., K. M. Baldwin, J. Cooksey, B. Samson and R. A. Sutter. Cardiovascular adaptation to twelve minutes of mild daily exercise in middle-aged sedentary men. *J. Amer. Geriatr. Soc.* 21:164–168, 1973.
86. Wilmore, J. H., J. Royce, R. N. Girandola, F. I. Katch and V. L. Katch. Physiological alterations resulting from a 10-week jogging program. *Med. Sci. Sports* 2(1):7–14, 1970.
87. Wilmore, J. H., J. Royce, R. N. Girandola, F. I. Katch and V. L. Katch. Body composition changes with a 10-week jogging program. *Med. Sci. Sports* 2:113–117, 1970.
88. Wilmore, J. H. Alterations in strength, body composition, and anthropometric measurements consequent to a 10-week weight training program. *Med. Sci. Sports* 6:133–138, 1974.
89. Wilmore, J. Inferiority of female athletes: myth or reality. *J. Sports Med.* 3:1–6, 1974.
90. Wilmore, J., R. B. Parr, P. A. Vodak, T. J. Barstow, T. V. Pipes, A. Ward and P. Leslie. Strength, endurance, BMR, and body composition changes with circuit weight training. *Med. Sci. Sports* 8:58–60, 1976. (Abstract)

Appendix 4:
The Use and Abuse of Anabolic-Androgenic Steroids in Sports

Based on a comprehensive survey of the world literature and a careful analysis of the claims made for and against the efficacy of anabolic-androgenic steroids in improving human physical performance, it is the position of the American College of Sports Medicine that:

1. The administration of anabolic-androgenic steroids to healthy humans below age 50 in medically approved therapeutic doses often does not of itself bring about any significant improvements in strength, aerobic endurance, lean body mass, or body weight.
2. There is no conclusive scientific evidence that extremely large doses of anabolic-androgenic steroids either aid or hinder athletic performance.
3. The prolonged use of oral anabolic-androgenic steroids (C_{17}-alkylated derivatives of testosterone) has resulted in liver disorders in some persons. Some of these disorders are apparently reversible with the cessation of drug usage, but others are not.
4. The administration of anabolic-androgenic steroids to male humans may result in a decrease in testicular size and function and a decrease in sperm production. Although these effects appear to be reversible when small doses of steroids are used for short periods of time, the reversibility of the effects of large doses over extended periods of time is unclear.
5. Serious and continuing effort should be made to educate male and female athletes, coaches, physical educators, physicians, trainers, and the general public regarding the inconsistent effects of anabolic-androgenic steroids on improvement of human physical performance and the potential dangers of taking certain forms of these substances, especially in large doses, for prolonged periods.

American College of Sports Medicine. 1977. Position Statement on The Use and Abuse of Anabolic-Androgenic Steroids in Sports.

Research Background for the Position Statement

This position stand has been developed from an extensive survey and analysis of the world literature in the fields of medicine, physiology, endocrinology, and physical education. Although the reactions of humans to the use of drugs, including hormones or drugs which simulate the actions of natural hormones, are individual and not entirely predictable, some conclusions can nevertheless be drawn with regard to what desirable and what undesirable effects may be achieved. Accordingly, whereas positive effects of drugs may sometimes arise because persons have been led to expect such changes ("placebo" effect) (8), repeated experiments of a similar nature often fail to support the initial positive effects and lead to the conclusion that any positive effect that does exist may not be substantial.

1. Administration of testosterone-like synthetic drugs which have anabolic (tissue building) and androgenic (development of male secondary sex characteristics) properties in amounts up to twice those normally prescribed for medical use have been associated with increased strength, lean body mass and/or body weight in some studies (6,19,20,26,27,33,34,36) but not in others (9,10,12,13,21,35,36). One study (13) reported an increase in the amount of weight the steroid group could lift compared to controls but found no difference in isometric strength, which suggests a placebo effect in the drug group, a learning effect or possibly a differential drug effect on isotonic compared to isometric strength. An initial report of enhanced aerobic endurance after administration of an anabolic-androgenic steroid (20) has not been confirmed (6,9,19,21,27). Because of the lack of adequate control groups in many studies it seems likely that some of the positive effects on strength that have been reported are due to "placebo" effects (3,8), but a few apparently well-designed studies have also shown beneficial effects of steroid administration on muscular strength and lean body mass. Some of the discrepancies in results may also be due to differences in the type of drug administered, the method of drug administration, the nature of the exercise programs involved, the duration of the experiment, and individual differences in sensitivity to the administered drug. High protein dietary supplements do not insure the effectiveness of the steroids (13,21,36). Because of the many failures to show improved muscular strength, lean body mass, or body weight after therapeutic doses of anabolic-androgenic steroids it is obvious that for many individuals any benefits are likely to be small and not worth the health risks involved.

2. Testimonial evidence by individual athletes suggests that athletes often use much larger doses of steroids than those ordinarily prescribed by physicians and those evaluated in published research. Because of the health risks involved with the long-term use of high doses and requirements for informed consent it is unlikely that scientifically acceptable evidence will be forthcoming to evaluate the effectiveness of such large doses of drugs on athletic performance.

3. Alterations of normal liver function have been found in as many as 80 percent of one series of 69 patients treated with C_{17}-alkylated testosterone derivatives (oral anabolic-androgenic steroids) (29). Cholestasis has been observed histologically in the livers of persons taking these substances (31). These changes appear to be benign and reversible (30). Five reports (4,7,23,31,39) document the occurrence of peliosis hepatitis in 17 patients without evidence of significant liver disease who were treated with C_{17}-alkylated androgenic steroids. Seven of these patients died of liver failure. The first case of hepato-cellular carcinoma associated with taking an androgenic-anabolic steroid was reported in 1965 (28). Since then at least 13 other patients taking C_{17}-alkylated androgenic steroids have developed hepato-cellular carcinoma (5,11,14,15,16,17,18,25). In some cases dosages as low as 10–15 mg/day taken for only three or four months have caused liver complications (13,25).
4. Administration of therapeutic doses of androgenic-anabolic steroids in men often (15,22), but not always (1,10,19), reduces the output of testosterone and gonadotropins and reduces spermatogenesis. Some steroids are less potent than others in causing these effects (1). Although these effects on the reproductive system appear to be reversible in animals, the long-term results of taking large doses by humans is unknown.
5. Precise information concerning the abuse of anabolic steroids by female athletes is unavailable. Nevertheless, there is no reason to believe females will not be tempted to adopt the use of these medicines. The use of anabolic steroids by females, particularly those who are either prepubertal or have not attained full growth, is especially dangerous. The undesired side effects include masculinization (2,29,30), disruption of normal growth pattern (30), voice changes (2,30,32), acne (2,29,30,32), hirsutism (29,30,32), and enlargement of the clitoris (29). The long-term effects on reproductive function are unknown, but anabolic steroids may be harmful in this area. Their ability to interfere with the menstrual cycle has been well documented (29).

For these reasons, all concerned with advising, training, coaching, and providing medical care for female athletes should exercise all persuasions available to prevent the use of anabolic steroids by female athletes.

References

1. Aakvaag, A. and S. B. Stromme. The effect of mesterolone administration to normal men on the pituitary-testicular function. *Acta Endocrinol.* 77:380–386, 1974.
2. Allen, D. M., M. H. Fine, T. F. Necheles, and W. Dameshek. Oxymetholone therapy in aplastic anemia. *Blood* 32:83–89, July 1968
3. Ariel, G. and W. Saville. Anabolic steroids: the physiological effects of placebos. *Med. Sci. Sports* 4:124–126, 1972.
4. Bagheri, S. A. and J. L. Boyer. Peliosis hepatitis associated with androgenic-anabolic steroid therapy. *Ann. Int. Med.* 81:610–618, 1974.
5. Bernstein, M. S., R. L. Hunter and S. Yachrin. Hepatoma and peliosis hepatitis developing in a patient with Fanconi's anemia. *N. Engl. J. Med.* 284:1135–1136, 1971.
6. Bowers, R. and J. Reardon. Effects of methandro-stenolone (Dianabol) on strength development and aerobic capacity. *Med. Sci. Sports* 4:54, 1972.
7. Burger, R. A. and P. M. Marcuse. Peliosis hepatitis, report of a case. *Am. J. Clin. Path.* 22:569–573, 1952.

8. Byerly, H. Explaining and exploiting placebo effects. *Prosp. Biol. Med.* 19:423–436, 1976.
9. Casner, S., R. Early, and B. R. Carlson. Anabolic steroid effects on body composition in normal young men. *J. Sports Med. and Phys. Fit.* 11:98–103, 1971.
10. Fahey, T. D. and C. H. Brown. The effects of an anabolic steroid on the strength, body composition and endurance of college males when accompanied by a weight training program. *Med. Sci. Sports* 5:272–276, 1973.
11. Farrell, G. C., D. E. Joshua, R. F. Uren, P. J. Baird, K. W. Perkins, and H. Kraienberg. Androgen-induced hepatoma. *Lancet* 1:430–431, 1975.
12. Fowler, Jr., W. M., G. W. Gardner, and G. H. Egstrom. Effect of an anabolic steroid on physical performance of young men. *J. Appl. Physiol.* 20:1038–1040, 1965.
13. Golding, L. A., J. E. Freydinger, and S. S. Fishel. Weight, size and strength-unchanged by steroids. *Physician Sports Med.* 2:39–45, 1974.
14. Guy, J. T. and M. O. Auxlander. Androgenic steroids and hepato-cellular carcinoma. *Lancet* 1:148, 1973.
15. Harkness, R. A., B. H. Kilshaw, and B. M. Hobson. Effects of large doses of anabolic steroids. *Brit. J. Sport Med.* 9:70–73, 1975.
16. Henderson, J. T., J. Richmond, and M. D. Sumerling. Androgenic-anabolic steroid therapy and hepato-cellular carcinoma. *Lancet* 1:934, 1972.
17. Johnson, F. L. The association of oral androgenic-anabolic steroids and life threatening disease. *Med. Sci. Sports* 7:284–286, 1975.
18. Johnson, F. L., J. R. Feagler, K. G. Lerner, P. W. Majems, M. Siegel, J. R. Hartman, and E. D. Thomas. Association of androgenic-anabolic steroid therapy with development of hepato-cellular carcinoma. *Lancet* 2:1273–1276, 1972.
19. Johnson, L. C., G. Fisher, L. J. Sylvester, and C. C. Hofheins. Anabolic steroid: Effects on strength, body weight, O_2 uptake and spermatogenesis in mature males. *Med. Sci. Sports* 4:43–45, 1972.
20. Johnson, L. C. and J. P. O'Shea. Anabolic steroid: effects on stregth development. *Science* 164:957–959, 1969.
21. Johnson, L. C., E. S. Roundy, P. Allsen, A. G. Fisher, and L. J. Sylvester. Effect of anabolic steroid treatment on endurance. *Med. Sci. Sports* 7:287–289, 1975.
22. Kilshaw, B. H., R. A. Harkness, B. M. Hobson, and A. W. M. Smith. The effects of large doses of the anabolic steroid, methandrostenolone, on an athlete. *Clin. Endocr.* 4:537–541, 1975.
23. Kintzen, W. and J. Silny. Peliosis hepatitis after administration of fluoxymesterone. *Canad. Med. Assoc. J.* 83:860–862, 1960.
24. McCredie, K. B. Oxymetholone in refractory anaemia. *Brit. J. of Haemtology,* 17:265–273, 1969.
25. Meadows, A. T., J. L. Naiman, and M. V. Valdes-Dapena. Hepatoma associated with androgen therapy for aplastic anemia. *J. Pediatr.* 84:109–110, 1974.
26. O'Shea, J. P. The effects of an anabolic steroid on dynamic strength levels of weight lifters. *Nutr. Report Internat.* 4:363–370, 1971.
27. O'Shea, J. P. and W. Winkler. Biochemical and physical effects of an anabolic steroid in competitive swimmers and weight lifters. *Nutr. Report Internat.* 2:351–362, 1970.
28. Recant, L. and P. Lacy (eds.). Fanconi's anemia and hepatic cirrhosis. Clinopathologic Conference. *Am. J. Med.* 39:464–475, 1965.
29. Sanchez-Medal, L., A. Gomez-Leal, L. Duarte, and M. Guadalupe-Rico. Anabolic-androgenic steroids in the treatment of acquired aplastic anemia. *Blood* 34:283–300, 1969.
30. Shahidi, N. T. Androgens and erythropoiesis. *N. Engl. J. Med.* 289:72–79, 1973.
31. Sherlock, S. *Disease of the Liver and Biliary System,* 4th Edition, Philadelphia: F. A. Davis, p. 371, 1968.
32. Silink, J. and B. G. Firkin. An analysis of hypoplastic anaemia with special reference to the use of oxymetholone ("Adroyd") in its therapy. *Australian Ann. of Med.* 17:224–235, 1968.
33. Stanford, B. A. and R. Moffat. Anabolic steroid: effectiveness as an ergogenic aid to experienced weight trainers. *J. Sports Med. and Phys. Fit.* 14:191–197, 1974.
34. Steinbach, M. Uber den Einfluss anabolen Wirkstoffe und Korpergewicht Muskelkraft und Muskeltraining. *Sportarzt und Sport-medizin.* 11:485–492, 1968.
35. Samuels, L. T., A. F. Henschel, and A. Kays. Influence of methyltestosterone on muscular work and creatine metabolism in normal young men. *J. Clin. Endocrinol. Metab.* 2:649–654, 1942.
36. Stromme, S. B., H. D. Meen, and A. Aakvaag. Effects of an androgenic-anabolic steroid on strength development and plasma testosterone levels in normal males. *Med. Sci. Sports* 6:203–208, 1974.
37. Ward, P. The effect of an anabolic steroid on strength and lean body mass. *Med. Sci. Sports* 5:277–282, 1973.
38. Zak, F. G. Peliosis hepatitis. *Am. J. Pathol.* 26:1–15, 1950.
39. Ziegenfuss, J. and R. Carabasi. Androgens and hepatocellular carcinoma. *Lancet* 1:262, 1973.

Appendix 5:
Weight Loss In Wrestlers

Despite repeated admonitions by medical, educational and athletic groups (2,8,17,22,33), most wrestlers have been inculcated by instruction or accepted tradition to lose weight in order to be certified for a class that is lower than their preseason weight (34). Studies (34,40) of weight losses in high school and college wrestlers indicate that from 3–20% of the preseason body weight is lost before certification or competition occurs. Of this weight loss, most of the decrease occurs in the final days or day before the official weigh-in (34,40) with the youngest and/or lightest members of the team losing the highest percentage of their body weight (34). Under existing rules and practices, it is not uncommon for an individual to repeat this weight losing process many times during the season because successful wrestlers complete in 15–30 matches/ year (13).

Contrary to existing beliefs, most wrestlers are not "fat" before the season starts (35). In fact, the fat content of high school and college wrestlers weighing less than 190 pounds has been shown to range from 1.6 to 15.1 percent of their body weight with the majority possessing less than 8% (14,28,31). It is well known and documented that wrestlers lose body weight by a combination of food restriction, fluid deprivation and sweating induced by thermal or exercise procedures (20,22,34,40). Of these methods, dehydration through sweating appears to be the method most frequently chosen.

Careful studies on the nature of the weight being lost show that water, fats and proteins are lost when food restriction and fluid deprivation procedures are followed (10). Moreover, the proportionality between these constituents will change with continued restriction and deprivation. For example, if food restriction is held constant when the volume of fluid being consumed is decreased, more water will be lost from the tissues of the body than before the fluid restriction occurred. The problem becomes more acute when thermal or exercise dehydration occurs because electrolyte losses will accompany the water losses (16). Even when 1–5 hours are allowed for purposes of rehydration after the weigh-in, this time interval is insufficient for fluid and electrolyte homeostasis to be completely reestablished (11,37,39,40).

American College of Sports Medicine. 1976. Position Stand on Weight Loss In Wrestlers.

Since the "making of weight" occurs by combinations of food restriction, fluid deprivation and dehydration, responsible officials should realize that the single or combined effects of these practices are generally associated with 1) a reduction in muscular strength (4,15,30); 2) a decrease in work performance times (24,26,27,30); 3) lower plasma and blood volumes (6,7,24,27); 4) a reduction in cardiac functioning during sub-maximal work conditions which are associated with higher heart rates (1,19,23,24,27), smaller stroke volumes (27), and reduced cardiac outputs (27); 5) a lower oxygen consumption, especially with food restriction (15,30); 6) an impairment of thermoregulatory processes (3,9,24); 7) a decrease in renal blood flow (21,25) and in the volume of fluid being filtered by the kidney (21); 8) a depletion of liver glycogen stores (12); and 9) an increase in the amount of electrolytes being lost from the body (6,7,16).

Since it is possible for these changes to impede normal growth and development, there is little physiological or medical justification for the use of the weight reduction methods currently followed by many wrestlers. These sentiments have been expressed in part within Rule 1, Section 3, Article 1 of the *Official Wrestling Rule Book* (18) published by the National Federation of State High School Associations which states, "The Rules Committee recommends that individual state high school associations develop and utilize an effective weight control program which will discourage severe weight reduction and/or wide variations in weight, because this may be harmful to the competitor. . . ." However, until the National Federation of State High School Associations defines the meaning of the terms "severe" and "wide variations," this rule will be ineffective in reducing the abuses associated with the "making of weight."

Therefore, it is the position of the American College of Sports Medicine that the potential health hazards created by the procedures used to "make weight" by wrestlers can be eliminated if state and national organizations will:

1. Assess the body composition of each wrestler several weeks in advance of the competitive season (5,14,28,31,38). Individuals with a fat content less than five percent of their certified body weight should receive medical clearance before being allowed to compete.
2. Emphasize the fact that the daily caloric requirements of wrestlers should be obtained from a balanced diet and determined on the basis of age, body surface area, growth and physical activity levels (29). The minimal caloric needs of wrestlers in high schools and colleges will range from 1200 to 2400 KCal/day (32); therefore, it is the responsibility of coaches, school officials, physicians and parents to discourage wrestlers from securing less than their minimal needs without prior medical approval.
3. Discourage the practice of fluid deprivation and dehydration. This can be accomplished by:
   a. Educating the coaches and wrestlers on the physiological consequences and medical complications that can occur as a result of these practices.
   b. Prohibiting the single or combined use of rubber suits, steam rooms, hot boxes, saunas, laxatives, and diuretics to "make weight."
   c. Scheduling weigh-ins just prior to competition.
   d. Scheduling more official weigh-ins between team matches.

4. Permit more participants/team to compete in those weight classes (119–145 pounds) which have the highest percentages of wrestlers certified for competition (36).
5. Standardize regulations concerning the eligibility rules at championship tournaments so that individuals can only participate in those weight classes in which they had the highest frequencies of matches throughout the season.
6. Encourage local and county organizations to systematically collect data on the hydration state (39,40) of wrestlers and its relationship to growth and development.

References

1. Ahlman, K. and M. J. Karvonen. Weight reduction by sweating in wrestlers and its effect on physical fitness. *J. Sports Med. Phys. Fit.* 1:58–62, 1961.
2. AMA Committee on the Medical Aspects of Sports, Wrestling and Weight Control. *JAMA* 201:541–543, 1967.
3. Bock, W. E., E. L. Fox and R. Bowers. The effect of acute dehydration upon cardiorespiratory endurance. *J. Sports Med. Phys. Fit.* 7:62–72, 1967.
4. Bosco, J. S., R. L. Terjung and J. E. Greenleaf. Effects of progressive hypohydration on maximal isometric muscular strength. *J. Sports Med. Phys. Fit.* 8:81–86, 1968.
5. Clarke, K. S. Predicting certified weight of young wrestlers: a field study of the Tcheng-Tipton method. *Med. Sci. Sports* 6:52–57, 1974.
6. Costill, D. L. and K. E. Sparks. Rapid fluid replacement following thermal dehydration. *J. Appl. Physiol.* 34:299–303, 1973.
7. Costill, D. L., R. Cote, E. Miller, T. Miller and S. Wynder. Water and electrolyte replacement during repeated days of work in the heat. *Aviat. Space Environ. Med.* 46:795–800, 1975.
8. Eriksen, F. G. Interscholastic wrestling and weight control: Current plans and their loopholes. *Proceedings of the Eighth National Conference on The Medical Aspects of Sports.* Chicago: AMA, 1967, pp. 34–39.
9. Grande, F., J. E. Monagle, E. R. Buskirk and H. L. Taylor. Body temperature responses to exercise in man on restricted food and water intake. *J. Appl. Physiol.* 14:194–198, 1959.
10. Grande, F. Nutrition and energy balance in body composition studies. *Techniques for Measuring Body Composition,* edited by J. Brozek and A. Henschel. Washington, D.C., National Acad. Sci. & Nat. Res. Council, pp. 168–188, 1961.
11. Herbert, W. G. and P. M. Ribisl. Effects of dehydration upon physical work capacity of wrestlers under competitive conditions. *Res. Quart.* 43:416–422, 1972.
12. Hultman, E. and L. Nilsson. Liver glycogen as glucose-supplying source during exercise. *Limiting Factors of Physical Performance,* edited by J. Keul. Stuttgart: Georg Thieme, pp. 179–189, 1973.
13. Iowa High School Athletic Association. *1975 Program for the 55th State Wrestling Tournament.,* pp. 7–9.
14. Katch, F. I. and E. D. Michael, Jr. Body composition of high school wrestlers according to age and wrestling weight category. *Med Sci. Sports* 3:190–194, 1971.
15. Keys, A. L., J. Brozek, A. Henschel, O. Mickelsen and H. L. Taylor. *The Biology of Human Starvation.* Minneapolis: U. of Minn. Press, Vol. 1, pp. 718–748, 1950.
16. Kozlowski, S. and B. Saltin. Effect of sweat loss on body fluids. *J. Appl. Physiol.* 19:1119–1124, 1964.
17. Kroll, W. Guidelines for rules and practices. *Proceedings of the Eighth National Conference on the Medical Aspects of Sports.* Chicago: AMA, pp. 40–44, 1967.
18. *The National Federation 1974–75 Wrestling Rule Book.* The National Federation Publications. Elgin, Illinois, p. 6.
19. Palmer, W. Selected physiological responses of normal young men following dehydration and rehydration. *Res. Quart.* 30:1054–1059, 1968.
20. Paul, W. D. Crash diets in wrestling. *J. Iowa Med. Soc.* 56:835–840, 1966.
21. Radigan, L. R. and S. Robinson. Effect of environmental heat stress and exercise on renal blood flow and filtration rate. *J. Appl. Physiol.* 2:185–191, 1949.
22. Rasch, P. G. and W. Kroll. *What Research Tells the Coach About Wrestling.* Washington: AAHPER, pp. 41–50, 1964.
23. Ribisl, P. M. and W. G. Herbert. Effect of rapid weight reduction and subsequent rehydration upon the physical working capacity of wrestlers. *Res. Quart.* 41:536–541, 1970.
24. Robinson, S. The effect of dehydration on performance. *Football Injuries.* Washington, DC: Nat. Acad. Sci., pp. 191–197, 1970.

25. Rowell, L. B. Human cardiovascular adjustments to exercise and thermal stress. *Physiol. Rev.* 54:75–159, 1974.
26. Saltin, B. Aerobic and anaerobic work capacity after dehydration. *J. Appl Physiol.* 19:1114–1118, 1964.
27. Saltin, B. Circulatory response to submaximal and maximal exercise after thermal dehydration. *J. Appl. Physiol.* 19:1125–1132, 1964.
28. Sinning, W. E. Body composition assessment of college wrestlers. *Med. Sci. Sports* 6:139–145, 1974.
29. Suggested Daily Dietary Requirements. National Research Council Data, published in Oser, B. O. *Hawk's Physiological Chemistry.* 14th Edition, New York: McGraw-Hill, pp. 1370–1371, 1965.
30. Taylor, H. L., E. R. Buskirk, J. Brozek, J. T. Anderson and F. Grande. Performance capacity and effects of caloric restriction with hard physical work on young men. *J. Appl. Physiol.* 10:421–429, 1957.
31. Tcheng, T. K. and C. M. Tipton. Iowa wrestling study: Anthropometric measurements and the prediction of a "minimal" body weight for high school wrestlers. *Med. Sci. Sports* 5:1–10, 1973.
32. Tipton, C. M. Unpublished calculations on Iowa High School Wrestlers using a height and weight surface area nomogram. (Consalazio, C. F., R. E. Johnson and L. J. Pecora. *Physiological Measurements of Metabolic Functions in Man.* New York: McGraw-Hill, 1963, p. 27, that was constructed from the Dubois-Meech formula published in Arch. Int. Med. 17:863–871, 1916) plus the metabolic standards for age used by the Mayo Foundation Standards that were published by Boothby, Berkson and Dunn in *Am. J. Physiol.* 116:467–484, 1936.
33. Tipton, C. M., T. K. Tcheng and W. D. Paul. Evaluation of the Hall Method for determining minimum wrestling weights. *J. Iowa Med. Soc.* 59:571–574, 1969.
34. Tipton, C. M. and T. K. Tcheng. Iowa wrestling study: Weight loss in high school students. *JAMA* 2114:1269–1274, 1970.
35. Tipton, C. M. Current status of the Iowa Wrestling Study. *The Predicament,* 12-30-73, p. 7.
36. Tipton, C. M., T. K. Tcheng and E. J. Zambraski. Iowa Wrestling Study: Weight classification systems. *Med. Sci. Sports* 8:101–104, 1976.
37. Vaccaro, P., C. W. Zauner and J. R. Cade. Changes in body weight, hematocrit and plasma protein concentration due to dehydration and rehydration in wrestlers. *Med. Sci. Sports* 7:76, 1975.
38. Wilmore, J. H. and A. Behnke. An anthropometric estimation of body density and lean body weight in young men. *J. Appl. Physiol.* 27:25–31, 1969.
39. Zambraski, E. J., C. M. Tipton, T. K. Tcheng, H. R. Jordan, A. C. Vailas and A. K. Callahan. Changes in the urinary profiles of wrestlers prior to and after competition. *Med. Sci. Sports.* 7:217–220, 1975.
40. Zambraski, E. J., D. T. Foster, P. M. Gross and C. M. Tipton. Iowa wrestling study: Weight loss and urinary profiles of collegiate wrestlers. *Med. Sci. Sports* 8:105–108, 1976.

350

Appendix 6: Prevention of Heat Injuries During Distance Running

The Purpose of this Position Statement is:

(a) To alert local, national and international sponsors of distance running events of the health hazards of heat injury during distance running, and

(b) To inform said sponsors of injury preventive actions that may reduce the frequency of this type of injury.

The recommendations address only the manner in which distance running sports activities may be conducted to further reduce incidence of heat injury among normal athletes conditioned to participate in distance running. The Recommendations Are Advisory Only.

Recommendations concerning the ingested quantity and content of fluid are merely a partial preventive to heat injury. The physiology of each individual athlete varies; strict compliance with these recommendations and the current rules governing distance running may not reduce the incidence of heat injuries among those so inclined to such injury.

Research Findings

Based on research findings and current rules governing distance running competition, it is the position of the American College of Sports Medicine that:

1. Distance races (> 16 km or 10 miles) should *not* be conducted when the wet bulb temperature—globe temperature (adapted from Minard, D. Prevention of heat casualties in Marine Corps recruits. *Milit. Med.* 126:261, 1961. WB-GT = 0.7 [WBT] + 0.2 [GT] + 0.1 [DBT]) exceeds 28°C (82.4°F). (1,2)
2. During periods of the year, when the daylight dry bulb temperature often exceeds 27°C (80°F), distance races should be conducted before 9:00 A.M. or after 4:00 P.M. (2,7,8,9)

American College of Sports Medicine. 1975. Position Statement on Prevention of Heat Injuries During Distance Running.

351

3. It is the responsibility of the race sponsors to provide fluids which contain small amounts of sugar (less than 2.5 g glucose per 100 ml of water) and electrolytes (less than 10 mEq sodium and 5 mEq potassium per liter of solution). (5,6)
4. Runners should be encouraged to frequently ingest fluids during competition and to consume 400–500 ml (13–17 oz.) of fluid 10–15 minutes before competition. (5,6,9)
5. Rules prohibiting the administration of fluids during the first 10 kilometers (6.2 miles) of a marathon race should be amended to permit fluid ingestion at frequent intervals along the race course. In light of the high sweat rates and body temperatures during distance running in the heat, race sponsors should provide "water stations" at 3–4 kilometer (2–2.5 mile) intervals for all races of 16 kilometers (10 miles) or more. (4,8,9)
6. Runners should be instructed in how to recognize the early warning symptoms that precede heat injury. Recognition of symptoms, cessation of running, and proper treatment can prevent heat injury. Early warning symptoms include the following: piloerection on chest and upper arms, chilling, throbbing pressure in the head, unsteadiness, nausea, and dry skin. (2,9)
7. Race sponsors should make prior arrangements with medical personnel for the care of cases of heat injury. Responsible and informed personnel should supervise each "feeding station." Organizational personnel should reserve the right to stop runners who exhibit clear signs of heat stroke or heat exhaustion.

It is the position of the American College of Sports Medicine that policies established by local, national, and international sponsors of distance running events should adhere to these guidelines. Failure to adhere to these guidelines may jeopardize the health of competitors through heat injury.

The requirements of distance running place great demands on both circulation and body temperature regulation (4,8,9). Numerous studies have reported rectal temperatures in excess of 40.6°C (105°F) after races of 6 to 26.2 miles (9.6 to 41.9 kilometers) (4,8,9). Attempting to counterblanace such overheating, runners incur large sweat losses of 0.8 to 1.1 liters/m²/hr (4,8,9). The resulting body water deficit may total 6–10% of the athlete's body weight. Dehydration of these proportions severely limits subsequent sweating, places dangerous demands on circulation, reduces exercise capacity and exposes the runner to the health hazards associated with hyperthermia (heat stroke, heat exhaustion and muscle cramps) (2,3,9).

Under moderate thermal conditions, e.g., 65–70°F (18.5–21.3°C), no cloud cover, relative humidity 49–55%, the risk of overheating is still a serious threat to highly motivated distance runners. Nevertheless, distance races are frequently conducted under more severe conditions than these. The air temperature at the 1967 U.S. Pan American Marathon Trial, for example, was 92–95°F (33.6–35.3°C). Many highly conditioned athletes failed to finish the race and several of the competitors demonstrated overt symptoms of heat stroke (no sweating, shivering and lack of orientation).

The above consequences are compounded by the current popularity of distance running among middle-aged and aging men and women who may possess significantly less heat tolerance than their younger counterparts. In recent years, races of 10 to 26.2 miles (16 to 41.9 kilometers) have attracted several thousand runners. Since it is likely that distance running enthusiasts will continue to sponsor races under adverse heat conditions, specific steps should be taken to minimize the health threats which accompany such endurance events.

Fluid ingestion during prolonged running (two hours) has been shown to effectively reduce rectal temperature and minimize dehydration (4). Although most competitors consume fluids during races that exceed 1–1.5 hours, current international distance running rules prohibit the administration of fluids until the runner has completed 10 miles (16 kilometers). Under such limitations, the competitor is certain to accumulate a large body water deficit ($-$ 3%) before any fluids would be ingested. To make the problem more complex, most runners are unable to judge the volume of fluids they consume during competition (4). At the 1968 U.S. Olympic Marathon Trial, it was observed that there were body weight losses of 6.1 kg, with an average total fluid ingestion of only 0.14 to 0.35 liters (4). It seems obvious that the rules and habits which prohibit fluid administration during distance running preclude any benefits which might be gained from this practice.

Runners who attempt to consume large volumes of sugar solution during competition complain of gastric discomfort (fullness) and an inability to consume fluids after the first few feedings (4,5,6). Generally speaking, most runners drink solutions containing 5–20 grams of sugar per 100 milliliters of water. Although saline is rapidly emptied from the stomach (25 ml/min), the addition of even small amounts of sugar can drastically impair the rate of gastric emptying (5). During exercise in the heat, carbohydrate supplementation is of secondary importance and the sugar content of the oral feedings should be minimized.

References

1. Adolph. E. I. *Physiology of Man in the Desert.* New York: Interscience, 1947.
2. Buskirk, E. R. and W. C. Grasley. Heat Injury and Conduct of Athletes. Ch. 16 in *Science and Medicine of Exercise and Sport,* 2nd Edition. W. R. Johnson and E. R. Buskirk, Editors, New York; Harper and Row, 1974.
3. Buskirk, E. R., P. F. Iampietro and D. E. Bass. Work performance after dehydration: effects of physical conditioning and heat acclimatization. *J. Appl. Physiol.* 12:189–194, 1958.
4. Costill, D. L., W. F. Kammer and A. Fisher. Fluid ingestion during distance running. *Arch. Environ. Health* 21:520–525, 1970.
5. Costill, D. L. and B. Saltin. Factors limiting gastric emptying during rest and exercise. *J. Appl. Physiol.* 37(5):679–683, 1974.
6. Fordtran, J. A. and B. Saltin. Gastric emptying and intestinal absorption during prolonged severe exercise. *J. Appl. Physiol.* 23:331–335, 1967.
7. Mylire, L. G. Shifts in blood volume during and following acute environmental and work stresses in man. (Doctoral Dissertation). Indiana University: Bloomington, Indiana, 1967.
8. Pugh, L. G. C., J. I. Corbett and R. H. Johnson. Rectal temperatures, weight losses and sweating rates in marathon running. *J. Appl. Physiol.* 23:347–353, 1957.
9. Wyndham, C. H. and N. B. Strydom. The danger of an inadequate water intake during marathon running. *S. Afr. Med. J.* 43:893–896, 1969.

Appendix 7:
The Participation of the Female Athlete in Long-Distance Running

In the Olympic Games and other international contests, female athletes run distances ranging from 100 meters to 3,000 meters, whereas male athletes run distances ranging from 100 meters through 10,000 meters as well as the marathon (42.2 km). The limitation on distance for women's running events has been defended at times on the grounds that long-distance running may be harmful to the health of girls and women.

Opinion Statement

It is the opinion of the American College of Sports Medicine that females should not be denied the opportunity to compete in long-distance running. There exists no conclusive scientific or medical evidence that long-distance running is contraindicated for the healthy, trained female athlete. The American College of Sports Medicine recommends that females be allowed to compete at the national and international level in the same distances in which their male counterparts compete.

Supportive Information

Studies (10,20,32,41,54) have shown that females respond in much the same manner as males to systematic exercise training. Cardiorespiratory function is improved as indicated by significant increases in maximal oxygen uptake (4,6,13,16,30). At maximal exercise, stroke volume and cardiac output are increased after training (30). At standardized submaximal exercise intensities after training, cardiac output remains unchanged, heart rate decreases, and stroke volume increases (6,30,31). Also, resting heart rate decreases after training (30). As is the case for males, relative body fat content is reduced consequent to systematic endurance training (33,35,51).

American College of Sports Medicine. 1979. Opinion Statement on The Participation of the Female Athlete in Long-Distance Running.

Long-distance running imposes a significant thermal stress on the participant. Some differences do exist between males and females with regard to thermoregulation during prolonged exercise. However, the differences in thermal stress response are more quantitative than qualitative in nature (36,38,47). For example, women experience lower evaporative heat losses than do men exposed to the same thermal stress (29,40,53) and usually have higher skin temperatures and deep body temperatures upon onset of sweating (3,18,45). This may actually be an advantage in reducing body water loss so long as thermal equilibrium can be maintained. In view of current findings (10,11,15,40,48,49,50), it appears that the earlier studies which indicated that women were less tolerant to exercise in the heat than men (36,53) were misleading because they failed to consider the women's relatively low level of cardiorespiratory fitness and heat acclimatization. Apparently, cardiorespiratory fitness as measured by maximum oxygen uptake is a most important functional capacity as regards a person's ability to respond adequately to thermal stress (9,11,15,47). In fact, there has been considerable interest in the seeming cross-adaptation of a life style characterized by physical activity involving regular and prolonged periods of exercise hyperthermia and response to high environmental temperatures (1,37,39). Women trained in long-distance running have been reported to be more tolerant of heat stress than non-athletic women matched for age and body surface area (15). Thus, it appears that trained female long-distance runners have the capacity to deal with the thermal stress of prolonged exercise as well as the moderate-to-high environmental temperatures and relative humidities that often accompany these events.

The participation of males and females in road races of various distances has increased tremendously during the last decade. This type of competition attracts the entire spectrum of runners with respect to ability—from the elite to the novice. A common feature of virtually all of these races is that a small number of participants develop medical problems (primarily heat injuries) which frequently require hospitalization. One of the first documentations of the medical problems associated with mass participation in this form of athletic competition was by Sutton and co-workers (46). Twenty-nine of 2,005 entrants in the 1971 Sydney City-to-Surf race collapsed; seven required hospitalization. All of the entrants who collapsed were males, although 4% of the race entrants were females. By 1978 the number of entrants increased approximately 10 fold with females accounting for approximately 30% of the entrants. In the 1978 race only nine entrants were treated for heat injury and again all were males (43). In a 1978 Canadian road race, in which 1,250 people participated, 15 entrants developed heat injuries—three females and 12 males, representing 1.3% and 1.2% of the total number of female and male entrants, respectively (27). Thus, females seem to tolerate the phsyiological stress of road race competition at least as well as males.

Because long-distance running competition sometimes occurs at moderate altitudes, the female's response to an environment where the partial pressure of oxygen is reduced (hypoxia) should be considered. Buskirk (5) noted that, although there is little information about the physiological responses of women to altitude, the proportional reduction in performance at Mexico City during the Pan American and Olympic Games was the same for males and females. Drinkwater et al. (13) found that women mountaineers exposed to hypoxia demonstrated a similar decrement in maximal oxygen uptake as that predicted for men. Hannon et al. (23,24) have found that females tolerate the effects of altitude better than males because there appears to be both a lower frequency and shorter duration of mountain sickness in women. Furthermore, at altitude women experience less alteration in such variables as resting heart rate, body weight, blood volume, electrocardiograms, and blood chemistries than men (23,24). Although one study has reported that women and men experience approximately the same respiratory changes with altitude exposure (44), another (22) reports that women hyperventilate more than men, thereby increasing the partial pressure of arterial oxygen and decreasing the partial pressure of arterial carbon dioxide. Thus, females tolerate the stress of altitude at least as well as men.

Long-distance running is occasionally associated with various overuse syndromes such as stress fracture, chondromalacia, shinsplints, and tendinitis. Pollock et al. (42) have shown that the incidence of these injuries for males engaged in a program of jogging was as high as 54% and was related to the frequency, duration, and intensity of the exercise training. Franklin et al. (19) recently reported the injury incidence of 42 sedentary females exposed to a 12-week jogging program. The injury rate for the females appeared to be comparable to that found for males in other studies although, as the investigators indicated, a decisive interpretation of presently available information may be premature because of the limited orthopedic injury data available for women. It has been suggested that the anatomical differences between men's and women's pelvic width and joint laxity may lead to a higher incidence of injuries for women who run (26). There are no data available, however, to support this suggestion. Whether or not the higher intensity training programs of competitive male and female long-distance runners result in a difference in injury rate between the sexes is now known at this time. It is believed, however, that the incidence of injury due to running surfaces encountered, biomechanics of back, leg and foot, and to foot apparel (28).

Of particular concern to female competitors and to the American College of Sports Medicine is evidence which indicates that approximately one-third of the competitive female long-distance runners between the ages of 12 and 45 experience amenorrhea or oligomenorrhea for at least brief periods (7,8). This phenomenon appears more frequently in those women with late onset of menarche, who have not experienced pregnancy, or who have taken contraceptive hormones. This same phenomenon also occurs in some competing gymnasts, swimmers, and professional ballerinas as well as sedentary individuals who have experienced some instances of undue stress or severe psychological trauma (25). Apparently, amenorrhea and oligomenorrhea may be caused by many factors characterized by loss of body weight (7,21,25). Running long distances may lead to decreased serum levels of pituitary gonadotrophic hormones in some women and may directly or indirectly lead to amenorrhea or oligomenorrhea. The role of running and the pathogenesis of these menstrual irregularities remains unknown (7,8).

The long-term effects of these types of menstrual irregularities for young girls that have undergone strenuous exercise training are unknown at this time. Eriksson and coworkers (17) have reported, however, that a group of 28 young girl swimmers, who underwent strenuous swim training for 2.5 years, were normal in all respects (e.g., childbearing) 10 years after discontinuing training.

In summary, a review of the literature demonstrates that males and females adapt to exercise training in a similar manner. Female distance runners are characterizied by having large maximal oxygen uptakes and low relative body fat content (52). The challenges of the heat stress of long-distance running or the lower partial pressure of oxygen at altitude seem to be well tolerated by females. The limited data available suggest that females, compared to males, have about the same incidence of orthopedic injuries consequent to endurance training. Disruption of the menstrual cycle is a common problem for female athletes. While it is important to recognize this problem and discover its etiology, no evidence exists to indicate that this is harmful to the female reproductive system.

References

1. Allan, J. R. The effects of physical training in a temperate and hot climate on the physiological response to heat stress. *Ergonomics* 8:445–453, 1965.
2. Astrand, P. O., L. Engström, B. Eriksson, P. Kalberg, I. Nylander, and C. Thofen. Girl Swimmers. *Acta Paediat. Scand.* Suppl. 147, 1963.
3. Bittel, J. and R. Henane. Comparison of thermal exchanges in men and women under neutral and hot conditions. *J. Physiol. (Lond.)* 250:475–489, 1975.
4. Brown, C. H., J. R. Harrower, and M. F. Deeter. The effects of cross-country running on pre-adolescent girls. *Med. Sci. Sports* 4:1–5, 1972.
5. Buskirk, E. R. Work and fatigue in high altitude In: *Physiology of Work Capacity and Fatigue*. E. Simonson (Ed.), Springfield, Illinois: Charles C. Thomas, pp. 312–324, 1971.
6. Cunningham, D. A. and J. S. Hill. Effect of training on cardiovascular response to exercise in women. *J. Appl. Physiol.* 39:891–895, 1975.
7. Dale, E., D. H. Gerlach, D. E. Martin, and C. R. Alexander. Physical fitness profiles and reproductive physiology of the female distance runner. *Phys. and Sportsmed.* 7:83–95, 1979(Jan).
8. Dale, E., D. H. Gerlach, and A. L. Withite. Menstrual dysfunction in distance runners. *Obst. Gyne.* 54:47–53, 1979.
9. Dill, B. D., L. F. Soholt, D. C. McLean, T. F. Drost, Jr., and M. T. Loughran. Capacity of young males and females for running in desert heat. *Med. Sci. Sports* 9:137–142, 1977.
10. Drinkwater, B. L. Physiological responses of women to exercise. In: *Exercise and Sports Sciences Reviews*, J. H. Wilmore (Ed.), New York, NY: Academic Press, Vol. I, pp. 125–153, 1973.
11. Drinkwater, B. L., J. E. Denton, I. C. Kupprat, T. S. Talag, and S. M. Horvath. Aerobic power as a factor in women's response to work in hot environments. *J. Appl. Physiol.* 41:815–821, 1976.
12. Drinkwater, B. L., J. E. Denton, P. B. Raven and S. M. Horvath. Thermoregulatory response of women to intermittent work in the heat. *J. Appl. Physiol.* 41:57–61, 1976.
13. Drinkwater, B. L., L. J. Folinsbee, J. F. Bedi, S. A. Plowman, A. B. Loucks, and S. M. Horvath. Response of women mountaineers to maximal exercise during hypoxia. *Aviat. Space Environ. Med.* 50:657–662, 1979.
14. Drinkwater, B. L., I. C. Kupprat, J. E. Denton, J. L. Crist, and S. M. Horvath. Response of prepubertal girls and college women to work in the heat. *J. Appl. Physiol.: Respirat. Environ. Exercise Physiol.* 43:1046–1053, 1977.
15. Drinkwater, B. L., I. C. Kupprat, J. E. Denton, and S. M. Horvath. Heat tolerance of female distance runners. *Annals NY Acad. Sci.* 301:777–792, 1977.
16. Eddy, D. O., K. L. Sparks, and D. A. Adelizi. The effect of continuous and interval training in women and men. *Europ. J. Appl. Physiol.* 37:83–92, 1977.
17. Eriksson, B. O., I. Engström, P. Karlberg, A. Lundin, B. Saltin, and C. Thofen. Long-term effect of previous swimtraining in girls. A 10-year follow-up on the "Girl Swimmers." *Acta Paediat. Scand.* 67:285–292, 1978.
18. Fox, R. H., B. E. Lofstedt, P. M. Woodward, E. Eriksson, and B. Werkstrom. Comparison of thermoregulatory function in men and women. *J. Appl. Physiol.* 26:444–453, 1969.
19. Franklin, B. A., L. Lussier, and E. R. Buskirk. Injury rates in women joggers. *Phys. and Sportsmed.* 7:105–112, 1979(Mar).
20. Fringer, M. N. and G. A. Stull. Changes in cardiorespiratory parameters during periods of training and detraining in young adult females. *Med. Sci. Sports* 6:20–25, 1974.
21. Frisch, R. E. Fatness and the onset and maintenance of menstrual cycles. *Res. In Reprod.* 6:1, 1977.
22. Hannon, J. P. Comparative altitude adaptability of young men and women. In: *Environmental stress: individual human adaptations.* L. J. Folinsbee et al. (Eds.), San Francisco: Academic Press, pp. 335–350, 1978.

23. Hannon, J. P., J. L. Shields, and C. W. Harris. A comparative review of certain responses of men and women to high altitude. In: *Proceedings symposia on arctic biology and medicine. VI. The physiology of work in cold and altitude.* C. Helfferich, (Ed.), Fort Wainwright, Alaska: Arctic Aeromedical Laboratory, pp. 113–245, 1966.

24. Hannon, J. P., J. L. Shields, and C. W. Harris. Effects of altitude acclimatization on blood composition of women. *J. Appl. Physiol.* 26:540–547, 1969.

25. Harris, D. V. (quoted in) Secondary amenorrhea linked to stress. *Phys. and Sportsmed.* 6:24, 1978(Oct).

26. Haycock, C. E., and J. V. Gillette. Susceptibility of women athletes to injury: Myths vs. Reality. *JAMA* 236:163–165, 1976.

27. Hughson, R. L. and J. R. Sutton. Heat stroke in "run for fun." *Br. Med. J.* 2(No. 6145): 1158, 1978, (Oct).

28. James, S. L., B. J. Bates, and L. R. Osternig. Injuries to runners. *Am. J. Sports Med.* 6:40–50, 1978(Mar-Apr).

29. Kawahata, A. Sex differences in sweating. In: *Essential problems in climatic physiology,* M. Yoshimura, K. Ogata and S. Ito (Eds.), Kyoto: Nankodo, pp. 169–184, 1960.

30. Kilbom, A. Physical training in women. *Scand. J. Clin. Lab. Invest.* 28:1–34, Suppl. 119, 1971.

31. Kollis, J., H. L. Barlett, P. Oja, and C. L. Shearburn. Cardiac output of sedentary and physically conditioned women during submaximal exercise. *Aust. J. Sports Med.* 9:63–68, 1977.

32. Lamb, D. R. *Physiology of exercise: responses and adaptations.* New York: Macmillan Publishing Co., Inc., p. 252, 1978.

33. Mayhew, J. L. and P. M. Gross. Body composition changes in young women with high resistance weight training. *Res. Q. Am. Assoc. Health Phys. Ed.* 56:433–440, 1974.

34. Moody, D. L., J. Kollias, and E. R. Buskirk. The effect of a moderate exercise program on body weight and skinfold thickness in overweight college women. *Med. Sci. Sports* 1:75–80, 1969.

35. Moody, D. L., J. H. Wilmore, R. N. Girandola, and J. P. Royce. The effects of a jogging program on the body composition of normal and obese high school girls. *Med. Sci. Sports* 4:210–213, 1972.

36. Moromoto, T., Z. Slabochova, R. K. Naman, and F. Sargent, II. Sex differences in physiological reactions to thermal stress. *J. Appl. Physiol.* 22:526–532, 1967.

37. Nadel, E. R., K. B. Pandolf, M. F. Roberts, and J. A. J. Stolwijk. Mechanisms of thermal acclimation to exercise and heat. *J. Appl. Physiol.* 37:515–520, 1974.

38. Nunneley, S. A. Physiological responses of women to thermal stress: A Review. *Med. Sci. Sports* 10:250–255, 1978.

39. Pandolf, K. B. Effects of physical training and cardiorespiratory physical fitness on exercise-heat tolerance: recent observations. *Med. Sci. Sports* 11:60–65, 1979.

40. Paolone, A. M., C. L. Wells, and G. T. Kelly. Sexual variations in thermoregulation during heat stress. *Aviat. Space Environ. Med.* 49:715–719, 1978.

41. Pollock, M. L. The quantification of endurance training programs. In: *Exercise and sport science reviews.* J. H. Wilmore (Ed.). New York, NY: Academic Press, Vol. 1, pp. 155–188, 1973.

42. Pollock, M. L., L. R. Gettman, C. A. Milesis, M. D. Bah, L. Durstine, and R. B. Johnson. Effects of frequency and duration of training on attrition and incidence of injury. *Med. Sci. Sports* 9:31–36, 1977.

43. Richards, R., D. Richards, P. Schofield, V. Ross, and J. Sutton. Reducing the hazards in Sydney's *The Sun* City-to-Surf Runs, 1971–1979. *Med. J. Aust.* 2:453–457, 1979.

44. Shields, J. L., J. P. Hannon, C. W. Harris and W. S. Platner. Effects of altitude acclimatization on pulmonary function in women. *J. Appl. Physiol.* 25:606–609, 1968.

45. Stolwijk, J. A. J. Responses to the thermal environment. *Fed. Proc.* 36:1655–1658, 1977.

46. Sutton, J., M. J. Coleman, A. P. Millar, L. Lararus, and P. Russo. The medical problems of mass participation in athletic competition. *Med. J. Aust.* 2:127–133, 1972.

47. Wells, C. L. Responses of physically active and acclimatized men and women to work in a desert environment. *Med. Sci. Sports* (accepted for publication, 1980).

48. Wells, C. L. Sexual differences in heat stress response. *Phys. and Sportmed.* 5:79–90, 1977 (Sept).

49. Wells, C. L., and S. M. Horvath. Metabolic and thermoregulatory responses of women to exercise in two thermal environments. *Med. Sci. Sports* 6:8–13, 1974.

50. Wells, C. L., and A. M. Paolone. Metabolic responses to exercise in three thermal environments. *Aviat. Space Environ. Med.* 48:989–993, 1977.

51. Wilmore, J. H. Alterations in strength, body composition and anthropometric measurements consequent to a 10-week weight training program. *Med. Sci. Sports* 6:133–138, 1974.

52. Wilmore, J. H., and C. H. Brown. Physiological profiles of women distance runners. *Med. Sci. Sports* 6:178–181, 1974.

53. Wyndham, C. H., J. F. Morrison, and C. G. Williams. Heat reactions of male and female Caucasians. *J. Appl. Physiol.* 20:357–364, 1965.

54. Yaeger, S. A., and P. Brynteson. Effects of varying training periods on the development of cardiovascular efficiency of college women. *Res. Q. Am. Assoc. Health Phys. Educ.* 41:589–592, 1970.

Appendix 8: Granola Recipe

Ingredients	Amount	Calories
Whole rolled oats	8 cups	6,922
Wheat germ	1 cup	876
Whole bran	½ cup	340
Whole walnuts	1 cup	1,458
Raw peanuts	1 cup	1,272
Sunflower seeds	2 cups	2,508
Sesame seeds	1 cup	1,261
Safflower oil	2 cups	3,960
Honey	1 cup	681
	TOTAL	19,348

Combine dry ingredients in a shallow baking pan. Heat oil and honey together in a saucepan and pour over dry ingredients, mixing well. Bake at 350° for 1 hour, stirring every 15 minutes. Makes 55 servings of ¼ cup each. 350 calories per serving.

Glossary

abduction Moving a body part (limb or limb segment) *away* from the midline of the body.

addiction A term used in drug education to refer to a state of physical or psychological dependence on a drug. Characteristics of addiction include an overpowering need to continue taking the drug, a tendency to increase dosage, and a psychological and physical dependence on the drug. Drug addiction has very definite, negative effects on the individual and on society.

adduction Moving a body part (limb or limb segment) *toward* the midline of the body.

aerobic power From the exercise physiology standpoint, is the amount of oxygen that a person can inhale during a progressive work (exercise) task.

aggression An intent to harm, in a physical or psychological way, one's opponent. There are generally two types of aggression; one is *reactive aggression,* and involves a specific attempt to harm or inflict injury against an opponent. The second type is *instrumental aggression,* defined as a striving to attain a goal. In instrumental aggression, the opponent becomes secondary, and the primary focus is on an attempt to achieve victory and not to harm the opponent.

amenorrhea Absence of monthly menstruation cycles in the female. *Primary amenorrhea* indicates that the young girl has not yet begun to menstruate, or have her monthly cycle or period. *Secondary amenorrhea* is a cessation of the monthly periods after menstruation has started, and continued for several months.

anabolic steroids A category of banned drugs, which includes synthetically produced testosterone derivatives. These drugs are purported to have an enhancing metabolic proficiency in the muscular system. There are many adverse side-effects related to taking anabolic steroids.

anaerobic Metabolism in which the individual is burning foodstuffs without sufficient oxygen supply present as in intense, all-out exercise.

anaerobic power A short-term (one to five minutes) work test of extreme intensity, in which the individual cannot consume enough oxygen during the work task and goes into oxygen debt. A major characteristic of an anaerobic power test is the accumulation of lactate in the muscle or blood as a result of the severe work intensity. After this short period of time, work diminishes, as exhaustion is reached, resulting in cessation of the work task.

anterior The front surface of the body.

anxiety In sport, this generally refers to a fear—real or imagined—about an upcoming event, which may lead the individual to perform in a somewhat less than optimum fashion.

ATP Adenosine triphosphate, a high-energy phosphate compound, which is one of the major forms of energy immediately available to the working cell.

attribution theory A psychological construct defined by Weiner in the early 1970s in an attempt to explain the success or failure outcome, as perceived by the individual. A phase of achievement motivation, the attribution theory considers such factors as ability and effort, internal characteristics of the individual, task difficulty and luck, and external characteristics in the situation—and how these four factors interact with the individual's perceived outcome of the event.

autogenic training A method of mental relaxation training used by the athlete to lessen the pre-event anxiety of competition.

basal metabolic rate (BMR) The amount of energy needed by the body to sustain life-supporting functions (breathing, heartbeat, digestion, etc.).

blood doping The extraction and storage of certain amounts of blood from the athlete, followed by the reintroduction of the withheld blood back into the athlete's system at a later date, with the hope of improving performance.

bone scan A type of X ray test used to detect a fracture or stress fracture of a bone. A low dose of radioactive substance is injected into the person. The radioactive material is circulated throughout the body and seems to concentrate in an area at which the bone is irritated. A specialized camera can then identify this irritated area of bone, and the radiologist, or orthopedic physician, can then make a proper diagnosis.

brand drug The name given to a drug by the labeler, or manufacturer of the drug (e.g., Bayer® brand aspirin, Valium® brand tranquilizer, or Dianabol® brand steroid).

bursitis An inflammation of the bursa, a fluid-filled sac lying beneath the tendons in the vicinity of joints, which lubricates and facilitates movement in that area.

Calorie The amount of heat energy necessary to raise one kilogram of water one degree centigrade. A large calorie (kilo-calorie, KC or C) is equivalent to 1000 small calories.

carbohydrate loading Dietary manipulation practiced by an athlete in preparing for an endurance event. It involves a few days of depletion of carbohydrate sources within the body, in addition to consuming a diet low in carbohydrates. About three days before the event, the athlete goes on a high-carbohydrate, low-calorie diet, while cutting back on the intensity of the workouts, in an attempt to supercompensate, or superpack the muscles with glycogen.

cardiac muscle A special type of muscle tissue found only in the heart, consisting mainly of a network of intermingled fibers. Cardiac muscle is unique in that it contracts rhythmically and automatically, without any outside stimulation, throughout the individual's lifetime.

cardiac output The stroke volume of the heart multiplied by the heart rate.

cardiologist A heart specialist.

chondromalacia An irritation of the cartilage lining behind the patella (knee cap). It is an overuse syndrome, very often caused by poor alignment of the patella with the lower extremity.

corrective therapist (CT) With a background in physical education, and advanced master's degree work, the CT performs in affiliation with hospitals, particularly in veteran's hospitals, to improve the physical work capacity of the patients.

creatine phosphate (CP) A high energy source, found within the muscle cell.

dentist (DDS or DMD) A doctor who treats conditions of the mouth, teeth, and gums.

dermatologist A medical doctor who is a skin specialist.

DMSO Dimethylsulfoxide, a by-product of paper manufacturing. This chemical appears to enter the bloodstream very quickly, and may be used in relieving pain and speeding up the healing process in musculoskeletal problems, such as tendinitis, muscle strains, and slight sprains.

doctor of philosophy (PhD) The PhD in Exercise Physiology is someone who studies the acute and chronic response to exercise and generally becomes involved in the training, conditioning, and preparation of the athlete for sport. Most of these people are found doing research and teaching at medical schools and universities.

doping As defined by the International Olympic Committee, doping refers to the use of a drug or drug substance by an athlete, with the intention of gaining an artificial and unfair improvement in performance.

dynamic flexibility Moving flexibility. It is the type of flexibility that an individual exhibits by bending over quickly at the waist in an attempt to touch the toes.

dysmenorrhea Pain or discomfort during the menstrual cycle. It generally occurs either just prior to flow of the menses, during actual flow, or in the immediate post-menstrual period. Common complaints include pain in the lower back, abdominal cramps, a feeling of fullness in the abdomen, headache, and nausea (sometimes vomiting).

endocrinologist An MD who specializes in diseases of the glands of internal secretion (e.g., diabetes).

endurance The ability to continue or to sustain a repetitive athletic movement, such as running.

exercise A prescribed work task, which generally includes intensity, duration, and frequency of the work bout. Exercise can be measured very accurately in a scientific manner and is prescribed for training and conditioning the individual and in rehabilitating the individual after injury or illness.

extension The opening of a joint surface, such as that which occurs when the hand begins close to the shoulder and is brought away from the shoulder in an opening movement at the elbow.

family practitioner MD who specializes in providing comprehensive health care for all members of the family, regardless of age and sex. In some areas, the family practitioner is called a general medical practitioner.

fartlek training A training program devised in Scandinavia wherein the athlete runs over an unstructured course, varying the speed. (Fartlek means "speed play.")

fasciitis An inflammation of the fascia, the tough white fibrous connective tissue.

fast twitch muscle fibers Muscles in which the contraction and relaxation phase is very quick—approximately forty to eighty milliseconds.

flexibility The range of movement, which can occur at a body joint or at a series of joints (such as the spine).

flexion Decreasing the joint angle, such as occurs at the elbow as when the hand is moved up toward the shoulder.

gastroenterologist An MD who specializes in diseases of the digestive tract.

generic drug A category of drug. The generic name specifies the chemically active ingredient in the drug, such as aspirin, tranquilizers, or steroids. The generic name is the public, established name for the drug.

glycolytic capacity The ability to engage in intense, vigorous, all-out activity, utilizing stored muscle glycogen (a sugar) via anaerobic metabolism.

golgi tendon organs Special sensory receptors found in tendons, which perceive the amount of tension generated in muscle contractions.

goniometer A protractor-like device which has two pivoting arms about a central point. The goniometer is used for measurement of joint or angular motion.

gynecologist An MD who specializes in the female reproductive system.

habit forming (habituation) Repeated consumption of a drug by an individual. Characteristics of habituation include a desire to continue consuming the drug, but with little or no tendency to increase dosage; some degree of psychic dependence on the drug, but an absence of physical dependence (e.g., the tobacco habit).

heat cramps Painful, involuntary spasms of the skeletal muscle. These may be caused by a dehydrated condition, and generally indicate that the athlete should refrain from further activity until properly rested and rehydrated.

heat exhaustion Extreme weakness, stupor, headache, and nausea, as a result of extreme exertion in a hot, humid environment. Profuse sweating is usually present in the heat exhaustion victim. Treatment involves restoring body fluid and removing the individual to a cooler environment.

heat fatigue A syndrome involving extreme weakness and tiredness in the athlete who has been performing in a very hot, humid environment. Rest and consumption of large amounts of fluid generally resolve this condition.

heat stroke A medical emergency characterized by extremely high core body temperature (105–107°F). Generally, a breakdown in the body's temperature regulatory mechanism is at fault. Clinical symptoms may include extremely hot body skin condition, unconsciousness, perspiration, low blood pressure, rapid pulse, dilated pupils, irregular breathing, general feelings of confusion, headache, and extreme hotness. This is a medical emergency, and proper medical treatment (lowering body temperature) must be administered or death may occur.

herniated disk Also called a ruptured disk. This happens when there is extreme pressure on an invertebral disk, causing a rupture of the inside of the disk (nucleus pulposus). Treatment involves rest, traction, injection of an enzyme into the disk, or surgery.

high density lipoprotein A sub-type of cholesterol found in the blood of humans. This type of lipoprotein is believed to be an effective carrier of the particles of cholesterol and does not allow for harmful deposits of cholesterol within the arteries. Proper diet and endurance activity seem to raise the high density lipoprotein portion of cholesterol in the blood.

hip pointer A bruise that occurs to the anterior/superior iliac spine (the upper front part of the hip) due to a blow to this area as would occur in football, or any contact sport.

hyperplasia An increase in the number of cells, for example, an increase in the number of fat cells in an individual who is rapidly gaining weight.

hypertrophy An increase in the size of a cell, for example, a muscle cell, due to increased overload strength training.

hypothermia A lowering of the core temperature of the human body to values of 95°F, or lower. Hypothermia is generally due to prolonged exposure to very cold environmental temperatures, or an abnormality of the brain's thermostat. If the lowering of body temperature is not curtailed, death may ensue.

internist (MD) A general medical doctor who specializes in the diagnosis and medical treatment of diseases of adults.

isokinetic A type of human movement in which the person is using an apparatus to accurately control the speed of the movement while the resistance to the movement is varied in accordance with the variable resistance applied by the machine (i.e., Cybex and Nautilus machines).

isometric A type of muscle contraction in which the muscle strains, but there is *no movement* because the resistance to be overcome is too great.

isotonic Movement at a particular joint in which there is no change in resistance (a barbell is moved), but the speed of muscle contraction varies as the movement occurs.

joint receptors Specialized sensory receptors, found in all movable joints of the skeleton, which provide movement information to the brain.

life quality The total impact of the environment on life, taking into account the physical environment, the social environment, the psychological environment, and the emotional health of the individual.

low density lipoprotein A second type of lipoprotein found in the blood. It tends to increase with age and with a diet that is high in saturated fats and cholesterol.

maximal oxygen consumption (VO₂ max) The capacity to take in and consume oxygen during a severe physical work task. Generally considered to be the best measure of a person's aerobic fitness.

medical doctor (MD) Individual who has completed medical school, plus three to seven years of graduate medical education. This generally includes a period of internship, followed by medical residency or association at a medical facility. MDs must be licensed by the state in which they practice.

mitochondria Small, specialized organelles, which serve as the major site of aerobic energy production within the muscle cell.

Morton's foot An abnormally long second metatarsal bone of the foot, causing the shorter first metatarsal to be exposed to undue stress and pronation (turning in of the foot) in running. It may lead to an irritation and a stress fracture of the second metatarsal, or other leg injuries.

motor unit The lower motor neuron (the alpha motor neuron) and all of the single muscle fibers (cells) innervated by that single motor nerve cell.

muscle spindle Sensory receptors, found in all skeletal muscle, which provide involuntary feedback to the individual regarding movement.

myositis ossificans A muscle/bone problem which occurs after a severe blow through the muscle, impacting on the bone. A resultant new growth of calcium occurs, painfully penetrating into the muscle itself. It may have to be surgically removed. Rest is indicated.

myotatic A type of muscle stretch. Generally, a muscle is stretched during the period in which it is contracting, resulting in a greater expression of strength than the muscle was capable of during an isometric contraction.

myotatic strength training Muscle stretch training in which an applied stretch is forcibly produced in a contracting muscle, leading to greater expressions of muscle force and strength. It is a very dangerous procedure to use in unsupervised situations.

NAIRS (National Athletic Injury/Illness Reporting System) A national classification and codifying system for the numbers and severity of athletic injuries. Formulated in 1948, it is based on the functional definition of an athletic injury. It attempts to categorize reportable injuries into those which require that the athlete visit a trained professional for some sort of treatment.

neurologist An MD who specializes in disorders of the brain and nervous system.

nurse practitioner (RN, or NP) A registered nurse with advanced training in nursing education. The nurse practitioner may perform physical examinations, do certain diagnostic tests, advise patients, and develop basic treatment programs— working very closely under the supervision of an MD.

occupational therapist (OT) Assists patients with disabilities to function more independently.

oncologist An MD who specializes in tumors and cancer.

ophthalmologist An MD who specializes in treating the eye.

optician A person who can supply, fit, and adjust glasses and contact lenses, which may have been prescribed by an ophthalmologist or an optometrist. The optician cannot examine or test eyes, or prescribe glasses or drugs.

optometrist A person having a bachelor's degree, plus three years of training in a school of optometry and who is trained to prescribe, supply, and adjust glasses and contact lenses.

orthopedist Surgeon and medical doctor who operates and treats problems of muscles, bones, joints, ligaments, and tendons.

Osgood-Schlatter's disease An irritation to the quadriceps tendon at the point where it inserts into the tibia (shin bone). It generally occurs in the young, growing athlete.

osteopath (DO) The doctor of osteopathic medicine receives training similar to that of an MD and provides general health care to individuals, as well as to families. The DO may manipulate the musculoskeletal system to treat specific problems and may perform surgery and recommend drugs.

over-the-counter drugs (OTC) These are types of drugs that may be issued without a doctor's prescription. Generally, if directions on the label are followed, these drugs are relatively safe for the adult population.

oxidative A type of metabolism in which the individual consumes sufficient oxygen for the actual physical activity being engaged in.

physical therapist (RPT, or LPT) Individual who helps sick or disabled people improve strength, mobility, sensation, or other areas. The physical therapist may utilize heat therapy, cold therapy, water therapy, or a combination of these treatments to control pain, increase strength in muscles, and improve coordination.

physician assistant (PA) Usually works in doctors' offices or hospitals doing some tasks which have been traditional for the MD. The PA does preliminary physical examinations, takes medical histories, carries out simple diagnostic tests, and develops brief treatment plans for patients. This is done under the close guidance and supervision of the physician.

placebo An inactive substance given to a patient at the request of the patient, who believes that there will be some physiological benefit from the drug. While the pill is inert (a bread or sugar pill) and can have no possible physiological effect on the person, if the individual believes that it will help, there may be a psychological improvement.

plantar fasciitis An inflammation of the plantar surface on the bottom of the foot. It is an overuse syndrome that occurs in runners when excessive trauma to the undersurface of the foot is caused by stiff shoes or too much speed work or hill work in the training program.

play Any self-rewarding activity that is not necessarily a part of the rigid daily function of life. Play is generally self-initiated and participated in during leisure hours. Play allows for complete freedom to engage in any unstructured activity which the individual desires. It is completely unserious in its nature, and seems to restore the individual for the next period of work.

podiatrist A doctor who specializes in diseases and ailments of the foot and whose practice is generally limited to surgery and concerns of the foot.

posterior The back, or dorsal, surface of the body.

prescription drugs Drugs which are ordered by a physician (MD) for a particular purpose in treating a specific disease or condition.

proprioception The individual's awareness of joint position and movement which occurs in the body. Special receptors, termed muscle spindles, joint receptors, and Golgi tendon organs, provide proprioceptive information to the individual.

psychiatrist An MD who treats individuals with emotional and mental difficulties.

psychologist Called doctors because they generally have a PhD degree, psychologists counsel people with mental and emotional problems.

registered dietician (RD) An individual who provides dietary counseling and nutritional advice. Most work in hospitals or doctors' offices or sports medicine clinics. They generally have a bachelor's degree, do an approved internship, and must pass a proficiency examination.

rheumatologist An MD who specializes in arthritis and rheumatism.

shin splints Pain occurring in the lower portion of the lower limb due to a bone problem, a muscle problem, or other soft tissue or blood vessel irritation in that area.

skeletal muscle Also termed striated muscle, this is the voluntary muscle which provides form and structure to the human body. The innervation of skeletal muscle is through the voluntary motor system.

slow twitch muscle fibers Muscle fibers in which the contraction and relaxation phase occurs over a longer period of time, generally over one hundred milliseconds.

smooth muscle Muscle fibers found in blood vessels and throughout the walls of hollow, visceral organs (e.g., the stomach). Smooth muscle receives innervation from the autonomic (automatic) nervous system. It is involuntary muscle.

spondylolisthesis A condition in the lower back caused by a forward slipping of some of the vertebral bodies in the spine, causing impingement on the spinal nerve.

spondylolysis A stress fracture of one of the vertebra in the spine caused by excessive bending or jarring to the backbone.

sport A highly complex, competitive situation, sport is very organized and structured in our society. Sporting activities take place within certain definite boundaries and within certain time constraints. There are always rules that the competitors must abide by. There is always a risk in the sporting activity—the winning and the losing nature of competition. Sports may be for the individual person, such as running, swimming, and cross-country skiing, or they may be also of a team nature, such as football, basketball, and field hockey.

sports medicine The scientific and medical aspects of exercise and sports. Sports medicine covers the training and conditioning of a person for competitive sport, and includes the medical aspects of prevention, treatment, and rehabilitation of sport injuries.

sprain An overstretching or tearing of a ligament. Graded according to degrees of one, two, or three, the higher number indicates a more severe sprain.

static flexibility Non-moving flexibility in which the individual takes the joint to the end of the range-of-motion and holds it in that position for a given period of time—often six to sixty seconds.

strain A muscle pull, stretching or tearing of a muscle because the muscle is taken beyond its normal length. Strains are graded according to classes, from one to three, with the higher number representing the more severe type of tear or rupture of the muscle.

strength The ability of a skeletal muscle to move a specified resistance one time.

stress fracture Results when the bone breaks down at a faster rate than that at which new bone is being produced. If the athlete continues to abuse the bone, a complete fracture may develop. Rest is the main treatment for a stress fracture.

stroke volume The capacity of the heart, in milliliters of blood that can be pumped during severe work tasks. Stroke volume equals cardiac output divided by heart rate.

subungual hematoma A mass of blood which forms under the nail on the finger or on the toe, as a result of a blow to that portion of the anatomy. An extremely painful condition, it may have to be drained by a surgeon.

tendinitis An irritation of a tendon, due to an overuse type of injury.

tennis elbow An inflammation in the tendons or at the point of insertion of the flexor and extensor muscle mass at the elbow. It is an overuse problem caused by too much physical activity in too short a period of time.

training threshold A level of intensity of heart rate at which the individual must stress the system in order to receive an endurance training benefit.

urologist An MD who specializes in the urinary system, including the bladder and kidneys.

well-being The absence of any injury or illness. Also implies a higher level of fitness, in terms of physical, psychological, social, and emotional factors.

Index